Revolutionizing Healthcare Services

The increasing prominence of generative AI across various industries presents an abundance of opportunities for integration within the healthcare sector. From generating valuable insights about patients to automating operations, streamlining patient care, and implementing preventive technologies, the use of generative AI has the potential to usher in a new era of productivity and profitability for stakeholders within the healthcare ecosystem.

Revolutionizing Healthcare Services: Unleashing Innovation through Generative AI explores the current and potential applications of generative AI in the healthcare sector. It covers regulatory frameworks, ethical considerations, practical applications, and real-world use cases. The book also provides a forward-looking perspective to help the healthcare industry keep pace with the integration of generative AI and its applications. In addition, it looks at the future potential of generative AI in conjunction with blockchain, machine learning, and predictive modeling to create electronic health records that can be shared across the healthcare ecosystem. By examining the detailed insights on how to integrate generative AI models with existing healthcare systems, the potential to enhance patient care services can be brought to the forefront. Practical strategies are also discussed to seamlessly integrate generative AI into healthcare services, ensuring prompt, reliable, and efficient care while prioritizing urgent needs.

This book aims to equip healthcare professionals with the knowledge and tools needed to leverage generative AI for superior patient care delivery. It is designed to appeal to a wide range of audiences, including healthcare professionals, generative AI developers, data scientists, healthcare practitioners, patients, educators, policymakers, and those with the knowledge and tools needed to leverage generative AI for superior patient care delivery. The coverage, diverse perspective, and practical approach make it suitable for both beginners looking for an introduction to generative AI and experienced experts.

Artificial Intelligence in Smart Healthcare Systems
Series Editors: Vishal Jain and Jyotir Moy Chatterjee

Designing Intelligent Healthcare Systems, Products, and Services Using Disruptive Technologies and Health Informatics
Teena Bagga, Kamal Upreti, Nishant Kumar, Amirul Hasan Ansari, and Danish Nadeem

Next Generation Healthcare Systems Using Soft Computing Techniques
D. Rekh Ram Janghel, Rohit Raja, and Korhan Cengiz

Machine Learning and Artificial Intelligence in Healthcare Systems: Tools and Techniques
Edited by Tawseef Ayoub Shaikh, Saqib Hakak, Tabasum Rasool, and Mohammed Wasid

IoT in Healthcare Systems: Applications, Benefits, Challenges and Case Studies
Edited by Piyush Kumar Shukla, Aditya Patel, Prashant Kumar Shukla, Prashant Parashar, and Basant Tiwari

6G-Enabled IoT and AI for Smart Healthcare: Challenges, Impact, and Analysis
Edited by Ashish Kumar, Rachna Jain, Meenu Gupta, and Sardar M. N. Islam

Immersive Virtual and Augmented Reality in Healthcare: An IoT and Blockchain Perspective
Rajendra Kumar, Vishal Jain, Garry Han, and Abderezak Touzene

Machine Learning in Healthcare and Security: Advances, Obstacles, and Solutions
Edited by Prashant Pranav, Archana Patel, and Sarika Jain

Handbook on Augmenting Telehealth Services: Using Artificial Intelligence
Edited by Sonali Vyas, Sunil Gupta, Monit Kapoor, and Samiya Khan

Handbook of AI-Based Models in Healthcare and Medicine: Approaches, Theories and Application
Edited by Bhanu Chander, Koppala Guravaiah, B. Anoop, and G. Kumaravelan

Smart Technologies in Healthcare Management: Pioneering Trends and Applications
Edited by Nidhi Sindhwani, Ajay Rana, Sarvesh Tanwar, and Ramani Kannan

Deep Learning in Medical Image Analysis: Recent Advances and Future Trends
Edited by R. Indrakumari, T. Ganesh Kumar, D. Murugan, and Sherimon P.C.

AIoT Innovations in Digital Health: Emerging Trends, Challenges, and Solutions
Edited by Inam Ullah, Salma El Hajjami, Shashi Kant Gupta, Hameedur Rahman, Thiagarajan Yogamoorthi, Inam Ullah, and Muhammad Adnan Khan

Revolutionizing Healthcare Services: Unleashing Innovation through Generative AI
Edited by Babita Singla, Kumar Shalender, Nripendra Singh, and Sandhir Sharma

For more information about this series please visit: https://www.routledge.com/Artificial-Intelligence-in-Smart-Healthcare-Systems/book-series/CRCAISHS

Revolutionizing Healthcare Services

Unleashing Innovation through Generative AI

Edited by
Babita Singla, Kumar Shalender,
Nripendra Singh, and Sandhir Sharma

CRC Press
Taylor & Francis Group
Boca Raton London New York

CRC Press is an imprint of the
Taylor & Francis Group, an **informa** business

Designed cover image: Shutterstock

First edition published 2025
by CRC Press
2385 NW Executive Center Drive, Suite 320, Boca Raton FL 33431

and by CRC Press
4 Park Square, Milton Park, Abingdon, Oxon, OX14 4RN

CRC Press is an imprint of Taylor & Francis Group, LLC

ISBN: 978-1-032-87158-5 (hbk)
ISBN: 978-1-032-87177-6 (pbk)
ISBN: 978-1-003-53127-2 (ebk)

DOI: 10.1201/9781003531272

Typeset in Times
by KnowledgeWorks Global Ltd.

Contents

Series Preface

The progress of the healthcare sector is incremental as it learns from associations between data over time through the application of suitable big data and Internet of Things (IoT) frameworks and patterns. Many healthcare service providers are employing IoT-enabled devices for monitoring patient healthcare, but their diagnosis and prescriptions are instance-specific only. However, these IoT-enabled healthcare devices are generating volumes of data (Big-IoT Data), that can be analyzed for more accurate diagnosis and prescriptions. A major challenge in the above realm is the effective and accurate learning of unstructured clinical data through the application of precise algorithms. Incorrect input data leading to erroneous outputs with false positives shall be intolerable in healthcare as patient's lives are at stake. This new book series addresses various aspects of how smart healthcare can be used to detect and analyze diseases, the underlying methodologies, and related security concerns. Healthcare is a multidisciplinary field that involves a range of factors like the financial system, social factors, health technologies, and organizational structures that affect the healthcare provided to individuals, families, institutions, organizations, and populations. The goals of healthcare services include patient safety, timeliness, effectiveness, efficiency, and equity. Smart healthcare consists of m-health, e-health, electronic resource management, smart and intelligent home services, and medical devices. The IoT is a system comprising real-world things that interact and communicate with each other via networking technologies. The wide range of potential applications of IoT includes healthcare services. IoT-enabled healthcare technologies are suitable for remote health monitoring, including rehabilitation, assisted ambient living, etc. In turn, healthcare analytics can be applied to the data gathered from different areas to improve healthcare at a minimum expense.

This new book series is designed to be a first-choice reference at university libraries, academic institutions, research and development centers, information technology centers, and any institutions interested in using, design, modelling, and analyzing intelligent healthcare services. Successful application of deep learning frameworks to enable meaningful, cost-effective personalized healthcare services is the primary aim of the healthcare industry in the present scenario. However, realizing this goal requires effective understanding, application, and amalgamation of IoT, Big Data and several other computing technologies to deploy such systems in an effective manner. This series shall help clarify the understanding of certain key mechanisms and technologies helpful in realizing such systems.

Vishal Jain
Jyotir Moy Chatterjee

Preface

The game-changing potential of generative AI is very much apparent in across the business sectors in different industry verticals. Technology has now also started to revolutionize the healthcare sector with a number of applications making a way to make patient care a seamless and convenient process. Using the smart algorithms which have been specifically trained on the specialized content, generative AI is proving beneficial for all the stakeholders in the healthcare sector. The applications of the technology are many and prominent among these include improving the diagnostic procedure related to patient care, streamlining the entire discovery of drugs and vaccines, and delivering superior services to the end patients. The technology is also proving relevant in enhancing the services related to the healthcare sector and allied segments by streamlining the processes with the help of automated technologies. Generative AI is also results in optimizing the various parameters related to the healthcare operation so that maximum results can be achieved with minimum use of the resources. It is proving specifically beneficial for resolving the clams in a speedy manner while offering enhanced benefits to the entire ecosystem. Generative AI is also proving extensively useful in automating the various processes and procedures involved in the healthcare system. Especially when it comes to sharing information between the important stakeholders of the healthcare sector, the use of generative AI can take the entire efficiency of the sector to a new level. That said, there are significant challenges associated with the use of generative AI in the field of healthcare sector. The challenges related to the sharing of data and keeping it safe from hackers are some of the issues that need to be addressed by all the stakeholders in the ecosystem. There are regulatory challenges too and policymakers must concert the issues with the healthcare ecosystem so that an open and constructive policy Framework can be designed for the sector. Generative AI has revolutionary potential and if used constructively, it can help the healthcare ecosystem to achieve new levels of efficiency and effectiveness. The time is opportune for all participating stakeholders to have open and constructive conversations regarding the use of generative AI so that systems, processes, procedures, and tools associated with the delivery of the healthcare ecosystem can make full use of the technology. It is also incumbent on the technology developers to come up with new-age innovations that can further enhance the utility and efficiency of the generative AI and make the technology more democratic and easy to use for the public at large. The challenge here is to ensure that the interface for the generative AI is made simpler than before and the technology comes across as an innovative solution without harming the prospects of data privacy.

Babita Singla, Kumar Shalender and Sandhir Sharma
Chitkara Business School, Chitkara University, Punjab, India

Nripendra Singh
PennWest University, USA

Editors

Babita Singla is a Professor at the Chitkara Business School, Chitkara University, Punjab, India. She earned a PhD in management and is UGC-NET qualified. Dr. Singla has over 14 years of experience in teaching, research, and administration. In her career, she has been involved in important academic and research assignments, such as being the guest editor of a reputed journal, organizing and conducting international and national-level conferences and faculty development programs, and providing guidance for research projects. Her research has been published by Scopus, Springer, SCI, etc., and Dr. Singla has presented research papers at various national and international conferences.

Kumar Shalender is a Post-Doctorate in the field of strategic and technology management. With 14 years of experience in business model development and diffusion of technology, Dr. Shalender is actively involved in system thinking, flexibility, and management of technology. He has written more than 70 research papers, including publications in esteemed journals in the fields of innovation, business model development, and sustainable business practices. Dr. Shalender is also a reviewer for several reputed publications.

Nripendra Singh is a Fulbright Fellow, which is a flagship program of the U.S. Department of State, and he has completed research at the Pennsylvania State University. He has published in reputed journals and has received a prestigious grant from the Pennsylvania State System of Higher Education (PASSHE-FPDC) integrating Clarion University, local businesses, and SBDC for student learning and the development of an entrepreneurial ecosystem as the Principal Investigator.

Sandhir Sharma earned a PhD in strategic management and has nearly 22 years of experience in higher education and five years in the telecom industry. With more than 94 research papers to his credit, Dr. Sharma has developed his core expertise in the area of strategy formulation. His research has been widely published in various newspapers. Currently, he is serving as Pro Vice Chancellor of the Chitkara Business School and as Visiting Faculty at Binus University, Indonesia, and the University of Applied Sciences, Osnabruck, Germany. Dr. Sharma has traveled around the globe to participate in academic events and is an active member of various management associations and university bodies.

Contributors

Manita Arora
Amity School of Business
Amity University
Uttar Pradesh, India

K D Balaji
Faculty of Management
SRM Institute of Science and Technology
Chennai, Tamil Nadu, India

Ananya Bhowmick
Department of Pharmaceutical Technology
Brainware University
Barasat, Kolkata

S. Catherine
Department of Management Studies
Saveetha Engineering College
Chennai, India

Priyanka Chakraborty
BCDA College of Pharmacy and Technology
Barasat, Kolkata

Amit Chaudhary
School of Pharmacy
Chitkara University
Baddi, Himachal Pradesh, India

Jyoti Chauhan
Amity College of Commerce and Finance
Amity University
Noida, Uttar Pradesh, India

Swati Chawla
Amity School of Business
Amity University
Noida, Uttar Pradesh, India

Pradeep Chintale
SEI Investment Company
Downingtown, Pennsylvania, USA

Sailee Chowdhury
BCDA College of Pharmacy and Technology
Barasat, Kolkata

Ramesh Kumari Dasgupta
Department of Pharmaceutical Technology
Brainware University
Barasat, Kolkata

Narayanage Jayantha Dewasiri
Sabaragamuwa University of Sri Lanka
Belihuloya, Sri Lanka

Sivaraman Eswaran
Electrical and Computer Engineering
Curtin University Malaysia
Sarawak, Malaysia

Shayeri Chatterjee Ganguly
Department of Pharmaceutical Technology
Brainware University
Barasat, Kolkata

Manoj Govindaraj
Department of Management Studies
Vel Tech Rangarajan
Dr. Sagunthala R&D Institute of Science and Technology
Avadi, Tamil Nadu, India

Nidhi Gupta
Amity School of Business
Amity University
Noida, Uttar Pradesh, India

Qamrul Islam
Faculty of Business Studies
Arab Open University
Kingdom of Saudi Arabia

Saranya J
SRM Institute of Science and Technology
Kattankulathur, Tamil Nadu, India

M. Jayakumar
Vel Tech Rangarajan
Dr. Sagunthala R&D Institute of Science and Technology
Avadi, Chennai, India

Leena Jenefa
Hindustan Institute of Technology and Science
Padur, Chennai, India

Thavamani Jeyaraj
Department of Mechanical Engineering
SRM IST
Kattankulathur, India

Shenson Joseph
J.P. Morgan Chase & Co
New York, New York, USA

Herat Joshi
Great River Health Systems
West Burlington, Iowa, USA

Sindu Bharathi S K
SRM Institute of Science and Technology
Kattankulathur, Tamil Nadu, India

Parvez Khan
Department of Business
Atria University
Bangalore, Karnataka, India

Jatin Kumar
School of Pharmacy
Chitkara University
Baddi, Himachal Pradesh, India

Cyril Lawrence
Department of Computer Science and Engineering
Christ University
Bangalore, India

Jenifer Lawrence
Department of Management Studies
Woldia University
Weldiya, Ethiopia

Jeevitha M.
School of Management
Hindustan Institute of Technology and Science
Padur, Chennai, India

Ramya M
SRM Institute of Science and Technology
Kattankulathur, Tamil Nadu, India

Neha Mishra
Chitkara Business School
Chitkara University
Punjab, India

Banani Mondal
Department of Pharmaceutical Technology
Brainware University
Barasat, Kolkata

Jayapandian Natarajan
Department of Computer Science and Engineering
Christ University
Bangalore, India

Shalmali Arun Patil
Amazon AWS
Seattle, Washington, USA

Mananage Shanika Hansini Rathnasiri
Sabaragamuwa University of Sri Lanka
Belihuloya, Sri Lanka

Ashok Kumar S.
School of Management
Hindustan Institute of Technology and Science
Padur, Chennai, India

Oliver Nesa Raj S
Department of Mechanical Engineering
SRM IST
Kattankulathur, India

Vishakha Saini
Global Research Institute of Pharmacy
Yamuna Nagar, Haryana, India

Dikshita Sen
Department of Computer Science and Engineering
Christ University
Bangalore, India

Saladi Jaswanth Seshasai
Faculty of Management
SRM Institute of Science and Technology
Chennai, Tamil Nadu, India

Kumar Shalender
Chitkara Business School
Chitkara University
Punjab, India

Aruna Sharma
School of Pharmacy
Chitkara University
Baddi, Himachal Pradesh, India

Shalaghya Sharma
CMS Business School
Jain University
Bangalore, India

Avneet Singh
Electrical Engineering and Computer Science Department
University of Toledo
Toledo, Ohio, USA

Gurmeet Singh
Chitkara Business School
Chitkara University
Punjab, India

Harjit Singh
Symbiosis Centre for Management Studies
Symbiosis International University
Pune, India

Jaswinder Pal Singh
Central Library
Chitkara University
Punjab, India

Nripendra Singh
Pennsylvania Western University
Clarion, Pennsylvania, USA

Rubee Singh
Institute of Business Management
GLA University
Mathura, Uttar Pradesh, India

Babita Singla
Chitkara Business School
Chitkara University
Punjab, India

Rubani Singla
Department of Computer Science Engineering
Chandigarh Group of Colleges
Jhanjeri, Punjab, India

Deepak Sood
Chitkara Business School
Chitkara University
Punjab, India

Kiran Sood
Chitkara University
Punjab, India

Rahul Tripathi
Jagannath University
Haryana, India

Parekh Hetvi Vimal
Department of Computer Science and Engineering
Christ University
Bangalore, India

1 Generative AI in Healthcare

Scope, Possibilities, and Adoption Roadmap

Nripendra Singh, Kumar Shalender, Babita Singla, and Rubani Singla

INTRODUCTION

The potential of generative intelligence in taking the effectiveness of the healthcare sector to a new level has just begun to emerge. Professionals across the ecosystem are finding the technology very useful not only in enhancing the efficiency of treatment procedures but also in offering superior value to the end patients. In this particular context, this chapter looks into the transformative potential of intelligence in taking the overall effectiveness of the healthcare sector to a new level. By looking into the different frameworks related to the application of generative artificial intelligence (AI) in the healthcare sector, the exploration of how technology can bring comprehensive change in the systems procedures and processes related to healthcare is discussed in detail in this particular chapter. In addition to taking the efficiency of the procedures to the next level, the emergence of generative intelligence is also leading to new inventions in the segment and promises to offer new-age solutions to the entire healthcare sector. The holistic benefits of the technology for the entire ecosystem related to the healthcare industry are also apparent from the fact that in the last few years, the industry has discovered many use cases of generative intelligence and successfully deployed them for the greater benefit of society. The most significant benefit of generative AI technology is the trust and transparency it has brought to the healthcare sector. For example, today there are many use cases related to natural language processing (NLP) and machine learning in the healthcare sector which are completely changing the very face of the way patient care is delivered in the healthcare sector (Aggarwal et al. 2020). From demonstrating the specific abilities in translating the procedure to diagnosing patients and ultimately delivering them the prescription, the use of generative AI is helping the entire system to perform to its optimum. The saving of crucial resources is another striking benefit that is related to generative AI as it allows physicians, doctors, and healthcare attendants to offer personalised services aligned with the specific needs and preferences of the patients. The role of generative AI in democratising knowledge, procedures, and personalised services is also very crucial. In addition, the various

DOI: 10.1201/9781003531272-1

applications related to the generative AI are also leading to the enhanced interoperability in the healthcare ecosystem that will prove beneficial for bringing healthcare services on one platform for enhanced benefits to patients. Against this specific background, this research deeply dives into the scope, possibilities, and adoption roadmap related to generative AI in the healthcare sector (Apell & Eriksson 2021). While the scope and possibilities are related to the different segments of the healthcare sector, the adoption roadmap is specifically related to generating more use cases of generative AI. By focusing on real-world applications of generative AI, the likelihood of making the technology mean day in the healthcare sector can be enhanced significantly.

GENERATIVE AI IN HEALTHCARE: SCOPE AND POSSIBILITIES

The primary application of generative AI in the healthcare sector pertains to taking the efficiency of the treatment procedure to the next level. This can be achieved by offering personalised services to patients by accurately diagnosing the key issue and accordingly devising the prescriptions that will specifically address the problems faced by them. This personalisation is a key, and by specifically catering to the needs and preferences of the patient and aligning the treatment procedure with the core problems faced by them, generative AI can help the healthcare sector to become more efficient and effective in their treatment procedures (Alugubelli 2016). This technology is also instrumental in scanning the records of patients and accordingly extrapolating the data to offer them that treatment procedure in advance that can help them save from future health issues that might arise with their age. This proactive diagnosis and preventive mechanism makes the technology wonderful to address the issues of patients and prepare them in advance to tackle issues. The application of generative AI is also witnessing traction in medical imaging, screening, and treatment procedures as these new-age innovations can help practitioners to offer superior treatment procedures to patients. This assistance is very useful as the overall consumption of time and resources can be reduced drastically with the help of generative AI. The medical imaging services offered by the generative AI are also instrumental in assisting technicians to diagnose the issues and accordingly offering treatment procedures for the same. In the field of new vaccines and drug discovery, the use of technology is proving to be a game changer. Especially when it comes to finding the interaction between the different molecules, their therapeutic impact can be analysed iteratively without involving the huge amount of resources that are required in the process. This ability of the technology to reiterate time and again and replicate the results is very much conducive to enhancing the speed and agility of the discovery process. The accuracy of the medical image analysis can be taken to a new level with the help of generative AI while the technology is equally beneficial for promoting awareness and education among the patients related to the different types of diseases and healthcare procedures (Bughin et al. 2017). The use of generative AI in promoting campaigns related to various healthcare procedures and ailments is also proving very critical for enhancing the awareness of people about the various kinds of procedures (Figure 1.1).

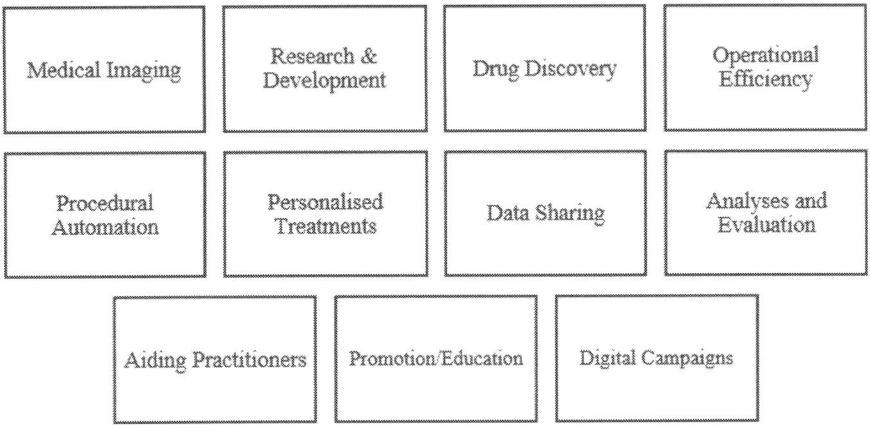

FIGURE 1.1 Generative AI scope and possibilities.

Source: Authors' conceptualization.

Especially when it comes to choosing the various digital media platforms and customising the message according to the language and culture of people, the use of generative AI is proving very beneficial in the process. The automation of the processes related to patient diagnosis and documentation is also coming across as one of the crucial applications of the generative in the healthcare sector. Not only do the processes save a lot of resources but also lead to the enhancement of the overall efficiency of the clinical procedures. Converting the patients' records into electronic formats which can be shared across the healthcare system by taking proper care and safety protocols is also helping the healthcare industry a lot (Davenport & Kalakota 2019). It is also very important to note that research and development activities in the healthcare sector have taken a giant leap because of the integration of generative AI and its associated procedures. The technology is also proving crucial for collecting analysing and evaluating complex data patterns and accordingly correlating the results to aid new research and breakthrough innovations in the healthcare sector. In fact, the delivery of the holistic benefits related to the use of the generated AI and its associated technologies is making a significant impact on the entire healthcare ecosystem leading to a win-win situation in the case. While all use cases of generative AI in the healthcare domain is prominent, the easy-to-use interface and speed at which the comfort and convenience are delivered right at the mobile phones of both patients and practitioners is really taking the game of generative AI in the field of healthcare to the next level. People at the reception centre or working in the CRM department of the healthcare units can readily take down notes and with the help of the generative AI can translate into very useful records that can be referred to in the future. These notes can be used for subsequent use in the future and can be edited modified and altered as per the discretion of stakeholders in the value chain. The utility of the technology in arranging disparate data and deriving information that can be utilised for decision-making is also being highlighted by the use cases of the technology. With the help of smart algorithms, the data can be structured and spectrums can be formed that can be utilised for looking into the behaviour of the patients. This information can also be correlated with the family history of the patients so that the subsequent issues that might manifest and impact their health inverse manner in the future can be taken care of in time.

GENERATIVE AI: BENEFITS AND ADOPTION ROADMAP

From enhancing efficiency to adding effectiveness and decision-making, generative AI can be easily considered a panacea for all challenges faced by the stakeholders in the healthcare ecosystem. The automation process can be achieved with the help of generative AI which can free up crucial time so that they start focusing on important and critical issues related to patient care (Dhiman et al. 2018). This automation of the manual work can also help in optimally utilising the resources and deploying the manpower to the functions where they are needed the most. The effectiveness of decision-making can be significant with new-age technologies such as AI, ML, and smart algorithms. Especially when it comes to the top management of healthcare facilities, the utilisation of generative AI can offer unique insights, fresh takes, and smart perspectives. Increasing pressure on the healthcare ecosystem and the speed at which competition is intensifying between the players is also making a strong case for the use of generative AI technology in the sector. The use of smart algorithms can enhance the value delivery process and by utilising all the resources available at one's disposal, the efficiency and effectiveness of the procedures can be taken a step ahead. The utility of generative AI is also making a strong case for itself in helping the healthcare sector decide the strategic vision of the entire industry (Esmaeilzadeh 2020). As the value delivery process continues to remain one of the strategic imperatives of the healthcare sector, the use of technology can help suppliers, pharmacies, practitioners, and policymakers to collaborate on a common platform and deliver superior value to end patients. Take the case of health insurance where the use of generative AI can help in the complete management and processing of claims (Grover & Shalender 2023). The entire process can be automated with the help of generating AI process and by converting the entire manual process into an automation exercise, the planes related to the health insurance can be dispersed without any problem or unnecessary delay. There are many models available in generative technology that can benefit from the help of advanced algorithms and smart machine-learning processes (Figure 1.2). Especially when it comes to determining the models of revenue and overprofitability with specific relation to the acquisition of the cost, the models related to the general can be of immense use (Mileva 2024).

With the help of generative AI technology, healthcare players can summarise the findings of the models, correlate the past information related to customer feedback, and come up with improved processes that can be utilised to make the entire ecosystem more vibrant and dynamic. Another important use case related to generative AI in the healthcare ecosystem is to off for personalised recommendations to patients in their own native language. The technology can also be used for generating the checklist and to ensure better understanding and coordination among the stakeholders, the instructions can also be automated with the help of smart algorithms (Padasalgi 2024). Relationship management is very crucial in the healthcare ecosystem and can

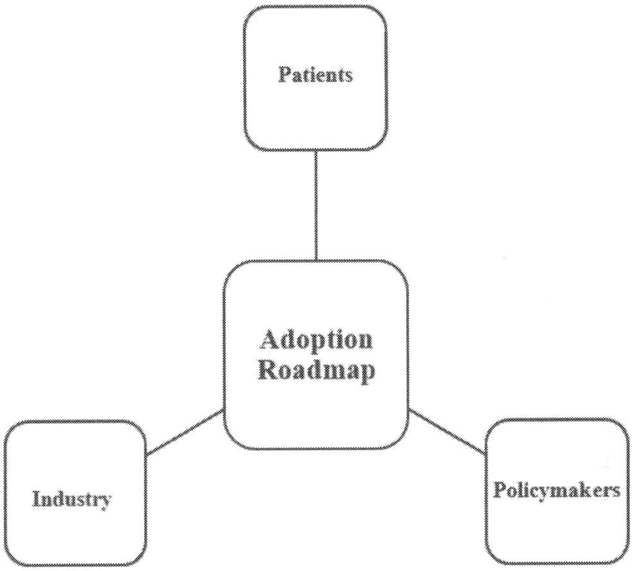

FIGURE 1.2 Recommended adoption framework.

Source: Authors' conceptualization.

be taken to the next level with the help of generative AI. The technology can automate the entire process of taking the feedback from the patients also which intern is very crucial for strategically improving the processes in the long run. The effectiveness of the human resource departments in clinics, hospitals, and infirmaries can also be aided with the help of generative AI technology (Manohar et al. 2020). In order to ensure the successful implementation of generative AI in the healthcare ecosystem, it is very important that patients, industry, and policymakers come together and develop a common platform for integrating new-age innovations in the sector. Patients need to be enthusiastic about the use of the technology and by furnishing information to the industry safely and securely, they can help in the successful adoption of the technology in the sector. All the information must be submitted to the players in the healthcare ecosystem in a safe and secure manner so that no leakage of the information will take place to hackers or players with malafide intent. The industry stakeholders, on the other hand, need to adopt the technology and allocate the requisite resources to operational mechanisms. In the integration, the support of the top management of the organisation is critically important. The positive attitude of the top management will result in seamless integration of the generative AI and will ultimately lead to complete integration of the technology (Shalender 2023). Policymakers need to play a decisively positive role in the integration of generative AI in the healthcare sector. The officials have already adopted an open and constructive mindset towards that technology and buy a lion administrators to a dog the generative AI in a seamless manner they can definitely take the overall efficiency of healthcare to the next level (Shalender 2022). Administrators can also offer benefits and subsidies related to the use of technology in healthcare and by encouraging the companies that are coming forward with the integration of generative AI; examples can be set for others to follow (Shroff 2024).

CONCLUSION AND DISCUSSION

Generative AI has the game-changing potential, and by integrating the technology into the processes and procedures of the healthcare systems, it can definitely revolutionise the sector by automating systems, aiding efficiency, and enhancing effectiveness. The technology is also beneficial for patients, and by helping them in early diagnosis and prevention of diseases, it can offer superior value to each and every stakeholder in the ecosystem (Singh 2024). The approach is also beneficial in analysing the entire ecosystem of healthcare in a complete and cohesive manner. The piecemeal approach associated with healthcare will not work in the future, and in order to offer affordable and quality healthcare to the masses, it is absolutely essential to use the generative AI to its full potential. This technology is also very helpful in evaluating the overall landscape of the healthcare and finding new use cases that can be integrated into the delivery of better healthcare services to the people at large. The importance of technology in making sure that health services are available to every person around the world is well recognised among policymakers today. Especially when it comes to developing economies, the need of the hour is to use technology in a manner so that the benefits can reach the last person standing in the row. In other words, the inclusion of the masses in the healthcare ecosystem can be achieved with the help of generative AI (Welch 2023). All the benefits related to generative AI in the healthcare ecosystem also need to be looked at from the prism of the safety and security of the data. It is important and critical for all the stakeholders in the healthcare ecosystem to ensure that data will not be shared with unauthorised participants, and accordingly a strong layer of security has to be offered. This can be ensured by putting in place a robust system capable of offering security to the data and making strong provisions that no information is shared before the prior consent of the patients. The ethical and moral implications related to the use of generative AI also need to be considered by the stakeholders in the ecosystem. They have to be addressed from the multifaceted approach, and the desired objective of the use of technology can be achieved by investing in collaborations and partnerships across the board. Another important dimension that needs to be kept in mind is the overall evolution of generative AI technology and its convergence with allied tools. For example, it is widely accepted that the application of generative AI will ultimately converge with other game-changing technologies such as augmented reality (AR), virtual reality (VR), and blockchain among others. The use of the technology has to be complemented with the help of other new-age innovations as the singular use of generative AI might not be good enough to deliver a whole host of benefits. The adoption of the technology at a large scale might not be feasible given the amount of resources the integration of the generative AI requires, and hence it is incumbent on the leading players in the healthcare ecosystem to come up with the most beneficial use cases of the technology and deploy them for others to learn from it. Priority must be given to the use cases where the technology is aiding the efficiency of the operational procedures rather than replacing human beings in their specific position and roles. The sensitivity of the healthcare ecosystem requires close coordination between the technology and the human element as one cannot be prioritised at the expense of the other. It is therefore the responsibility of the leading corporate houses in the healthcare ecosystem to come forward and use generative AI as an example for others to follow. Policymakers can also offer incentives for using the technology which will encourage other players to come forward and embrace the technology wholeheartedly.

REFERENCES

Aggarwal, A., Chand, P. K., Jhamb, D., & Mittal, A. (2020). Leader–Member exchange, work engagement, and psychological withdrawal behavior: The mediating role of psychological empowerment. Frontiers in Psychology, 11(423). https://doi.org/10.3389/fpsyg.2020.00423

Alugubelli, R. (2016). Exploratory study of artificial intelligence in healthcare. International Journal of Innovations in Engineering Research and Technology, 3(1), 1–10.

Apell, P., & Eriksson, H. (2021). Artificial intelligence (AI) healthcare technology innovations: The current state and challenges from a life science industry perspective. Technology Analysis & Strategic Management, 35(2), 179–193.

Bughin, J., Hazan, E., Ramaswamy, S., Allas, T., Dahlström, P., Henke, N., & Trench, M. (2017). Artificial intelligence: The next digital frontier? New York, NY: McKinsey Global Institute.

Davenport, T., & Kalakota, R. (2019). The potential for artificial intelligence in healthcare. Future Healthcare Journal, 6(2), 94–98.

Dhiman, R., Chand, P. K., & Gupta, S. (2018). Behavioural aspects influencing decision to purchase apparels amongst young Indian consumers. FIIB Business Review, 7(3), 188–200. https://doi.org/10.1177/2319714518790308

Esmaeilzadeh, P. (2020). Use of AI-based tools for healthcare purposes: A survey study from consumers' perspectives. BMC Medical Informatics and Decision Making, 6. https://doi.org/10.1186/s12911-020-01191-1

Grover, A., & Shalender, K. (2023). Virtual world – Metaverse governance conceptual framework. Applied Data Science and Smart Systems AIP Conference Proceedings, 2916(1), 220001.

Manohar, S., Mittal, A., & Marwah, S. (2020). Service innovation, corporate reputation and word-of-mouth in the banking sector: A test on multigroup-moderated mediation effect. Benchmarking: An International Journal, 27(1), 406–429.

Mileva, G. (2024). 5 AI healthcare tools revolutionizing healthcare in hospitals and clinics. Available at https://influencermarketinghub.com/ai-healthcare-tools/

Padasalgi, S. R. (2024). Transforming healthcare: The power of AI in revolutionizing patient care and research. Available at https://health.economictimes.indiatimes.com/news/health-it/transforming-healthcare-the-power-of-ai-in-revolutionizing-patient-care-and-researchais-integration-into-healthcare-a-game-changer/107183802

Shalender, K. (2022). Key variables in team dynamics in small businesses and start-ups. In New teaching resources for management in a globalised world. World Scientific Publishing, Singapore, pp. 141–153. https://doi.org/10.1142/9789811239212_0007

Shalender, K. (2023). Skill development for society 5.0: A focus on the new-age skilling process. In Trivedi, S., Aggarwal, R., & Sharma, S. (Eds.), Innovations and sustainability in society 5.0. Hauppauge, NY: Nova Science Publishers, pp. 43–52.

Shroff, K. (2024). Artificial intelligence (AI) revolutionizing healthcare: A look at the present and future! Available at https://www.dsij.in/dsijarticledetail/artificial-intelligence-ai-revolutionizing-healthcare-a-look-at-the-present-and-future-37593

Singh, H. (2024). How AI and ML are revolutionising healthcare industry. Available at https://www.entrepreneur.com/en-in/news-and-trends/how-ai-and-ml-are-revolutionising-healthcare-industry/472959

Singla, B., Shalender, K., & Sharma, S. (2023). Consumers' preferences towards digital payments while online and offline shopping post COVID-19. In Mehta, K. Sharma, R., & Yu, P. (Eds.), Revolutionizing financial services and markets through FinTech and Blockchain. IGI Global Scientific Publishing, pp. 288–297. https://doi.org/10.4018/978-1-6684-8624-5.ch019

Singla, B., & Kumar, S. (Eds.). (2024). AI Healthcare Applications and Security, Ethical, and Legal Considerations. Hershey, PA: IGI Global, 2024. https://doi.org/10.4018/979-8-3693-7452-8

Singla, B., Kumar, S., & Katja, S. (Eds.). (2024). Revolutionizing the Healthcare Sector with AI. Hershey, PA: IGI Global. https://doi.org/10.4018/979-8-3693-3731-8

Welch, A. (2023). Artificial intelligence is helping revolutionize healthcare as we know it. Available at https://www.jnj.com/innovation/artificial-intelligence-in-healthcare

2 Dynamics of AI Challenges in Hospital Operations

From Bytes to Better Health

Sindu Bharathi S K, Saranya J, and Ramya M

INTRODUCTION

The growing discipline of artificial intelligence (AI) is expanding at a rapid pace across many industries due to its potential to revolutionise the global economy and determine which initiatives are crucial. According to Jarrett et al. (2021), in the field of medical, AI is the use of intelligent techniques, and technologies include machine learning and deep learning which associate auxiliary diagnosis, risk prediction, illness triage, health management, and hospital administration. Vaishya et al. (2020) magnified how the COVID-19 issue highlights how artificial intelligence could potentially use for a range of functions, including diagnostic and treatment decision assistance. Consequently, the healthcare sector has decided to use fresh information technology-based solutions and procedures meant to save costs and provide answers to these growing challenges. AI has great potential to revolutionise public health, save costs, and improve patient care. It helps with illness diagnosis, treatment plan customising, and patient outcome projections (Zhang et al., 2008). In addition, technology acceptance model (TAM) investigates elements driving AI adoption in companies (Chatterjee et al., 2021). Strategic uses for AI abound in the hospital sector (Hobbs et al., 2020; Rust, 2021; Sanaei & Sobhani, 2018; Sobhani et al., 2018). Though efficiently building and implementing artificial intelligence to solve different challenges in industry has been one of the most complicated areas of research, in both academia and industry, these applications have not been substantially investigated. Existing literature on healthcare workers' intent to adopt AI is mostly grounded on a single theory of technology adoption of TAM, which stands as technology adoption model that looked into how factors such as AI technical characteristics (Habermann, 2021) and individual psychological cognition (Adenuga et al., 2017; Bawack & Kamdjoug, 2018; Fan et al., 2020) affect the intension. The techno turbulence moderates the relationship between responsible AI and operational performance in the healthcare industry. Healthcare service providers must create ethical AI in order to create value propositions and enhance operational performance (Huang & Rust, 2021).

DOI: 10.1201/9781003531272-2

LITERATURE REVIEW AND HYPOTHESIS DEVELOPMENT

Applying the Unified Theory of Acceptance and Use of Technology (UTAUT) in the setting of the hospital sector in the city of Chennai, the theoretical structure of the present research effort is analogous. Researchers aspire to gain insight into how AI adoption behaviour mediates the relationship between organisational and technological readiness, innovativeness, perceived risk (PR), and operational effectiveness. This study further seeks to examine whether the techno turbulence component moderates the association with adoption of artificial intelligence behaviour and operational efficacy. These correlations between variables lead to the formulation of several hypotheses. The conceptual structure for AI adoption behaviour is exhibited in Figure 2.1.

ORGANISATIONAL READINESS AND AIAB

Organisational traits like the size of the business, senior management, etc. have a bearing on the implementation of novel innovations (Wade & Hulland, 2004). According to Iacovou et al. (1995), organisational readiness is "the availability of the appropriate organisational amenities for utilization." The present work incorporates managerial backing, business size, and the resources as facets of institutional

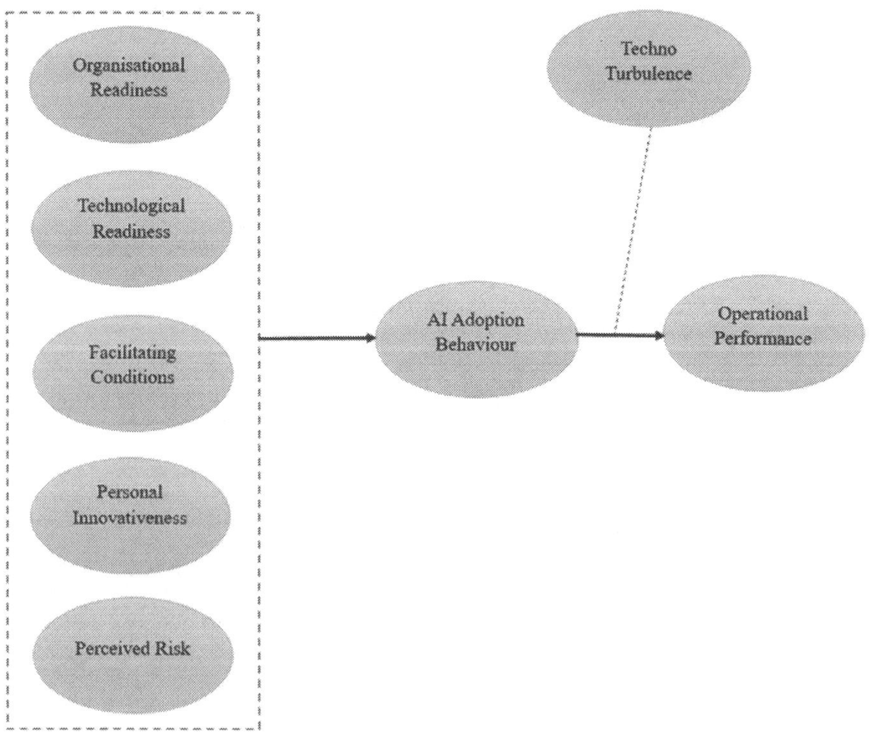

FIGURE 2.1 Conceptual Research Framework

Source: Authors' own.

readiness, relying on prior work on contemporary innovation (Duan, 2010; Hung et al., 2014; Idris, 2015; Yan et al., 2009; Yang et al., 2015; Zahi et al., 2010).

Managerial Backing

Engaging a top-level leader for Information Technology (IT) implementations is crucial for success (Ifinedo, 2005). According to resource-based theory, experiencing strong support from top management is indispensable (Alsyouf & Ishak, 2018). Without such backing, an organisation not just fails to strengthen its competitiveness but also becomes more likely to resist adopting new innovations (Wade & Hulland, 2004). Having strong support from the executive level is vital for the effective adoption of contemporary technology. Research has shown that when leaders articulate a concise goal, provide necessary funding, and allocate resources, it greatly enhances the chances of successful implementation (Hung et al., 2014; Yang et al., 2015; Zahi et al., 2010). As an illustration, in studies on IS/IT adoption, it was found that the endorsement of cloud-based computing (Yang et al., 2015) and e-business (Ifinedo, 2005) was positively influenced by managerial backing. Deploying AI to spearhead a corporate revolution is typically a calculated risk (Gartner, 2017b). Thus, this hypothesis is put forth:

H1a: Managerial backing positively influence AI adoption in organisation

Business Size

According to Rogers (2003), a company's propensity to embrace new technologies is proportional to its size. According to numerous studies (Aboelmaged, 2014; Duan, 2010; Zahi et al., 2010), larger firms are more likely to make investments in emerging technologies. According to Duan (2010), the capacity for incorporating technology is greater in large businesses. Similarly, it was noted by Zahi et al. (2010) that big enterprises are subject to increased pressure from rivals, and by Aboelmaged (2014) that the reason bigger enterprises possess greater financial and technological resources is the reason size matters (Singla, 2021; Singla, 2023). Based on this research, we can therefore hypothesise:

H2a: Business size has a positive influence on AI adoption in organisation

Resources

In addition to considering components related to organisational readiness, it requires attention to additionally take into account the availability of people businesses, and technological resources when implementing a novel concept at the business threshold (Iacovou et al., 1995). Technological capabilities incorporate hardware for computers, facts, and networking purposes, which are crucial for embracing novel advances (Aboelmaged, 2014). Within the realm of AI, numerous contemporary AI systems initially rely on conventional learning with machines computation, and subsequently acquire intelligence through training (Ransbotham et al., 2017). According to a recent survey by Narrative Science (2016), 59% of institutions proficient in big data are likewise utilising AI algorithms. Resources were categorised by Hung et al. (2014) as either manpower or technology. The latest study conducted by Gartner (2017a) indicates that most businesses have difficulty implementing AI and intelligent machines due to an overemphasis on advances in technology in place of sufficient abilities and processes. Extensive empirical studies in the field of information systems have consistently demonstrated that businesses that possess ample human, enterprise, and technological resources are more likely to embrace innovative practices, which include the adoption of web pages (Hung et al., 2015), e-maintenance (Aboelmaged, 2014), and electronic commerce (Wang et al., 2008). The findings from this study suggest that resources have a positive impact on AI readiness.

H3a: Human, enterprise, and technology resources positively influence AI adoption in organisations

Technological Readiness and AIAB

According to Lai (2007), technology readiness refers to individuals' willingness to adopt and utilise contemporary innovations to achieve their goals both in their personal lives and professional settings. They debated the dual nature of one's perception of the technology, acknowledging its advantages as well as drawbacks. The four elements of technology readiness—innovation, insecurity, discomfort, and optimism—are brought about by it.

Having a positive outlook on technology and recognising its benefits can greatly enhance job productivity and personal efficiency, both in the job environment and at their homes. The innovative nature category pertains to individuals who are enthusiastic about conducting trials with technological advances and are keen to be at the forefront of trying to develop novel goods and services based on the most recent innovations. The unease component refers to a feeling of inadequate proficiency with technology and a diminished sense of self-worth when using the most recent technological advancements. While it is unrelated to the extent of unpleasantness that indicates unease regarding technological advancements in broad terms, the factor of insecurity involves a lack of trust in technology-based transactions and worries about the functionality of the technology.

Two key factors that can enhance the readiness for employing technology are optimism and innovativeness, which play an integral part in driving technological adoption. On the contrary hand, the remaining two parameters, discomfort and insecurity, are seen as obstacles that can hinder the willingness to use the technology (Lai, 2007).

H2: Techno readiness positively influence AI adoption in organisations

Facilitating Conditions and AIAB

According to Venkatesh et al. (2003), it refers to the level of confidence that one has in the availability and effectiveness of the technological and associated structure that will facilitate the use of the fresh system. The concept of facilitating conditions (FC) encompasses the perception of having authority over one's conduct and being compatible with different paradigms, as proposed by Lee and Lin in 2008. An explicit correlation has been shown regarding FC and behavioural intent (BI) (Venkatesh et al., 2012).

Empirical studies have shown that there is a notable correlation between the utilisation of technology among people and the effects of FC on BI (Chiu et al., 2012). The usage of electronic filing by American taxpayers has shown that FC has a substantial role in deciphering the BI of the payers. This observation was made by Schaupp et al. (2010) and further established by Carter et al. in 2012. Based on these conversations, the subsequent hypothesis is developed.

H3: Facilitating Conditions (FC) have positive and significant impact on AI adoption behaviour

Personal Innovativeness and AIAB

Being innovative means actively seeking out new and unique concepts or techniques. In a study conducted by Thakur and Srivastava (2014), it was found that individual inventiveness played a significant role in influencing the decisions of individuals, as opposed to those who don't when it came to implementing m-payments in India. Conversely, innovativeness was determined by Kasilingam (2020) to function as the key predictor of BI to utilise chatbots; users' willingness to adopt chatbots will be impacted by how helpful and simple they find it to be, in addition to how confident they are in the technological reliability and safety. Innovation plays a crucial role in the entire adoption procedure, as it has an essential effect on adoption attitude. Therefore, we put forth the following hypothesis:

H4: Innovativeness positively influences AI adoption behaviour to use chatbots in organisations

Perceived Risk on AIAB

Perceived risk (PR) is recognised as the belief that those who use PR will experience negative consequences when they pursue a particular objective (Warkentin et al., 2002). AI is a form of technology that operates through the web. PR is the combination of feelings of uncertainty about one's actions coupled with concerns about the environment around them. The hostile structure of web-based functions contributes to behavioural uncertainty, whereas the erratic nature of online resources is accountable for ambient insecurity (Zhang & Maruping, 2008). Research has shown that decreasing PR has a notable effect on customer perceptions. According to a study by Teo and Liu (2007), the theoretical framework on electronic commerce suggests that PR has a detrimental and significant effect on users' behaviour. Hence, the following hypothesis is proposed,

H5: Perceived risk has positive and significant influence on AI adoption behaviour in organisations

DATA ANALYSIS

Of the participants in this study from Table 2.1, 44% were women and 56% were men, according to the data available. By age, 31% of respondents were between the ages of 20 and 25, 25% between the ages of 25 and 30, 20% between the ages of 30 and 35, 12% between the ages of 35 and 40, 7% between the ages of 40 and 45, and 5% over the age of 45. The majority of respondents fell into the age range of 25 to 30 years. Respondents with one to three years' experience accounted for the majority (37%), while those with more than ten years' experience (10%) made up the least percentage. In comparison to other categories, 29% of respondents with monthly salaries between 20,000 and 40,000 was higher.

The coefficient used to assess internal consistency and dependability is mostly estimated using Cronbach's alpha value. In this regard, the findings show that the scale had an exceptional level of consistency and reliability within the range of 0.810 in Table 2.2. The degree of sampling for each variable in the model is assessed using

TABLE 2.1
The Respondents' Demographic Characteristics

S. No.	Demographic Variable	Category	Frequency	Percentage (%)
1	Gender	Male	176	56
		Female	139	44
		Total	315	100
2	Age	20–25	98	31
		25–30	79	25
		30–35	63	20
		35–40	38	12
		40–45	23	7
		Above 45	14	5
		Total	315	100
3	Work Experiences	<One year	61	19
		One to three years	115	37
		Three to six years	65	21
		Six to ten years	41	13
		>Ten years	33	10
		Total	315	100
4	Monthly Salary	<20000	41	13
		20,001–40,000	94	29
		40,001–60000	74	24
		60,001–80,000	68	22
		80,001–1,00,000	27	9
		>1,00,000	11	3
		Total	315	100

Source: Authors' calculation (2024).

TABLE 2.2
Reliability and Validity

Reliability Statistics		
Cronbach's Alpha	**Cronbach's Alpha Based on Standardised Items**	**N of Items**
0.810	0.807	39

Source: Authors' calculation (2024).

the KMO Bartlett test. The sample adequacy is quite good with 39 items from the instrument, as shown by the computed value of 0.826.

R-Square is the percentage of variance in the dependent variable (operational performance) that can be anticipated based on the independent variables (organisational readiness technological readiness, facilitating conditions, personal innovativeness, PR, AI adoption behaviour, techno turbulence). The value 78.8% from Table 2.3 indicates that operational performance can be determined based on the independent variables. The Durbin-Watson statistic (1.834) can be used to test the output of a regression model for autocorrelation; it shows that there is no autocorrelation between the variables.

The *p* value (0.000) from Table 2.4 infers that there is an existence of the link between the exogenous and endogenous variable as it is < 0.05.

Regression analysis's variance inflation factor (VIF) is a measure for multicollinearity. All the VIF values are lesser than 5. Hence it indicates that all the variables are free from multicollinearity. The regression equation from Table 2.5 can be observed as,

$$\begin{aligned}\text{Operational Performance} = {} & 1.127 + 0.131\ (\text{Organisational Readiness}) \\ & + 0.166\ (\text{Technological Readiness}) \\ & + 0.057\ (\text{Facilitating Conditions}) \\ & + 0.210\ (\text{Personal Innovativeness}) \\ & + 0.001\ (\text{Perceived Risk}) \\ & + 0.196\ (\text{AI Adoption Behavior}) \\ & + 0.233\ (\text{Techno Turbulence})\end{aligned}$$

TABLE 2.3
Regression

Model Summary[b]

Model	R	R Square	Adjusted R Square	Std. Error of the Estimate	Durbin-Watson
1	0.698[a]	0.788	0.731	2.43882	1.827

Source: Authors' calculation (2024).

[a] Predictors: (Constant), TECHNO_TURBULENCE, PERC_RISK, AI_ADOPTIONBEH, FACI_CONDITIONS, TECH_READINESS, PERS_INNOVATIVENESS, ORG_READINESS

[b] Dependent variable: OPER_PERFORMANCE

TABLE 2.4
Significance Table of ANOVA

ANOVA[a]						
Model		Sum of Squares	df	Mean Square	F	Sig.
1	Regression	602.529	7	86.076	14.472	0.000[b]
	Residual	1825.991	307	5.948		
	Total	2428.521	314			

Source: Authors' calculation (2024).

[a] Dependent variable: OPER_PERFORMANCE

[b] Predictors: (Constant), TECHNO_TURBULENCE, PERC_RISK, AI_ADOPTIONBEH, FACI_CONDITIONS, TECH_READINESS, PERS_INNOVATIVENESS, ORG_READINESS

TABLE 2.5
Regression Coefficients

	Unstandardised Coefficients		Std Coefficients			Collinearity Statistics	
Model	B	Std. Error	Beta	t	Sig.	Tolerance	VIF
1 (Constant)	1.127	1.541		0.731	0.465		
ORG_READINESS	0.131	0.053	0.135	2.451	0.015	0.809	1.236
TECH_READINESS	0.166	0.051	0.176	3.237	0.001	0.825	1.213
FACI_CONDITIONS	0.057	0.056	0.052	1.029	0.304	0.944	1.059
PERS_INNOVATIVENESS	0.210	0.064	0.170	3.273	0.001	0.913	1.095
PERC_RISK	0.001	0.055	0.001	0.017	0.987	0.966	1.035
AI_ADOPTIONBEH	0.196	0.066	0.148	2.963	0.003	0.976	1.024
TECHNO_TURBULENCE	0.233	0.057	0.216	4.101	0.000	0.879	1.137

Source: Authors' calculation (2024).

Histogram shown in Figure 2.2 displays the distribution of residuals to assess the normality of errors.

To sum up, there are a few, however slight, outliers from the norm. Assuming that the residuals are approximately normally distributed, most analysts would draw this conclusion.

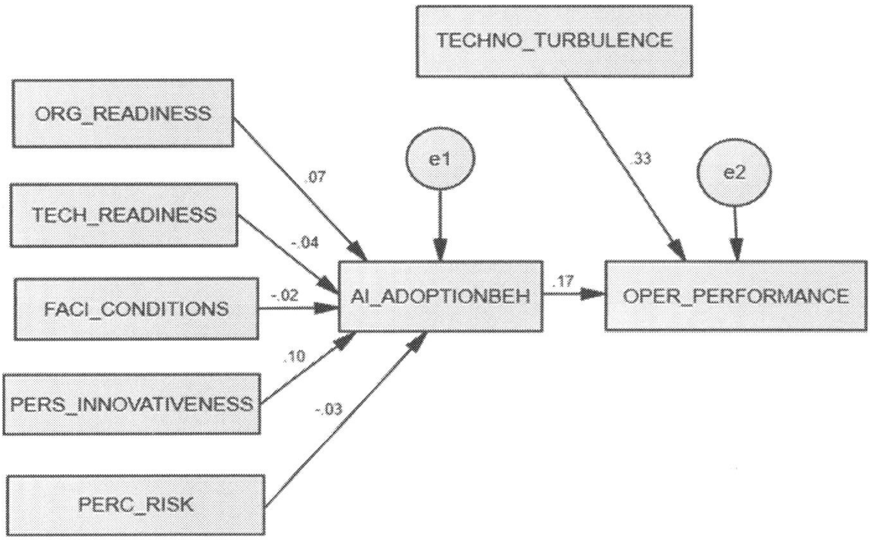

FIGURE 2.2 Histogram of Regression Analysis

Source: Authors' conceptualizations.

Path Analysis

Path analysis in Figure 2.3 is a statistical technique used to examine the direct and indirect relationships between variables in a model.

As per Table 2.6, the first hypothesis has a favourable impact on AIAB, which positively influences organisational readiness of managerial backing, business size and resources ($\beta = 0.51$, $p = 0.001$) and technological readiness ($\beta = 0.128$, $p = 0.007$), which leads to the approval of hypotheses 1a, 2a, 3a, and 2. As per Hypothesis 3,

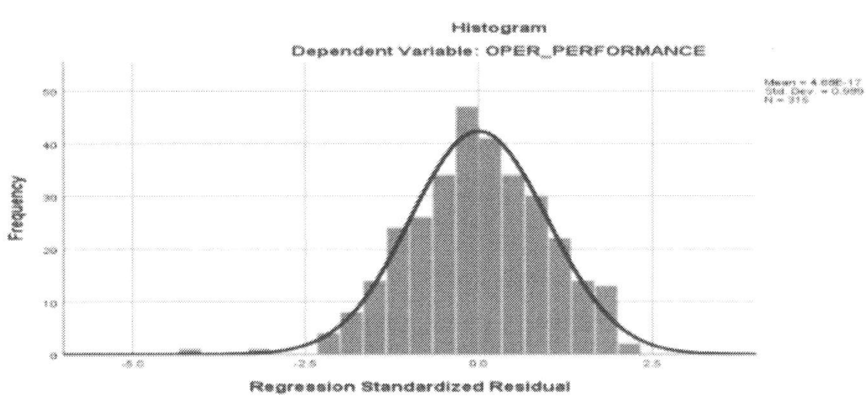

FIGURE 2.3 Path Analysis

Source: Authors' conceptualizations.

TABLE 2.6
Regression Weights: (Group Number 1—Default Model)

Dependent Variable	Path	Independent Variable	Estimate	S.E.	C.R.	p
AI_ADOPTIONBEH	<---	ORG_READINESS	0.051	0.042	2.225	0.001
AI_ADOPTIONBEH	<---	TECH_READINESS	0.128	0.041	2.695	0.007
AI_ADOPTIONBEH	<---	FACI_CONDITIONS	0.216	0.047	0.329	0.142
AI_ADOPTIONBEH	<---	PERS_INNOVATIVENESS	0.013	0.054	4.713	0.005
AI_ADOPTIONBEH	<---	PERC_RISK	0.027	0.047	2.572	0.008
OPER_PERFORMANCE	<---	AI_ADOPTIONBEH	0.217	0.069	3.123	0.002
OPER_PERFORMANCE	<---	TECHNO_TURBULENCE	0.352	0.056	6.238	***

Source: Authors' calculation (2024).

facilitating conditions showed negligible results, indicating that the AIAB has no positive influence ($\beta = 0.216$, $p = 0.142$). Consequently, Hypothesis 3 was found to be "not supported." Hypotheses 4 and 5 have a favourable influence on AIAB including personal innovativeness ($\beta = 0.13$, $p = 0.005$), perceived risk ($\beta = 0.217$, $p = 0.008$), which leads to the approval of hypotheses 4 and 5. Hypotheses 7 and 8 also found to be significant on operational performance by AIAB ($\beta = 0.217$, $p = 0.002$) and techno turbulence ($\beta = 0.352$, $p = 0.000$).

Based on the GFI value of 0.924 and the AGFI score of 0.917 in Table 2.7, which both exceed 0.9, the current instance has an exceptional model fit rating. Indicating a perfect match, the RMSEA and RMR values of 0.072 and 0.068, respectively, are less than 0.08. Further evidence that it is a perfect fit comes from the computed NFI value (0.965) and CFI value (0.908). Ultimately model fit is determined.

TABLE 2.7
Model Fit Summary

Indices	Value	Suggested Value
Chi-square value	7.897	-
DF	4	-
p value	0.107	> 0.05 (Hair et al., 1998)
Chi-square value/DF	2.002	< 5.00 (Hair et al., 1998)
GFI	0.924	> 0.90 (Hu and Bentler, 1999)
AGFI	0.917	> 0.90 (Hair et al. 2006)
NFI	0.965	> 0.90 (Hu and Bentler, 1999)
CFI	0.908	> 0.90 (Hooper et al., 2008)
RMR	0.068	< 0.08 (Hair et al. 2006)
RMSEA	0.072	< 0.08 (Hair et al. 2006)

Source: Authors' calculation (2024).

DISCUSSION AND FINDINGS

A number of respondents based on gender included 56% of male respondents and 44% female respondents. The majority of respondents fell into the age range of 25 to 30 years. Respondents with one to three years' experience accounted for the majority (37%), while those with more than ten years' experience (10%) made up the least percentage. In comparison to other categories, 29% of respondents with monthly salaries between 20,000 and 40,000 was higher. Recurrent chores cause administrative problems for hospitals. AI handles patient communication, scheduling, and revenue cycle management among other tasks. Higher preparedness strengthens the probability of innovation adoption while decreasing the possibility of failure. Organisations that anticipate an unambiguous business rationale for the application of AI, and a readiness to allocate resources towards talent acquisition and ongoing development better positioned to implement AI. Sharing knowledge and machine learning models among organisations helps to promote collaborative networks. Organisational readiness refers to people's tendency to adopt and implement cutting-edge technology. It is composed of up of two dimensions—motivators and inhibitors—that include innovativeness and optimism, which favourably influence technology usage, whereas inhibitors include insecurity and discomfort, which positively impact technology adoption. Patients are more inclined to accept AI if they believe it is trustworthy and reliable. The ease with which patients can utilise AI tools influences their willingness to accept AI adoption behaviour (Caputo et al., 2019). Patients are more inclined to accept AI technologies that are easy to use and intuitive. Our results help healthcare organisations develop an AI adoption behaviour while improving operational performance discovering how such technological improvements work. Our findings indicate that responsible AI influences a healthcare firm's value development and operational performance.

CONCLUSION

In a nutshell, this research puts up seven hypotheses. Among them, one was eliminated. On the other hand, there is ongoing research in terms of this, which is intended to provide additional information on the theories that were eliminated. For the purpose of bridging these inconsistencies, an extensive structure for the adoption behaviour of artificial intelligence applications was constructed and then implemented over an expanded spectrum of examples utilising the model of UTAUT. When it comes to technological preparedness, robust organisational backing may address uncertainty and uncomfortable aspects. The results of the study reveal that the presence of technological disruption has a profound moderating implications for the association that exists between the adoption behaviour of artificial intelligence and the operational accomplishments of the business.

In addition to this, it makes a contribution to the comprehension of the widespread adoption behaviours of artificial intelligence in healthcare facilities (Zhang et al., 2020). It is possible for decision-makers to capitalise on the use of the outcomes of this research in order to create customised rules that would make it easier for the staff working in healthcare settings to embrace artificial intelligence (AI)

(Nam et al., 2023; Chen et al., 2020). The presented research improves our consciousness of the technical setting, organisational preparedness, and external variables that influence the integration of AI in healthcare businesses in Chennai, thereby making a worthwhile contribution to the healthcare industry (Cheung et al., 2008).

IMPLICATIONS

As a result, being able to thoughtfully allocate their resources towards AI benefits economic growth and improves their competitive advantage. Policymakers might utilise the insights of this study to craft policies that promote the implementation of AI in hospitals, therefore contributing to the preservation of patients' lives. Realising the pressing need of government support, policy initiatives may focus on addressing barriers such as exorbitant costs and issues related to protecting intellectual property rights (Duan et al., 2024). To increase the level of confidence and acceptance of AI-assisted diagnosis and treatment among healthcare professionals, hospital managers ought to alter their management techniques. In addition to conveying the hospitals' support for the use of AI-assisted diagnosis and treatment, hospital administrators should encourage healthcare personnel to adopt the usage of AI-assisted diagnosis and treatment by communicating this support to them. Hospitals ensure training in AI technology to its allied healthcare staff in order to aid them in rapidly comprehending AI-assisted diagnosis and therapy. For the purpose of encouraging healthcare staff to use AI-assisted diagnosis and treatment, hospital administrators should also consider linking employees' job performance to their salaries and opportunities for advancement.

LIMITATION AND FUTURE DIRECTION

Several restrictions limit the scope of this investigation. To begin, an experiment with a cross-sectional approach was carried out as part of this investigation in order to investigate and assess hypothesis within the context of health facilities. Noting that the results of longitudinal studies carried out in other developing countries could provide conclusions that are different from one another is a crucial aspect to keep in consideration. Additionally, the current study was conducted solely with the purpose of examining healthcare organisations, although a number of other fields of service were not examined in order to gain a deeper understanding of the adoption of AI and its implications on various aspects of performance. Secondly, the findings of the current research provide evidence that the decision to use AI can have profound effects on the efficiency and effectiveness of hospitals. The hospital setting provides more evidence that AI has a significant impact on the creation of financial, environmental, and operational performance. Nevertheless, there is a requirement for further research to investigate the other variables that have an impact on the long-term sustainability of hospital settings.

Recognising that the population used for the investigation was solely collected from hospitals in the vicinity of Chennai is an essential point to emphasise. It is also recommended that various businesses be mindful when trying to implement the results of this research, knowing that there may be intrinsic variances that might impact the degree to whether these parameters impact their specific industries. Additionally, other organisations should take this into consideration. In addition, when it pertains to the use of AI, future research must additionally consider moral issues as a component of sustainable human resource practices. Guidelines relating to sustainability can be adhered to by ensuring that AI technologies are employed and regulated in a responsible manner.

REFERENCES

Abbass, H. A. (2019). Social integration of artificial intelligence: Functions, automation allocation logic and human-autonomy trust. *Cognitive Computation*, *11*(2), 159–171.

Aboelmaged, M. G. (2014). Predicting e-readiness at firm-level: An analysis of technological, organizational and environmental (TOE) effects on e-maintenance readiness in manufacturing firms. *International Journal of Information Management*, *34*(5), 639–651.

Adenuga, K. I., Iahad, N. A., & Miskon, S. (2017). Towards reinforcing telemedicine adoption amongst clinicians in Nigeria. *International Journal of Medical Informatics*, *104*, 84–96.

Akter, S., Wamba, S. F., Gunasekaran, A., Dubey, R., & Childe, S. J. (2016). How to improve firm performance using big data analytics capability and business strategy alignment? *International Journal of Production Economics*, *182*, 113–131.

Alsyouf, A., & Ishak, A. K. (2018). Understanding EHRs continuance intention to use from the perspectives of UTAUT: Practice environment moderating effect and top management support as predictor variables. *International Journal of Electronic Healthcare*, *10*(1–2), 24–59.

Autry, C. W., Grawe, S. J., Daugherty, P. J., & Richey, R. G. (2010). The effects of technological turbulence and breadth on supply chain technology acceptance and adoption. *Journal of Operations Management*, *28*(6), 522–536.

Aydiner, A. S., Tatoglu, E., Bayraktar, E., Zaim, S., & Delen, D. (2019). Business analytics and firm performance: The mediating role of business process performance. *Journal of Business Research*, *96*, 228–237.

Bawack, R. E., & Kamdjoug, J. R. K. (2018). Adequacy of UTAUT in clinician adoption of health information systems in developing countries: The case of Cameroon. *International Journal of Medical Informatics*, *109*, 15–22.

Bodlaj, M., & Čater, B. (2019). The impact of environmental turbulence on the perceived importance of innovation and innovativeness in SMEs. *Journal of Small Business Management*, *57*, 417–435.

Brougham, D., & Haar, J. (2018). Smart technology, artificial intelligence, robotics, and algorithms (STARA): Employees' perceptions of our future workplace. *Journal of Management & Organization*, *24*(2), 239–257.

Butner, K., & Ho, G. (2019). How the human-machine interchange will transform business operations. *Strategy & Leadership*, *47*(2), 25–33.

Caputo, F., Cillo, V., Candelo, E., & Liu, Y. (2019). Innovating through digital revolution: The role of soft skills and Big Data in increasing firm performance. *Management Decision*, *57*(8), 2032–2051.

Caputo, A., Pizzi, S., Pellegrini, M. M., & Dabić, M. (2021). Digitalization and business models: Where are we going? A science map of the field. *Journal of Business Research*, *123*, 489–501.

Carter, L., Schaupp, L. C., Hobbs, J., & Campbell, R. (2012). E-government utilization: Understanding the impact of reputation and risk. *International Journal of Electronic Government Research (IJEGR)*, *8*(1), 83–97.

Chatterjee, S., Rana, N. P., Dwivedi, Y. K., & Baabdullah, A. M. (2021). Understanding AI adoption in manufacturing and production firms using an integrated TAM-TOE model. *Technological Forecasting and Social Change*, *170*, 120880.

Chen, H. L., Vicki Widarso, G., & Sutrisno, H. (2020). A chatbot for learning Chinese: Learning achievement and technology acceptance. *Journal of Educational Computing Research*, *58*(6), 1161–1189.

Chen, L., Feldmann, A., & Tang, O. (2015). The relationship between disclosures of corporate social performance and financial performance: Evidences from GRI reports in manufacturing industry. *International Journal of Production Economics*, *170*, 445–456.

Cheung, N., Klein, R., Wang, J. J., Cotch, M. F., Islam, A. F., Klein, B. E., & Wong, T. Y. (2008). Traditional and novel cardiovascular risk factors for retinal vein occlusion: The multiethnic study of atherosclerosis. *Investigative Ophthalmology & Visual Science*, *49*(10), 4297–4302.

Chiu, C. M., Hsu, M. H., Lai, H., & Chang, C. M. (2012). Re-examining the influence of trust on online repeat purchase intention: The moderating role of habit and its antecedents. *Decision Support Systems*, *53*(4), 835–845.

Choi, Y. J., Baek, J. H., Park, H. S., Shim, W. H., Kim, T. Y., Shong, Y. K., & Lee, J. H. (2017). A computer-aided diagnosis system using artificial intelligence for the diagnosis and characterization of thyroid nodules on ultrasound: Initial clinical assessment. *Thyroid*, *27*(4), 546–552.

Duan, G. R. (2010). Analysis and Design of Descriptor Linear Systems (Vol. 23). Springer Science & Business Media. DOI 10.1007/978-1-4419-6397-0

Duan, Y., Edwards, J. S., & Dwivedi, Y. K. (2019). Artificial intelligence for decision making in the era of Big Data–evolution, challenges and research agenda. *International Journal of Information Management*, *48*, 63–71.

Duan, Y., Zhou, F., Li, X., Geng, L., & Yue, S. (2024). Is better readiness the key to deeper learning in distance education? A cross-sectional online study. *Heliyon*, *10*(9), 1–8.

Dubey, R., Gunasekaran, A., Childe, S. J., Blome, C., & Papadopoulos, T. (2019). Big data and predictive analytics and manufacturing performance: Integrating institutional theory, resource-based view and big data culture. *British Journal of Management*, *30*(2), 341–361.

Eisenhardt, K. M., & Martin, J. A. (2000). Dynamic capabilities: What are they? *Strategic Management Journal*, *21*(10–11), 1105–1121.

Fan, J., Fang, L., Wu, J., Guo, Y., & Dai, Q. (2020). From brain science to artificial intelligence. *Engineering*, *6*(3), 248–252.

Gartner. (2017a). Hype cycle for artificial intelligence, 2017. Retrieved from https://www.gartner.com/document/3770467?ref=solrAll&refval=193456093&qid=063144043355fa4bde62ca5985043d81#

Gartner. (2017b). Predicts 2018: artificial intelligence. Retrieved from https://www.gartner.com/document/3827163/meter/charge

Habermann, J. (2021). Psychological impacts of COVID-19 and preventive strategies: A review. 1–16

Hair, J. F., Anderson, R. E., Tatham, R. L., & Black, W. C. (1998). *Multivariate data analysis* (5th ed.). Prentice Hall.

Hair, J. F., Black, W. C., Babin, B. J., Anderson, R. E. & Tatham, R. L. (2006). *Multivariate data analysis*. Pearson Prentice Hall.

Hobbs, G., Manchester, R. N., Dunning, A., Jameson, A., Roberts, P., George, D., & Whiting, M. (2020). An ultra-wide bandwidth (704 to 4 032 MHz) receiver for the Parkes radio telescope. *Publications of the Astronomical Society of Australia*, *37*, e012.

Hooper, D., Coughlan, J., & Mullen, M. R. (2008). Structural equation modelling: Guidelines for determining model fit. *Electronic Journal of Business Research Methods*, *6*(1), 53–60.

Hu, L. T., & Bentler, P. M. (1999). Cutoff criteria for fit indexes in covariance structure analysis: Conventional criteria versus new alternatives. *Structural Equation Modeling: A Multidisciplinary Journal*, *6*(1), 1–55.

Huang, M. H., & Rust, R. T. (2021). A strategic framework for artificial intelligence in marketing. *Journal of the Academy of Marketing Science*, *49*, 30–50.

Hung, S. C., Hung, S. W., & Lin, M. J. J. (2015). Are alliances a panacea for SMEs? The achievement of competitive priorities and firm performance. *Total Quality Management & Business Excellence*, *26*(1-2), 190–202.

Hung, W. H., Chang, L. M., Lin, C. P., & Hsiao, C. H. (2014). E-readiness of website acceptance and implementation in SMEs. *Computers in Human Behavior*, *40*, 44–55.

Iacovou, C. L., Benbasat, I., & Dexter, A. S. (1995). Electronic data interchange and small organizations: Adoption and impact of technology. *MIS Quarterly*, *19*(4) 465–485.

Idris, A. O. (2015). Assessing a theoretically-derived e-readiness framework for e-commerce in a Nigerian SME. *Evidence Based Information Systems Journal*, *1*(1), 1–20.

Ifinedo, P. (2005). Measuring Africa's e-readiness in the global networked economy: A nine-country data analysis. *International Journal of Education and Development Using ICT*, *1*(1), 53–71.

Jarrett, D. E., Lio, P., & Ercole, A. (2021). How artificial intelligence and machine learning can help healthcare systems respond to COVID-19. *Machine Learning*, *110*(1), 1–14.

Kasilingam, D. L. (2020). Understanding the attitude and intention to use smartphone chatbots for shopping. *Technology in Society*, *62*, 101280.

Lai, M. L. (2007). Professional students' technology readiness, prior computing experience and acceptance of an e-learning system/Lai Ming Ling and Chong Moi Moi. *Malaysian Accounting Review*, *6*(1), 85–99.

Lee, A. J., & Lin, W. H. (2008). Twelve-week biomechanical ankle platform system training on postural stability and ankle proprioception in subjects with unilateral functional ankle instability. *Clinical biomechanics*, *23*(8), 1065–1072.

Lingmont, D. N., & Alexiou, A. (2020). The contingent effect of job automating technology awareness on perceived job insecurity: Exploring the moderating role of organizational culture. *Technological Forecasting and Social Change*, *161*, 120302.

Lu, R., Wu, X., Wan, Z., Li, Y., Zuo, L., Qin, J., ... & Zhang, C. (2020). Development of a novel reverse transcription loop-mediated isothermal amplification method for rapid detection of SARS-CoV-2. *Virologica Sinica*, *35*, 344–347.

Nam, T. (2019). Technology usage, expected job sustainability, and perceived job insecurity. *Technological Forecasting and Social Change*, *138*, 155–165.

Nam, J. G., Hwang, E. J., Kim, J., Park, N., Lee, E. H., Kim, H. J., & Goo, J. M. (2023). AI improves nodule detection on chest radiographs in a health screening population: A randomized controlled trial. *Radiology*, *307*(2), e221894.

Oztemel, E., & Gursev, S. (2020). Literature review of industry 4.0 and related technologies. *Journal of Intelligent Manufacturing*, *31*(1), 127–182.

Panichayakorn, T., & Jermsittiparsert, K. (2019). Mobilizing organizational performance through robotic and artificial intelligence awareness in mediating role of supply chain agility. *International Journal of Supply Chain Management*, *8*(5), 757–768.

Ramanathan, U., Subramanian, N., & Parrott, G. (2017). Role of social media in retail network operations and marketing to enhance customer satisfaction. *International Journal of Operations & Production Management*, *37*(1), 105–123.

Ransbotham, S., Kiron, D., Gerbert, P., & Reeves, M. (2017). Reshaping business with artificial intelligence: Closing the gap between ambition and action. *MIT Sloan Management Review*, *59*(1), 1–17.

Rogers, E. M. (2003). Diffusion networks. *Networks in the Knowledge Economy*, *10*, 134–161.

Rust, R. T., Rand, W., Huang, M. H., Stephen, A. T., Brooks, G., & Chabuk, T. (2021). Real-time brand reputation tracking using social media. *Journal of Marketing*, *85*(4), 21–43.

Sanaei, M. R., & Sobhani, F. M. (2018). Information technology and e-business marketing strategy. *Information Technology and Management*, *19*, 185–196.

Schaupp, L. C., Carter, L., & McBride, M. E. (2010). E-file adoption: A study of US taxpayers' intentions. *Computers in Human Behavior*, *26*(4), 636–644.

Singla, B. (2023). Promotional strategies for organized retail. *International Journal of Asian Business and Information Management*, *14*(1), 1–11. DOI: 10.4018/IJABIM.325229

Singla, B., Dyczek, B., Soto, R. M. H., & Mukthar, K. J. (2021). Whatever is seen is sold: Merchandise mantra. *Webology*, *18*(Special Issue 03), 451–461. https://doi.org/10.14704/web/v18si03/web18106

Srinivasan, R., & Swink, M. (2018). An investigation of visibility and flexibility as complements to supply chain analytics: An organizational information processing theory perspective. *Production and Operations Management*, *27*(10), 1849–1867.

Sobhani, M. R., Abrisham, S. M. J., Jahanbakhti, H., Pahlavanhossein, H., & Shokraneh, S. (2018). Studying outcomes of hardware removal in patients admitted to Yazd Shahid Sadoughi Hospital from April 2010 to May 2015. *SSU_Journals*, *26*(4), 355–362.

Stone, M., Aravopoulou, E., Ekinci, Y., Evans, G., Hobbs, M., Labib, A., Laughlin, P., Machtynger, J., & Machtynger, L. (2020). Artificial intelligence (AI) in strategic marketing decision-making: A research agenda. *The Bottom Line*, *33*(2), 183–200.

Teo, T. S. H., & Liu, J. (2007). Consumer trust in e-commerce in the United States, Singapore and China. *Omega*, *35*(1), 22–38.

Thakur, R., & Srivastava, M. (2014). Adoption readiness, personal innovativeness, perceived risk and usage intention across customer groups for mobile payment services in India. *Internet Research*, *24*(3), 369–392.

Vaishya, R., Javaid, M., Khan, I. H., & Haleem, A. (2020). Artificial intelligence (AI) applications for COVID-19 pandemic. *Diabetes & Metabolic Syndrome: Clinical Research & Reviews*, *14*(4), 337–339.

Venkatesh, V., Morris, M. G., Davis, G. B., & Davis, F. D. (2003). User acceptance of information technology: Toward a unified view. *MIS Quarterly*, *27*(3), 425–478.

Venkatesh, V., Thong, J. Y. L., & Xu, X. (2012). Consumer acceptance and use of information technology: Extending the Unified Theory of Acceptance and Use of Technology. *MIS Quarterly*, *36*(1), 157–178.

Wade, M., & Hulland, J. (2004). The resource-based view and information systems research: Review, extension, and suggestions for future research. *MIS Quarterly*, *28*(1), 107–142.

Wamba, S. F., Gunasekaran, A., Akter, S., Ren, S. J.-fan, Dubey, R., & Childe, S. J. (2017). Big data analytics and firm performance: Effects of dynamic capabilities. *Journal of Business Research*, *70*, 356–365.

Wang, M., Liu, J., Wang, H., Cheung, W. K., & Xie, X. (2008). On-demand e-supply chain integration: A multi-agent constraint-based approach. *Expert Systems with Applications*, *34*(4), 2683–2692.

Warkentin, M., Gefen, D., Pavlou, P. A., & Rose, G. M. (2002). Encouraging citizen adoption of e-government by building trust. *Electronic Markets*, *12*(3), 157–162.

Yan, T. D., Black, D., Bannon, P. G., & McCaughan, B. C. (2009). Systematic review and meta-analysis of randomized and nonrandomized trials on safety and efficacy of video-assisted thoracic surgery lobectomy for early-stage non–small-cell lung cancer. *Journal of Clinical Oncology*, *27*(15), 2553–2562.

Yang, J., Zhang, F., Jiang, X., & Sun, W. (2015). Strategic flexibility, green management, and firm competitiveness in an emerging economy. *Technological Forecasting and Social Change*, *101*, 347–356.

Zahi, R., Vialle, R., Abelin, K., Mary, P., Khouri, N., & Damsin, J. P. (2010). Spinopelvic fixation with iliosacral screws in neuromuscular spinal deformities: results in a prospective cohort of 62 patients. *Child's Nervous System*, *26*, 81–86.

Zhang, K., Liu, X., Shen, J., Li, Z., Sang, Y., Wu, X., & Zha, Y., et al. (2020). Clinically applicable AI system for accurate diagnosis, quantitative measurements, and prognosis of COVID-19 pneumonia using computed tomography. *Cell*, *181*(6), 1423–1433.

Zhang, X., & Maruping, L. M. (2008). Household technology adoption in a global marketplace: Incorporating the role of espoused cultural values. *Information Systems Frontiers*, *10*, 403–413.

3 The Application of Artificial Intelligence and Robotics in Healthcare Services

Leena Jenefa, M. Jayakumar, S. Catherine, Ashok Kumar S., Rahul Tripathi, and Jeevitha M.

INTRODUCTION

Emerging healthcare technologies, such as digital healthcare and the advanced artificial intelligence (AI) techniques, have altered the medical scenario like clinical treatment for patients like uterus problem, overbleeding, and cancer by addressing gaps in the present healthcare delivery system. The introduction of AI techniques and robotics tools in healthcare service sector has providing huge offering to patients suffering from various health issues by providing opportunities to enhance patient care along with systematic processes and helping to direct to the concern medical professionals. AI tools helped in all advanced technical advancements for managing to imitate individual cognitive processes like knowledge and problem-solving (Bajwa et al. 2021).

The technology robots have a role in medical diagnosis, surgery, rehabilitation, patient monitoring, and medication development. The knowledge and data generated by AI solutions may be used by both people and other technologies. Currently, the area of biomedical research and clinical practice is confronting hurdles due to the size and complexity of the data created by sequencing technologies, as well as the question of how to derive novel diagnoses and therapies from this data. It is required to gather, assess, and apply the outcomes of investigations, which are typically disguised within clinical data warehouses (Granić, 2022). So many institutions are using AI in the field of medicine to take fast decision-making mechanisms in healthcare sector. AI helped to analyze and follow up the patient health chart and identify the illness and send the report to the doctor to follow-up action.

The use of Robot plays an important role in production in manufacturing units and used in healthcare sector too. It opened an eye for all businesses and helps to diagnose the patient, having virtual consultations and identifying the problem, helping in surgical procedures, following the care of the patient and automated advanced equipment to simplify the process in the hospitals (Abdi et al., 2018). In addition to that, these robots with high and advanced technology are providing follow-up and

DOI: 10.1201/9781003531272-3

sending messages to the patients. The robotic systems have high potential to support clinical practice in the hospital (Duffy et al., 2022). These innovations have the potential to transform how medicine is performed.

There are enormous increases in using AI application or tools having a significant role and applicable in all issues in healthcare sector from consultation to implementation. The use of AI helps reduce the risk and critical thinking comparable to that of a human being. AI-inbuilt chatbots have numerous and virtual assistants to the patients using online services in healthcare to provide individualized assistance and information to patients. These intelligent devices can answer medical queries, offer self-care advice, and triage patients based on symptoms (Al-Emran and Arpaci, 2021). This enhances healthcare accessibility while simultaneously reducing the pressure on providers. AI has demonstrated potential in predictive analytics and patient monitoring. AI techniques are used to analyze huge volumes of patient data to segregate, analyze illness and risk factors, allowing healthcare practitioners to react early, and avoid unpleasant occurrences. AI-powered wearables and remote monitoring systems continuously monitor vital indicators and warn patients of crucial changes in their health state (Babita, 2023).

AI tools are used everywhere to reduce human labor like replacing the physicians and nurses, who work for patient in healthcare. AI tools have the possibility to change the healthcare. AI technologies enable computers to accomplish things that humans generally do, such as learn new things, intellectual, and analyzing. Under the different classifications in the field of computer science and networking, these tools create advanced technology by using advanced computers by doing numerous activities that would normally need human brain (Gereon, 2018). Nowadays, organizations are using automated discussion by using visual speech, recognition of the issues, and taking decision-making by using machine language translation. AI is being used in all disciplines in all the sectors like medicine, supply chain, logistics, marketing, and architecture. In health sector, it is used as pre operation consultant, patient communication, preparing medical documents like basic prescriptions, and virtual remote patient treatment (Dhamnani et al., 2019).

AI is ready to assist healthcare division from administrative works to clinical documentation and patient management, by providing medical advice and patient monitoring for health check-up. Understanding the panorama of roles that robots play in healthcare is critical for informing future research and development (Singla et al., 2021).

The robots in healthcare are mostly focused on remote presence and task execution away from human presence (Table 3.1). Robots will help people to be more

TABLE 3.1
Robotics in Healthcare

Sl. No.	Robotics in Healthcare
1.	Patient care
2.	Surgical procedures
3.	Diagnosis
4.	Rehabilitation

present and flexible. This will help provide consistent, change-resistant, and adaptable services. Advanced infrastructure is required for robot adoption. Investment in the systems that enable robots to function is critical (White et al., 2021).

With continual technical breakthroughs, robots may be designed to perform new dimension of work assigned by the human. The roles used in this detailed analysis are based on robotic influence used in clinical context; however, there are special robots with inbuilt techniques used for pre-clinical assessment that may be used for future. The AI techniques are highly demanded for further research that is needed to determine the efficacy and highly used in hospital services.

This chapter will address some of the primary benefits of AI in health services. The chapter reviews the existing and potential uses of AI in healthcare. Advancements in AI present promising potential for the healthcare business. Advanced technologies, like machine learning, have significantly improved healthcare delivery. These developments might considerably improve patient care, diagnostics, administrative operations, and medical research and innovation.

Technological Advancements Artificial Intelligence Applications in Healthcare

AI is automated machine learning set up by modifying the medical practices. AI applications in medical sector are incorporated in all the areas including clinical practices, automatic diagnostic, rehabilitation, pre- and post-surgical operations, and predictive procedures. AI is having an influence in clinical decision-making, and early diagnosis can help radiologists spot problems more quickly. It helps to make treatment easily. AI has significant impact on medication discovery and development (Staehler et al., 2015). AI systems analyze the biological data to find the prospective therapeutic, optimize drug design, and speed up clinical trials in the healthcare unit. This might speed up the procedure by using high automatic instruments and improve the delivery of innovative treatment for patients. AI has made significant contributions to human being by helping in healthcare sector, but its promise for the future is much more exciting. Machine learning applications are making a huge impact on healthcare that allows to study from data and analyze it. It helped the healthcare sector in different ways like image analysis, diagnosis the patient, and follow up for consultation. The algorithms used for machine learning can analyze the medical treatment records including magnetic resonance imaging (MRI) scans reports and able to deduct the basic and fundamental information to the patient. Machine learning can help to forecast the illness of the patient based on their past history. Machine learning has transformed healthcare by improving image processing, diagnosis, and treatment planning capabilities (Croghan et al., 2018). These algorithms are able to deduct with accurately and categorize the different diseases like tumors and other disorders. Training on the huge informations allowed the machine learning tools to detect the minor issues that human being may be unable to identify. This can help radiologists and healthcare workers provide more accurate and faster diagnoses, resulting in better patient care. Machine learning algorithms can help forecast illness progression and therapy response. Machine learning algorithms help to analyze the data of the in and out patient information, including description, doctors' advice, records, counseling, and family history of the patient information, etc. to detect the problem identification and risk factors for specific conditions. AI technology in healthcare has accelerated medication discovery. In contrast, it automates target identification. These technologies will identify the modern advice and medications for health services and to treat the patients effectively (Chakradhar et al., 2017).

Radiotherapy

AI has improved tumor segmentation and organ risk assessment, saving radiation oncologists a significant amount of time. AI techniques used in various areas like treatment planning and optimization and forecasting provide accurate data in a fast manner.

Radiotherapy radiation robots can help in the delivery of radiation. This robot can help with the use of radiation and visual guidance to treat problems including liver and orbital metastases (Mohr et al., 2001). Automatic modern techniques have several benefits and challenges, including reduced variability across in observers and reduced time savings in analyzing the clinical practice. Currently, it is understood that automated machines like x-ray devices should not be employed unattended with human being; however, correcting automatic machines helped the patients to reduce time in waiting for consultation (Weinstein et al., 2014; Burton et al., 2019).

Telepresence

Many industrialized and developing nations are experiencing with huge number of old people. These factors create both socio cultural and economic problems, related toward genetic illnesses, commonly linked with aging and inability to walk (Hwei and Octavius, 2021). Medical expenses and medication consultation are increasing, together with the increased frequency of chronic and young-generation related illness like depression, anxiety, etc. (Sekhon et al., 2021). Telepresence is a potential explanation in the domain of personal care innovation, encompassing several distant healthcare delivery technologies such as wearable health, and digital health (Gogia, 2019). Given the growing number of long-lasting illnesses and the limits of healthcare distribution, it has the latent to become a crucial technique for giving quality treatment.

A key characteristic of the telepresence robotic group is the capacity to provide humans with a distant presence via the robot. The robot may be utilized for things like remote ward rounds and surgical mentorship.

Health Services Management

The intense concentration, usage, and implementation of AI in medical exercise remain restricted, with numerous AI solutions for healthcare still in the project and development stages (Chen et al., 2022). AI approaches can benefit physicians, nurtures, and superintendents in their work. AI systems may give continual, potentially apprises from diverse sources, like periodicals, manuals, and medical practices (Badash et al., 2016).

Maternal Care

To identify the risk factors in expected mothers during scanning process and minimizing complications. Using electronic health data and AI, predict if expecting moms are at high risk of delivery complications.

AI-Powered Stethoscope

One advantage is that, unlike traditional stethoscopes, readings may be collected in loud surroundings for more accurate diagnosis. The digital gadget is user-friendly and requires no training to gather and transmit records to doctors. This reduces the risk of getting COVID-19 and improves access to medical care for chronically sick people. AI and machine learning enable computers to identify trends and problems in healthcare data.

Wearable Health Technologies

A smart device, such as a tablet, might serve as an interface between individuals and sensors. Additionally, collected data is stored and analyzed on the cloud for geriatric care.

Wearable technology has introduced whole new and rapidly evolving tools to the popular field of personal devices. Wearable gadgets are now available for healthcare applications by helping them in analyzing data using standard protocols and technology like machine learning helps to forecast health-related issues for human being and for animals.

The combination of AI with wearable health technologies has revolutionized how patients and consumers monitor and manage their health. Innovation and emerging technology provide users with additional information about their own health and raise awareness, which may help them manage their sleep, stress, and other everyday activities better.

Robotic Surgery

Machine-like operating systems have transformed medical techniques by giving doctors more accuracy, dexterity, and vision. These devices enable reduce procedures in lesser scratches, less patient trauma, and shorter retrieval periods. Non-human surgery has applications in a variety of disciplines, including heart, gynecological, urine, and intestinal procedures (Vercelli et al., 2018; Luxton and Riek, 2019).

Rehabilitation

Automation has altered the area of reintegration by introducing cutting-edge gadgets. It can assist individuals with mobility disabilities. These offer regulated and repeated motions, helping affected role re-learn and improve physical strength (Goldzweig et al., 2013).

Wearable technology's inertial sensors can monitor workout performance and compliance (Yang et al., 2019). The study evaluated exercise adherence in healthy persons wearing an Apple iWatch throughout a rotator-cuff workout routine.

AI and robots are changing rehabilitation research and practice. Smart homes can help inhabitants with everyday tasks and inform caretakers when assistance is required. Smart mobile and wearable devices may gather and analyze data to help people improve their health and achieve individualized rehabilitation objectives (Esteva et al., 2017).

Medical Imaging and Diagnostics

Medical imaging and diagnostics rely heavily on robotics. Robotic devices help to get exact and high-resolution pictures, which allow for true finding and plan for treatment. Robot-procedures like robotic ultrasound, MRI treatments, and surgeries are the scope for treatment. Computerization in pathology employing automatic equipment and algorithms improves the efficacy and accurateness of investigative actions (Burton et al., 2019). One of the most potential uses of AI and robots in healthcare is medical diagnosis. AI-powered robotics provide unmatched precision and accuracy in medical diagnostics (Al-Qaysi et al., 2021).

The radiology experts are gradually using to detect illnesses early and reduce indicative errors in the situation of deterrence. Similarly, convenient tool for assessing ECG and echocardiogram charts are available to take decisions (Panch et al., 2019). It can evaluate massive volumes of persistent data, such as medicinal histories, imaging scans, and hereditary evidence, to detect trends and generate accurate diagnostic forecasts.

Assistive and Companion Robots

This technique is utilized to develop assistive robots for the aging and others with incapacities. It may contribute with everyday responsibilities and health circumstances by providing independent quality of life (Mathews et al., 2019).

Medicine Delivery

It is used for accurate and battered medicine distribution. This device outfitted inbuilt sensors, and microchips may travel the human being and administer pharmaceuticals to particular places, reducing adverse effects and enhancing treatment effectiveness (Weinstein et al., 2014; Yang et al., 2019; Amann et al., 2020). These technologies have the potential to transform medication administration and customized treatment.

Clinical Decision-Making

AI technologies helped doctors and medical researchers make clinical decisions. Algorithms can improve clinical rulings by fast moving up the procedure and care obtainable, letting down the cost of healthcare (Coeckelbergh, 2021). It can assist medicinal specialists and simplify their responsibilities. It has the ability to profoundly alter the healthcare business. Multiple improvements highlight its current condition in healthcare settings across a wide range of applications (Erikainen and

Chan, 2019). AI-powered algorithms enable doctors to deliver improved treatment for their patients.

Surgical Intervention

The use of AI and robots in surgery has improved accuracy, reduced errors, and improved patient outcomes (Ramanathan et al., 2024). AI-powered surgical robotics now allow healthcare practitioners to conduct difficult surgeries with greater precision and efficiency (Eubanks, 2018; AlQudah et al., 2021). The combination of AI and robots has revolutionized the surgical scene and has the potential to further innovate medical procedures. AI-enabled robotic tools provide surgeons with real-time input on tissue properties, vital signs, and operation parameters. AI algorithms assess patient data, including medical imaging, genetic information, and clinical history, to customize surgical procedures for each patient (Malik et al., 2019).

Medical Tourism through Artificial Intelligence

Medicinal tourism is measured as a luxury kind of travel. It includes how the marketing mix, including treatment location and pricing, impacts medical travel. The globe is undergoing a rapid technological revolution. The Computer Revolution and Artificial Intelligence led to widespread dominance in several sectors. The healthcare industry, including medical tourism, is no exception. AI may generate billions in foreign currency earnings for both the host country and the firms that provide these services, such as health service providers and hospitals. It offers two key benefits for patients and specialists (Eubanks, 2018).

AI models provide a variety of auditory and visual productions based on the input data. This expedient is capable of converting text information to acoustic form, audio form to video form, and video to high-resolution video.

BARRIERS TO USING AI IN INDIA

Aside from the numerous benefits of using robots in healthcare institutions, there is a risk of mistakes and mechanical malfunctions. There are various downsides to using robots in the healthcare field, particularly in India. In India, the huge burden of infectious illnesses such as TB, cancer, and heart failure is most emphasized. The outlay of acquiring and upholding the robots is quite exclusive.

Every enduring is exclusive, thus customizing healthcare service schemes is vital for both affected role and healthcare workers. As an effect, the existing healthcare system has to be further flexible in terms of contribution of mechanical facilities that are easily adequate to the patient's demands (Malik et al., 2019).

Expensive robotic interventions are not viable in small towns where they are genuinely required due to high workload and a shortage of health experts in government-owned health facilities (Brouwer et al., 2020). Due to its expanding popularity, there is a risk of an intensification in illogical demand for machine-like surgery in India.

The usage of robots in healthcare similarly raises significant medicolegal concerns. The surgical robot, like other computers, may be infected with viruses and fail to follow the surgeon's directions, resulting in a hazardous situation.

THEORETICAL FRAMEWORK

The researchers apply Technology Acceptance Model (TAM). It offers a theoretical framework for thoughtful elements that impact the acceptability of new and advanced technologies, such as machine learning and AI, in the healthcare sector (Figure 3.1). The researchers will investigate how healthcare professionals and patients view AI's usefulness in improving patient care and ease of use in clinical settings (Hawking, 2016).

RESEARCH QUESTIONS

a. How does AI impact healthcare delivery, including patient health and treatment quality?
b. How can we tackle the challenges of integrating AI into healthcare systems?

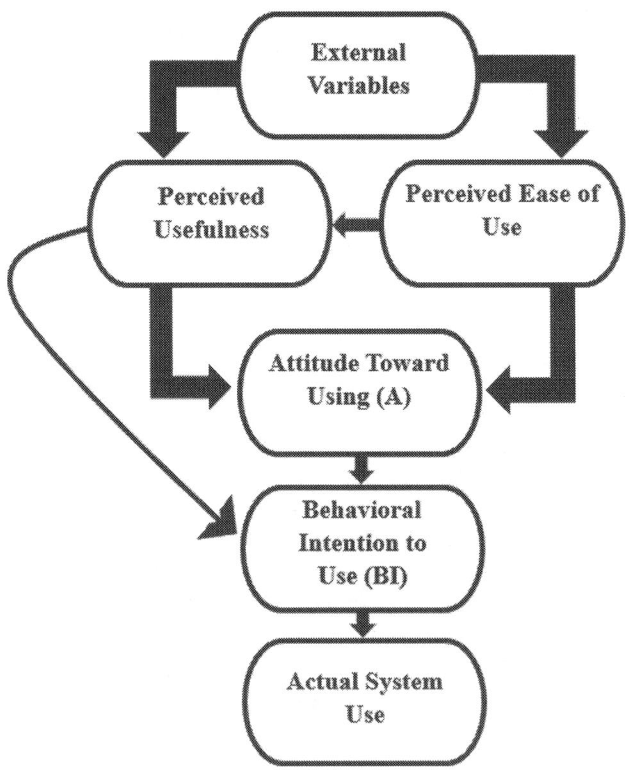

FIGURE 3.1 Technology Acceptance Model

Source: Authors' own.

AI is capable of tackling healthcare challenges even in resource-constrained situations; nevertheless, infrastructural and data protection problems still need to be solved (Shukla Shubhendu and Vijay, 2013). AI promises to change healthcare, but its fast use raises ethical and governance problems. Privacy of patients' data security is a crucial problem when trusting AI-based conclusions (Alcón et al., 2017; Boada et al., 2021). Due to increased usage of AI in healthcare, there are still significant gaps and limits in current research. This is still required to assess the usefulness and safety of AI applications in medical practice.

Hypothesis Framed

H1: Increased usage of AI in healthcare is projected to enhance patient outcomes due to its impact on diagnostic precision and tailored care.
H2: Possible problems of applying artificial intelligence in healthcare.

Challenges to Implementation in Real-World Healthcare

Experience is necessary for doctors to learn from their successes and mistakes before incorporating them into standard treatment and best practices. Doctors learn from peers, research papers, pharmaceutical companies, and personal experiences with patients.

Healthcare personnel have generally lagged behind other professions in adopting new technology for daily activities. Implementation is a crucial stage in healthcare innovation, as demonstrated by previous experiences. High-quality electronic health data is crucial for successful medical AI application. Medical data is often unstructured and loud, making it unsuitable for AI systems. AI technology has the potential to alter patient-healthcare professional relationships in unexpected ways. AI has significantly transformed several specializations, like image analysis. Patient-centered AI technologies have the ability to alter the clinician-patient relationship from a paternalistic one to a collaborative collaboration in decision-making through more openness and deeper talks. The information concerning derived risks of sickness, such as cancer or dementia, may have personal and ethical ramifications, which need to be explored. Clinical guidelines and care models should be modified to include AI-mediated healthcare connections (Luxton and Riek, 2019; Chen et al., 2022).

To ensure clinical interoperability and integration across diverse healthcare systems, AI manufacturers should collaborate with healthcare professionals and organizations to develop standard operating procedures for new AI tools.

Cost

Robotics systems may be expensive to purchase, maintain, and improve. Robotic technology may be costly for healthcare facilities, making it difficult to deploy.

Cost Effectiveness

Limited evidence exists to demonstrate the efficacy and cost-effectiveness of robots in healthcare. More study is needed to provide a robust evidence foundation for the benefits and effects of robots in healthcare applications.

Complexity of Healthcare Environment

The dynamic and complicated nature of healthcare environments makes it difficult for AI robotics systems to adapt successfully. Diverse patient populations, changing medical conditions, and the requirement for real-time decision-making necessitate complex AI algorithms and robotics capabilities (Anderson and Anderson, 2014).

Successful deployment of AI robots requires effective coordination with healthcare practitioners. Designing intuitive user interfaces and natural interaction modes are important issues. Addressing concerns about job displacement and ensuring AI robotics supplement rather than replace human skills is crucial (Fiorini et al., 2018).

Safety

Ensuring the safety and dependability of robotic systems is essential, especially in vital healthcare operations. Robotic systems require rigorous testing, validation, and regulatory compliance to reduce the possibility of mistakes, malfunctions, or negative outcomes.

Usage of Existing Infrastructure

Healthcare facilities may contain outdated systems and equipment that are incompatible with AI robotics technology. Successfully integrating AI robotics technologies into current processes and infrastructure needs careful planning and collaboration (Hoffman et al., 2016).

Easy Payment

Regulatory and reimbursement challenges may arise for healthcare robots, necessitating the development of tailored standards. Modifying payment methods for robots may be necessary to ensure equitable remuneration and promote wider adoption.

Data Privacy

AI requires correct data, yet healthcare data may be insufficient, inconsistent, or biased. Sharing medical data for AI research raises privacy issues for patients.

Training

Healthcare personnel require specific training to use and maintain robotic equipment successfully. Robotics technology has a high learning curve that requires constant training and education to maintain skill and competency.

Effective Use of AI Tools

Healthcare personnel may be resistant to the use of robots in patient care because of concerns about job displacement or perceived danger to the human touch. Effective implementation requires overcoming fears and cultivating a collaborative mentality.

Ethical

The employment of robots in healthcare might raise ethical concerns about patient permission, privacy, and less human connection. Implementing ethical principles and regulatory frameworks is crucial for maintaining patient confidence.

RISK OF AI IN HEALTHCARE

The research highlights potential hazards associated with implementing AI in healthcare (Table 3.2).

Patient Damage Caused by AI Faults

AI-guided clinical solutions in healthcare may fail and pose safety risks to end users, despite advancements in data availability and machine learning. Noise in input data can have a substantial influence on AI predictions. AI misclassifications can be caused by dataset shift. The statistical distribution of clinical data sometimes differs from the original dataset used (Dacko et al., 2017). This movement might be attributed to variances in demographic groups, hospital acquisition methods, or the use of devices from various manufacturers.

Misuse of Medical AI Technologies

Medical AI, like other health technology, has the potential of human mistake and misuse. The accuracy and robustness of AI algorithms depend on how they are utilized by end users, such as physicians, healthcare workers, and patients. Using AI technologies incorrectly might lead to inaccurate medical assessments and decisions, potentially causing harm to patients. Clinicians and the public must not only have access to medical AI tools, but also understand when and how to utilize them effectively. The growth of widely available medical AI apps raises the risk of misuse and harm to people and patients.

Bias in Medical AI and the Persistence of Disparities

Despite advancements in medical research and healthcare delivery, many nations still face significant discrepancies in medical treatment. Inequalities and inequities

TABLE 3.2
Risk of Using AI in Healthcare

Sl. No	Risks
1.	Patient damage caused by AI faults.
2.	Misapplication of medicinal AI technologies
3.	Unfairness in medical AI and the persistence of disparities
4.	Absence of transparency
5.	Secrecy and safety problems
6.	Shortcomings in AI responsibility

are mostly caused by characteristics such as gender, age, ethnicity, income, education, and location. Human prejudices, as well as structural factors like socioeconomic status and discrimination, contribute significantly to disparities. Research suggests that clinicians in the United States do not prioritize and respond to Black patients' pain complaints as promptly as they do to White patients (Kelley et al., 2020). Bias in healthcare is widespread and varies by country. Concerns have been raised that if AI solutions are not properly adopted, assessed, and controlled, they may perpetuate systemic gaps and biases that lead to healthcare inequities (Shukla Shubhendu and Vijay, 2013).

Lack of Transparency

Transparency is a significant challenge in developing and using AI systems in healthcare. AI's lack of trustworthiness is predicted, particularly in sensitive domains like medicine and healthcare, where peoples' well-being is at stake. Lack of credibility can hinder adoption of AI algorithms among patients, physicians, and healthcare systems.

Privacy and Security Problems

The COVID-19 pandemic has highlighted the growing use of AI in healthcare, raising concerns about data privacy, confidentiality, and protection for patients and people. This might have major repercussions including exposing and using sensitive data that violates peoples' rights or repurposing patient data for non-medical purposes.

Shortcomings in AI Accountability

Accountability is crucial for medical AI to gain acceptance, trust, and adoption in real world in the healthcare industry. Clinicians who believe they are held accountable for medical mistakes, regardless of who built the algorithms, are less inclined to use new techniques used by AI in their daily day-to-day practice. The major patients may lose faith if AI creators or users are not held accountable for potential damage. New processes and structures are needed to establish responsibility in medical AI, handle reclamations, compensations, and fines, and assure safety.

RESEARCH METHODOLOGY

The researcher used descriptive design. The research information was composed from healthcare administrators and patients from selected hospitals, clinics, and primary healthcare centers in South India by means of suitability sampling method. The first-hand data was composed through structural formal questionnaire using Likert scale and analyzed using SPSS version 20. The collected questionnaire was analyzed using statistical tools including Chi-square descriptive statistics and regression analyses.

DATA ANALYSIS

Cronbach Alpha Value

Sl. No	Particulars	Cronbach's Alpha Test
1	Delivering behavior using AI	0.85
2	Variety of amenities	0.84
3	Safe and good action	0.80
4	Providing trust about AI	0.715
5	Instant information	0.74

DEMOGRAPHIC ANALYSIS

Classification of the Respondents

		Classification of the Respondents				Total
		Patient	Doctors	Nurses	Hospital Administrators	
Gender	Male	45	30	53	44	172
	Female	31	32	55	30	148
Total		**76**	**62**	**108**	**74**	**320**

Source: Primary data.

Inference: Among 320 sample respondents, 108 are working in hospital and serving as nurse, followed by 76 sample respondents who belong to patient. Seventy-four respondents are working as administrators in the hospital.

Satisfaction Level of the Respondents

		The Level of Satisfaction of the Respondents				Total
		Highly Satisfied	Satisfied	Neither/Nor	Highly Not Satisfied	
Gender	Male	41	61	30	40	172
	Female	32	61	27	28	148
Total		**73**	**122**	**57**	**68**	**320**

Source: Primary data.

Inference: Among 320 respondents, a large amount of the respondents of 122 are pleased with usage of the AI in medical sector, 73 defendants belong to Highly satisfied.

Hypothesis Framed

H3: Association between Gender and respondents using AI.

Tests Output

Chi-Square Tests

	Value	Df	Asymp. Sig. (2-Sided)
Pearson C. Square	13.312[a]	3	.008
L.R	11.567	3	.014
Linear-by-Linear Association	6.413	1	.007
No. of V. Cases	320		

[a] 0 cells (0.0%) have expected count less than 5. The minimum expected count is 16.32.

Source: Computed data.

Inference: At 5% level, p-value is further than the 0.05. So, null hypothesis is recognized. The gender fairness may be spoken with the help of application of AI.

Hypothesis Framed

H4: Easy to adapt using AI tools used in Health Sector.

Association between Gender and Easy to Adapt Using AI Tools Used in Health Sector Association between Gender and Easy to Adapt Using AI Tools Used in Health Sector

Chi-Square Tests

	V	df	A. S. (2-Sided)
P. C. Square	13.312[a]	3	0.007
Likelihood ratio	11.317	3	0.005
Linear-by-linear association	6.921	1	0.007
N of valid cases	320		

Source: Computed data.

Inference: At 5% level, p-value is more than the 0.05. Hence, there is no substantial difference between gender and easy to adapt using AI tools used in health sector.

Regression analysis should not be used alone to determine causation; it does give useful linkages between variables. The Model Summary provides the answers of a multiple linear regression analysis used to investigate the relationships between outcomes and patient progress. It identifies that the usage of AI technology and with other variables. R-squared was 0.167, indicating that independent factors account

TABLE 3.3
Model Summary[a]

Models	R	R Square	A. R Square	Std. Error of the Estimate	Durbin-Watson
1	0.412[b]	0.167	−0.065	0.375	1.7632

[a] **Dependent Variable:**
Have you received positive outcomes in patient care while using AI technologies?

[b] **Predictors:** (Constant)
How do you think usage of AI technology need additional education and training?
How do you perceive the integration of AI in your healthcare system?
How you will protect the privacy and security of your patient data with the use of AI technologies?
How you can protect the data with unauthorized access with AI implementation?
In what setting are you primarily associated?
Do you think AI technology affect the patient care?
Do you think it is easy to take decisions with AI-powered tools?
How frequently you are using AI technologies in your healthcare?
Have you attended any training on AI technologies in healthcare?
How confident are you in the usage of AI-driven diagnoses and treatment?

for about 167% of the variation observed in favorable outcomes, as illustrated in Table 3.3.

The adjusted R-squared value is −0.065, which represents that this model may not be the best fit for this data. A negative adjusted R-squared value implies inaccuracy in describing connections between dependent and independent variables.

The average error of the estimate is 0.375, which is the average of the expected and actual findings. The Durbin-Watson cost is 1.7632, which is extremely near to 2, indicating that there is no substantial autocorrelation within the models. The overall results of the Model Summary show that the model's predictive capacity is restricted, as indicated by the low R-squared value. It is crucial to recall that the model's limitations might be caused by a variety of factors, including the complicated relationship between variables, sample size, or survey design.

CONCLUSION

The encounters to incorporating healthcare technologies into clinical practice are numerous.

The study will help healthcare professionals and policymakers maximize the benefits of AI in patient care. Addressing difficulties, providing proper information and training, and guaranteeing the successful integration of AI into healthcare settings may enhance patient outcomes as well as overall health quality.

The evidence foundation supporting the usage of robots in healthcare is growing, and they are being deployed in a variety of disciplines and situations. The forthcoming of robots rests in remote presence and the capacity to perform activities in difficult conditions and network capabilities to enable for effective adoption.

The study offered in-depth knowledge regarding AI adoption in healthcare by perceptions of its utility, accessibility, and ethical concerns. The study's findings have major implications for future healthcare practice, emphasizing the necessity of addressing ethics, education, and infrastructural preparation when facilitating AI acceptance in medical contexts. Usage of AI tool in healthcare sectors have positive and negative aspects. On the one hand, AI usage have high advanced and easy procedure, while at the same time it faces ethical issues.

AI can transform the healthcare sector by improving advanced and simplified procedure by reducing the expenses, and leads to increasing efficiency. Addressing ethical and regulatory problems is crucial for the safe and successful application of AI in healthcare.

AI systems can assist the nurses and the doctors by saving the time in consultation by inputting and arranging patient data into order. The diagnosing patients, medical records, medicine information, and test results were provided to the doctors for easy follow-up action. AI may also diagnose patients remotely by using conference and virtual reality to the remote area as well outside of the world.

The upcoming of AI in healthcare seems cheerful and talented, but much work is yet to be done. Experience allows clinicians to learn from their achievements and failures before implementing them into conventional therapy and best practices. Doctors learn from their peers, research publications, pharmaceutical firms, and personal patient encounters.

AI can assist healthcare workers with patient care and administrative responsibilities. While AI and healthcare advances are beneficial to the industry, their impact on tactics varies. Although AI can perform similar to or better than humans in certain activities, such as detecting illness, it is unlikely that AI will replace humans in all medical vocations.

REFERENCES

Abdi, Jordan, Ahmed Al-Hindawi, Tiffany Ng, and Marcela P. Vizcaychipi. "Scoping review on the use of socially assistive robot technology in elderly care." *BMJ open* 8, no. 2 (2018): e018815.

Alcón, Carmen Domínguez, Helen Kohlen, and Joan Tronto. *El futuro del cuidado: Compresión de la ética del cuidado y de la práctica enfermera*. Ediciones San Juan de Dios-Campus Docent, 2017.

Al-Emran, Mostafa, and Ibrahim Arpaci. "Intelligent systems and novel coronavirus (COVID-19): A bibliometric analysis." *Emerging technologies during the era of COVID-19 pandemic* (2021): 59–67.

Al-Qaysi, Noor, Norhisham Mohamad-Nordin, and Mostafa Al-Emran. "Factors affecting the adoption of social media in higher education: A systematic review of the technology acceptance model." *Recent advances in intelligent systems and smart applications*, no. 295 (2021): 571–584.

AlQudah, Adi A., Mostafa Al-Emran, and Khaled Shaalan. "Technology acceptance in healthcare: A systematic review." *Applied sciences* 11, no. 22 (2021): 10537.

Amann, Julia, Alessandro Blasimme, Effy Vayena, Dietmar Frey, and Vince I. MadaiPrecise4Q Consortium. "Explainability for artificial intelligence in healthcare:

A multidisciplinary perspective." *BMC medical informatics and decision making* 20 (2020): 1–9.

Anderson, Susan Leigh, and Michael Anderson. "Towards a principle-based healthcare agent." In *Machine medical ethics*, pp. 67–77. Cham: Springer International Publishing, 2014.

Badash, Ido, Karen Burtt, Carlos A. Solorzano, and Joseph N. Carey. "Innovations in surgery simulation: A review of past, current and future techniques." *Annals of translational medicine* 4, no. 23 (2016).

Bajwa, Junaid, Usman Munir, Aditya Nori, and Bryan Williams. "Artificial intelligence in healthcare: Transforming the practice of medicine." *Future healthcare journal* 8, no. 2 (2021): e188.

Boada, Júlia Pareto, Begoña Román Maestre, and Carme Torras Genís. "The ethical issues of social assistive robotics: A critical literature review." *Technology in society* 67 (2021): 101726.

Brouwer, Charlotte L., Djamal Boukerroui, Jorge Oliveira, Padraig Looney, Roel JHM Steenbakkers, Johannes A. Langendijk, Stefan Both, and Mark J. Gooding. "Assessment of manual adjustment performed in clinical practice following deep learning contouring for head and neck organs at risk in radiotherapy." *Physics and imaging in radiation oncology* 16 (2020): 54–60.

Burton, Ross J., Mahableshwar Albur, Matthias Eberl, and Simone M. Cuff. "Using artificial intelligence to reduce diagnostic workload without compromising detection of urinary tract infections." *BMC medical informatics and decision making* 19 (2019): 171.

Chakradhar, Shraddha. "Predictable response: Finding optimal drugs and doses using artificial intelligence." *Nature medicine* 23, no. 11 (2017): 1244–1248.

Chen, Yuanyuan, Dixiao Chen, Shuzhang Liang, Yuguo Dai, Xue Bai, Bin Song, Deyuan Zhang, Huawei Chen, and Lin Feng. "Recent advances in field-controlled micro–nano manipulations and micro–nano robots." *Advanced intelligent systems* 4, no. 3 (2022): 2100116.

Coeckelbergh, Mark. *Green leviathan or the poetics of political liberty: Navigating freedom in the age of climate change and artificial intelligence*. Routledge, 2021.

Croghan, Stefanie M., Paul Carroll, Paul F. Ridgway, Amy E. Gillis, and Sarah Reade. "Robot-assisted surgical ward rounds: Virtually always there." *BMJ health & care informatics* 25, no. 1 (2018).

Dacko, Scott G. "Enabling smart retail settings via mobile augmented reality shopping apps." *Technological forecasting and social change* 124 (2017): 243–256.

Dhamnani, Sunny, Dhruv Singal, Ritwik Sinha, Tharun Mohandoss, and Manish Dash. "RAPID: Rapid and precise interpretable decision sets." In *2019 IEEE International Conference on Big Data (Big Data)*, pp. 1292–1301. IEEE, 2019.

Duffy, Stephen W., Farah Seedat, Olive Kearins, Mike Press, Jackie Walton, Jonathan Myles, Daniel Vulkan, Nisha Sharma, and Anne Mackie. "The projected impact of the COVID-19 lockdown on breast cancer deaths in England due to the cessation of population screening: A national estimation." *British journal of cancer* 126, no. 9 (2022): 1355–1361.

Erikainen, Sonja, and Sarah Chan. "Contested futures: Envisioning personalized, stratified, and precision medicine." *New genetics and society* 38, no. 3 (2019): 308–330.

Esteva, Andre, Brett Kuprel, Roberto A. Novoa, Justin Ko, Susan M. Swetter, Helen M. Blau, and Sebastian Thrun. "Dermatologist-level classification of skin cancer with deep neural networks." *Nature* 542, no. 7639 (2017): 115–118.

Eubanks, Virginia. *Automating inequality: How high-tech tools profile, police, and punish the poor.* St. Martin's Press, 2018.

Fiorini, Nicolas, Robert Leaman, David J. Lipman, and Zhiyong Lu. "How user intelligence is improving PubMed." *Nature biotechnology* 36, no.10 (2018): 937–945.

Gereon, A "*Hands-on machine learning with scikit-learn and tensor flow.*" 'USA: O'Reily Media Inc, 2018.

Gogia, Shashi, ed. *Fundamentals of telemedicine and telehealth.* Academic Press, 2019.

Goldzweig, Caroline Lubick, Greg Orshansky, Neil M. Paige, Ali Alexander Towfigh, David A. Haggstrom, Isomi Miake-Lye, Jessica M. Beroes, and Paul G. Shekelle. "Electronic patient portals: Evidence on health outcomes, satisfaction, efficiency, and attitudes: A systematic review." *Annals of internal medicine* 159, no. 10 (2013): 677–687.

Granić, Andrina. "Educational technology adoption: A systematic review." *Education and information technologies* 27, no. 7 (2022): 9725–9744.

Hawking, Oppenheim M. Stephen. "Artificial intelligence could be the greatest disaster in human history." (2016). http://www.independent.co.uk/news/people/stephenhawking-artificial-intelligence-diaster-human-history-leverhulme-centre-cambridge-a7371106.html

Hoffman, Kelly M., Sophie Trawalter, Jordan R. Axt, and M. Norman Oliver. "Racial bias in pain assessment and treatment recommendations, and false beliefs about biological differences between blacks and whites." *Proceedings of the national academy of sciences* 113, no. 16 (2016): 4296–4301.

Hwei, Lie Rebecca Yen, and Gilbert Sterling Octavius. "Potential advantages and disadvantages of telemedicine: A literature review from the perspectives of patients, medical personnel, and hospitals." *Journal of community empowerment for health* 4, no. 3 (2021): 180–186.

Kelley, Leah Taylor, Jamie Fujioka, Kyle Liang, Madeline Cooper, Trevor Jamieson, and Laura Desveaux. "Barriers to creating scalable business models for digital health innovation in public systems: Qualitative case study." *JMIR public health and surveillance* 6, no. 4 (2020): e20579.

Luxton, David D., and Laurel D Riek. "Artificial intelligence and robotics in rehabilitation." In L. A. Brenner, S. A. Reid-Arndt, T. R. Elliott, R. G. Frank, & B. Caplan (Eds.), *Handbook of rehabilitation psychology*, 3rd ed., pp. 507–520. American Psychological Association, 2019. https://doi.org/10.1037/0000129-031

Malik, Paras, Monika Pathania, and Vyas Kumar Rathaur. "Overview of artificial intelligence in medicine." *Journal of family medicine and primary care* 8, no. 7 (2019): 2328–2331.

Mathews, Simon C., Michael J. McShea, Casey L. Hanley, Alan Ravitz, Alain B. Labrique, and Adam B. Cohen. "Digital health: A path to validation." *NPJ digital medicine* 2, no.1 (2019): 38.

Mohr, Friedrich W., Volkmar Falk, Anno Diegeler, Thomas Walther, Jan F. Gummert, Jan Bucerius, Stefan Jacobs, and Rüdiger Autschbach. "Computer-enhanced 'robotic' cardiac surgery: Experience in 148 patients." *The journal of thoracic and cardiovascular surgery* 121, no. 5 (2001): 842–853.

Panch, Trishan, Heather Mattie, and Leo Anthony Celi. "The 'inconvenient truth' about AI in healthcare." *NPJ digital medicine* 2, no. 1 (2019): 1–3.

Ramanathan, Karuppasamy, Leena Jenefa, and AL Rubaye Ahmed Hussein Radhi. "Redesigning of marketing mix elements affecting medical tourism through artificial intelligence (AI)." In *Reskilling the workforce for technological advancement*, pp. 222–240. IGI Global, 2024.

Sekhon, Harmehr, Kerman Sekhon, Cyrille Launay, Marc Afililo, Nathan Innocente, Ipsit Vahia, Soham Rej, and Olivier Beauchet. "Telemedicine and the rural dementia population: A systematic review." *Maturitas* 143 (2021): 105–114.

Shukla Shubhendu, S., and Jaiswal Vijay. "Applicability of artificial intelligence in different fields of life." *International journal of scientific engineering and research* 1, no. 1 (2013): 28–35.

Singla, B. "Promotional strategies for organized retail." *International journal of Asian business and information management* 14, no. 1 (2023): 1–11. https://doi.org/10.4018/ijabim.325229

Singla, B., B. Dyczek, R. M. H. Soto, and K. J. Mukthar. "Whatever is seen is sold: Merchandise mantra." *Webology* 18, no. Special Issue 03 (2021): 451–461. https://doi.org/10.14704/web/v18si03/web18106

Staehler, Michael, Markus Bader, Boris Schlenker, Jozefina Casuscelli, Alexander Karl, Alexander Roosen, Christian G. Stief, Axel Bex, Berndt Wowra, and Alexander Muacevic. "Single fraction radiosurgery for the treatment of renal tumors." *The journal of urology* 193, no. 3 (2015): 771–775.

Vercelli, Alessandro, Innocenzo Rainero, Ludovico Ciferri, Marina Boido, and Fabrizio Pirri. "Robots in elderly care." *DigitCult-scientific journal on digital cultures* 2, no. 2 (2018): 37–50.

Weinstein, Ronald S., Ana Maria Lopez, Bellal A. Joseph, Kristine A. Erps, Michael Holcomb, Gail P. Barker, and Elizabeth A. Krupinski. "Telemedicine, telehealth, and mobile health applications that work: Opportunities and barriers." *The American journal of medicine* 127, no. 3 (2014): 183–187.

White, Elizabeth M., Terrie Fox Wetle, Ann Reddy, and Rosa R. Baier. "Front-line nursing home staff experiences during the COVID-19 pandemic." *Journal of the American medical directors association* 22, no. 1 (2021): 199–203.

Yang, Xin, Yifei Wang, Ryan Byrne, Gisbert Schneider, and Shengyong Yang. "Concepts of artificial intelligence for computer-assisted drug discovery." *Chemical reviews* 119, no. 18 (2019): 10520–10594.

4 Advancing Healthcare with Responsible AI

Techniques, Barriers, and Best Practices

Herat Joshi and Shenson Joseph

INTRODUCTION

Healthcare organizations, which are the backbone of contemporary society, have enormous responsibility—that of ensuring the health and welfare of people and communities, but what they do is more complex than it may seem at an initial glance. Hospitals, clinics, and nursing homes are beacon of hope and provide the essential medical services to the needy. However, numerous challenges inhibit providing first-class healthcare including high costs, insufficient employees, and the perpetual necessity to replace new technology to enhance patient care and operational effectiveness (Oleka-Onyewuchi, 2023). Still amidst such obstacles, the practice of ethics in AI in healthcare institutions is a phenomenon that can potentially facilitate revolutionary development. The healthcare industry's potential uses for AI technologies are immense, as AI itself is progressing at an unbelievable pace. Applications include medication development, patient monitoring, and disease diagnosis and treatment planning (Haleem et al., 2022). But this integration must be handled carefully and cautiously, in order to prioritize patient safety, data privacy, and ethical decision making in the first place. There are multiple issues that contribute to the challenges of what happens when responsible AI is implemented in healthcare—algorithmic fairness, bias in data and models, transparency and accountability, and of course the thorny ethical and legal parameters that all merge together. Putting AI in the right places in healthcare institutions could change how we're going to approach and provide medical care in such a way that is completely unmatched. By combining sophisticated algorithms and machine learning models we can explore previously uncharted territory in drug development, disease diagnosis, treatment planning, and patient monitoring. Such AI technologies can enhance the diagnosis of disease with greater precision and can ensure that clinical approaches are more precise and that treatment regimens are customized to patient requirements. Also, the use of AI based on predictive analytics can also help predict possible health hazards and take preventive intervention steps, thus improving patient outcomes and quality of life. Responsible AI adoption can also help align different activities in healthcare systems towards better resource allocation, frees up admin burdens, and boosts cost efficiencies. Nevertheless, reaching this path to responsible implementation of AI

DOI: 10.1201/9781003531272-4

in healthcare is not straightforward. Algorithms are fair, and we minimize bias in data and models because if we don't, biased AI systems can perpetuate and amplify existing disparities in healthcare access and quality. On top of that, one can't afford to lose visibility and accountability in AI data-making decisions. There are also privacy and data security concerns so large, especially as healthcare data are inherently sensitive and a breach can have real consequences for patients. The implementation process also has to navigate the ethical and legal just as murky terrain of AI in healthcare. This chapter aims to study strategies for implementing responsible AI in healthcare organizations. The idea is to identify the potential benefits, challenges, and ethical considerations of integrating AI technologies into the practice of medicine in such a way to maintain patient safety, data privacy, and fairness. After all, responsible AI plays a pivotal role on the healthcare front. This gives you a foundational understanding of the topic so that you know why it's important and how it could affect you. After this section, we continue smoothly to the literature review, where available research and knowledge around responsible AI for healthcare are synthesized and analyzed.

LITERATURE REVIEW

In the literature review, we provide an overview of what has been written in the literature, and studies about responsible AI in healthcare. This is a comprehensive overview of this theme, which includes key themes, trends, and gaps in the existing work. After the literature review, we go on to healthcare organizations, their roles, and responsibilities to implement responsible AI.

HEALTHCARE ORGANIZATIONS

Healthcare organizations have an important role to play in delivering healthcare services by delivering quality of care to the individual and the community. There are many things healthcare organizations are responsible for such as allocating, coordinating, and delivering healthcare services (Ginter, Duncan, & Swayne, 2018). Basically, any entity that is responsible for the management, coordination, and provision of healthcare services forms a healthcare organization. The lots of these groups comprise a huge variety of institutions such as public health agencies, clinics, hospitals, and physician offices. Healthcare companies can be in the service of the public or commercial, as well as nonprofit organizations.

Significance of Healthcare Organizations

Healthcare organizations are important as the foundation of healthcare delivery. Essential services they provide include promoting health, preventing illness, diagnosing and treating medical conditions, and rehabilitating patients. Healthcare organizations are a platform for healthcare professionals to collaborate, provide resources, and deliver comprehensive care to individuals across the care continuum.

Functions of Healthcare Organizations

Healthcare organization does various important functions that help in achieving efficient and effective delivery of healthcare services. Service provision, coordination and continuity of care, quality improvement, resource allocation and management, and health promotion and disease prevention are these functions. Clinical services vary widely for healthcare organizations ranging from primary care to sophisticated treatments and diagnostic procedures, and surgical interventions (Greenwood-Lee, Jewett, Woodhouse, & Marshall, 2018). They want to deliver the wide spectrum of healthcare that people require, provide timely and appropriate care. As we dissect the roles of healthcare organizations in responsible AI adoption, we find that it is complex and challenging. This serves as the context for a more developed understanding of the intersection of responsible AI in the context of healthcare with regulatory and legal elements.

RESPONSIBLE AI IN HEALTHCARE

In some industries, including healthcare, the technology referred as artificial intelligence (AI) has changed game. Medical environments require that AI be made conscientious and moral as the AI develops. The strategy responsible for frontline priority in ethical and responsible AI technology deployment in healthcare systems is known as responsible AI in healthcare. Policy procedures should be focused on reducing AI biases and helping the sector take full advantage of the technology for delivering benefits to the society at large. Figure 4.1 synthesizes an overview of the essential

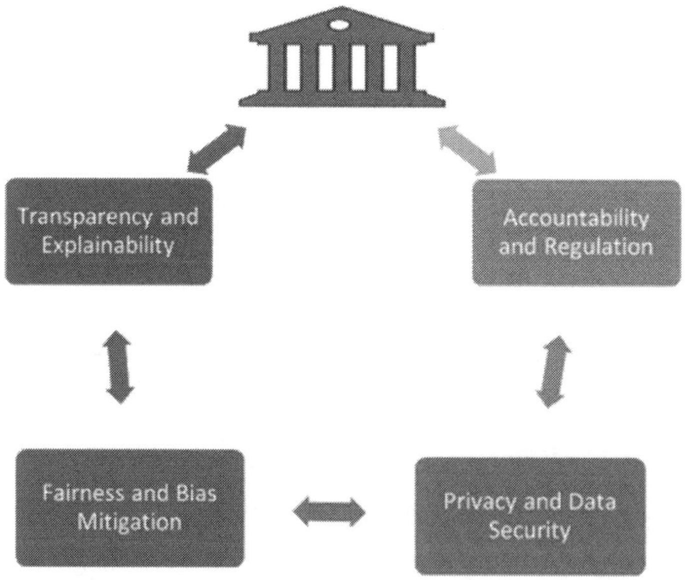

FIGURE 4.1 Conscientious AI in healthcare.

Source: Authors' own.

elements of AI in healthcare as applied to the creation and deployment of AI systems and algorithms with an emphasis on openness, justice, privacy, and equity.

Essential Elements of Conscientious AI in Healthcare

Transparency and Explainability: Figure 4.1 shows that responsible AI in healthcare requires openness in creating and applying AI algorithms. Like any other drug, patients and healthcare professionals need to know what data the prescriber for their AI system is relying on and how they use that data to make a decision. Explainability is essential in developing confidence and ensuring the accountability of clinical decisions made by means of AI.

Fairness and Bias Mitigation: Top AI algorithms in healthcare should not use bias to arrive at results and should also deliver fairness in healthcare outcomes. The evaluation- and strategy-based responsible AI in healthcare evaluates AI systems for their potential biases and implementing ways to remove the same. All patient populations should feel and be fair across race, ethnic background, gender, and socioeconomic status.

Privacy and Data Security: Figure 4.1 shows that in healthcare, responsible AI focuses on the security of sensitive health data and the patient's private healthcare. AI systems should behave morally and legally and protect patient data as it should be—secure and responsibly used. These are needed to ensure security and privacy of data, such that even if law enforcement tries to obtain access to your data, it will be virtually impossible.

Accountability and Regulation: What is important for responsible AI in healthcare is appropriate accountability procedures associated with the creation, application, and use of AI technologies. Healthcare institutions need to set up governance frameworks, rules, and guidelines to make sure that practice of ethical AI.

Regulatory frameworks should be put in place to monitor the ethical use of AI in healthcare and to make for liable of any injury associated consequence conceivable by AI frameworks.

Into responsible AI in healthcare we dive, exploring the many faces of responsible AI from patient care to outcomes, to risk mitigation. Naturally, we explore this to look into the regulatory and legal implications that govern the implementation of AI in the healthcare space.

IMPLICATIONS OF RESPONSIBLE AI IN HEALTHCARE

The concept of responsible AI in healthcare has significant implications for various stakeholders:

Patients and Healthcare Providers: Responsible AI in healthcare equips it with early and accurate diagnosis, tailored treatment plan, and powerful clinical decision support that can improve patient care. It can also help healthcare professionals overcome the fact that they have so much to do, and indulge them in things that are hard for doctors to do while being open to patient engagement.

Ethical Considerations: Responsible AI in healthcare prompts discussion of ethical conundrums as to how patient autonomy, informed consent, and the expectation that AI will, in the end, assume responsibility from human judgement. These conversations are important in order to ensure that AI technologies stay on the right side of moral standards and meet standards set for human rights.

Regulatory Bodies and Policymakers: What is needed to create responsible AI in healthcare are legal frameworks and guidelines on the use of AI in healthcare. If these frameworks already exist, they should at least encompass matters of responsible AI, bias, privacy, and how to properly utilize an AI algorithm. Policymakers are necessary to make sure AI serves the entire society, and to define the regulatory landscape.

The concept for responsible AI in healthcare is of being an ethical and accountable use of AI technologies within healthcare settings. Its goal is to optimize the advantages of AI with the risks and the biases of it, all obviously upon transparency and fairness and privacy and responsibility. To use safe AI in healthcare, the policymakers, regulatory agencies, technology developers, and healthcare practitioners must cooperate together. Responsible AI can be adopted by healthcare to leverage AI potential in the enhancement of clinical decision making, better patient outcomes, and fair healthcare delivery.

REGULATORY, LEGAL, AND ETHICAL IMPLICATIONS OF AI IN HEALTHCARE

AI provides an opportunity to revolutionize delivery of healthcare. But regulatory and legal implications must be thought about as well when using AI in healthcare organizations.

Regulatory Framework for AI in Healthcare

The landscape of the regulation of AI in healthcare is going through its own shaping as technologies continue to advance. The U.S. Food and Drug Administration (FDA), European Medicines Agency (EMA), and more and more regulatory bodies are looking to set guidelines and standards for how to develop, validate, and deploy AI systems in healthcare. The scope of these regulations is to ensure that the AI technologies are safe, effective, and reliable (Shneiderman, 2020).

For regulatory frameworks, another desirable feature is that of making sure that AI algorithms are not deployed into clinical practice without being tested and validated thoroughly. Robust clinical trials and validation studies to determine the diagnostic accuracy, reliability, and clinical applicability of AI algorithms in healthcare are needed to evaluate AI algorithms in healthcare, and make sure these technologies follow the standards to develop safe healthcare services (Magrabi et al., 2019).

Legal Considerations in AI Adoption

Healthcare institution also raises issues related to legal. Data security as well as patient privacy are important. Lacking weekends and other paid time off, it typically means that AI systems are trained and analyzed using massive amounts of patient data. Therefore, the significance of compliance increases with data protection laws such as the General Data Protection Regulation (GDPR) in Europe, HIPAA in USA, PIPEDA in Canada, Data Protection Act 2018 (DPA) is largely aligned with GDPR in Europe. Patient information privacy is part of the healthcare organizations' responsibility to ensure that the right consent mechanisms, data masking requirements, and safe data storing locations exist to protect patient information. But there's another legal consideration: liability with AI technologies. Now that AI systems are having an increased impact on patient care, many are becoming increasingly concerned over who is to blame for these decisions. When AI algorithms are used incorrectly by digital health systems, it's hard to identify who is liable. These issues have to be incorporated in legal framework, including the role and responsibility of the healthcare professional, manufacturers, and the regulating agency in the event of adverse outcomes in the adoption of AI.

Ethical Use of AI in Healthcare

Every integration of AI in healthcare is an ethical consideration. Developing and deploying AI technologies must do so guided by the principle of beneficence—to promote patient wellbeing—strictly adhering to ethical standards. The use of AI in healthcare is summarized in Table 4.1. In order for these systems to establish and maintain trust between healthcare providers and patients, it's important for these systems to be transparent about how decisions are made. Also important are problems with informed consent and with patient autonomy. Patients should be properly informed as to how AI is being used in their care, and even if they have been spared the indignity of a visit to the emergency department if they choose not to allow AI to help in their care, they must know that the doctor will not abandon them. Such collaborative decisions between healthcare professionals and patients are encouraged

TABLE 4.1
Ethical Use of AI in Healthcare

Aspect Summary	Summary
Regulatory Framework for AI in Healthcare	Regulatory bodies like FDA and EMA are establishing guidelines for AI development, focusing on safety and effectiveness through rigorous testing.
Legal Considerations in AI Adoption	Patient data privacy is governed by laws like GDPR and HIPAA and DPA, etc. The liability for AI use-related adverse outcomes needs clear legal framework.
Ethical Use of AI in Healthcare	AI development must prioritize patient well-being, avoid biases, ensure transparency, and respect patient autonomy through informed consent.

by the ethical guidelines as applied considering both the benefits and limitations in AI technologies.

The study demystifies the regulatory and legal issues surrounding the adoption of responsible AI, your guide through the complex and challenging labyrinth. This is a first step to deeper exploration of problems that healthcare companies encounter when trying to deploy responsible AI.

CHALLENGES IN IMPLEMENTING RESPONSIBLE AI IN HEALTHCARE SETTINGS

As is shown in Figure 4.2, the inclusion of AI in healthcare would completely change the way medical service delivery is performed. However, healthcare environments create challenges that need to be addressed as we deploy AI responsibly (Shaw et al., 2019).

Ethical Considerations

However, one of the greatest challenges faced in executing responsible AI in healthcare is the fact that ethical considerations are properly prioritized (Siala & Wang, 2022). The guidelines to create AI algorithms must be clear so they don't have any biases and discrimination. In an era when AI technologies begin to permeate healthcare, the principle of beneficence, i.e., the promotion of patient's wellbeing, should guide the creation and deployment of these technologies in the healthcare setting. Many ethics accordingly concern sustaining patient confidence and providing assurance of the just and fair application of AI.

Transparency and Explainability

For example, as Figure 4.2 shows, another issue in the execution of the responsible AI in the field of healthcare is with transparency and explainability (Arrieta et al., 2023). But healthcare providers, patients, and AI developers alike need to understand how AI algorithms make decisions and recommendations. Transparency in that AI system's decision-making process propels fostering confidence and collaboration

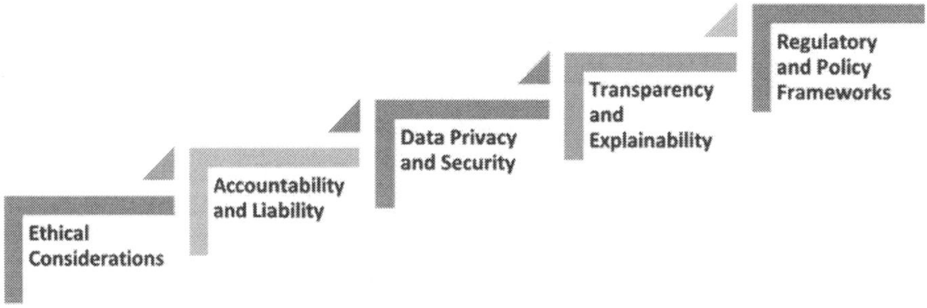

FIGURE 4.2 Responsible AI implementation challenges.

Source: Authors' own.

between healthcare professionals and patients. The edibility of explainable AI provides a window to understanding the rationale behind the outputs produced by AI systems leading to a more accurate reading and validation of the results.

Data Privacy and Security

That is, there needs to be the responsible implementation of AI in healthcare's data privacy and data security concerns (Murdoch, 2021). Training & Analysis entirely depends on extensive amounts of patient data on AI systems. It is needed to protect the patient's privacy from laws to enforce countries related to data protection. However, they need to ensure that appropriate consent mechanisms, secure storage, and data anonymization techniques are in place to protect this patient information from breach.

Accountability and Liability

Implementing responsible AI in healthcare faces great challenges of accountability and liability. When AI systems are making decisions that matter to patient care, there are inevitable questions about who should be responsible for bad outcomes. With regard to Figure 4.2, it's clear that there must be well defined roles and responsibilities for healthcare professionals, manufacturers, and regulatory bodies in the case of AI-related adverse events. Also, this helps to prevent mistaking accountability with liability (Siala & Wang, 2022).

Regulatory and Policy Frameworks

Figure 4.2 showed that further progress on developing robust regulatory and policy frameworks are necessary to safely realize AI in healthcare settings (O'Sullivan et al., 2019). Establishing guidelines and standards for AI technologies in healthcare is essentially the major work of regulatory bodies. They should also ensure that AI systems deploy safely, effectively, and reliably because the presumption of perfect failure modes is one thing, but that doesn't render the systems' application useful, necessary, or even desirable. As shown above in Figure 4.2, numerous challenges are posed when implementing responsible AI in healthcare settings, including being able to ethically handle them in responsible AI implementation in healthcare. Addressing these challenges will help healthcare organizations to utilize the full power of AI within the ethics and protections of patient's trust, privacy, and well-being. We explore the issues of data privacy, algorithmic bias, and organizational readiness as we get into the practical challenges. These challenges point to the urgent need to develop sound approaches and advice for fostering successful adoption of responsible AI into healthcare organizations (Rakova et al., 2021).

FUTURE DIRECTIONS AND RECOMMENDATIONS FOR SUCCESSFUL ADOPTION OF RESPONSIBLE AI

There is a great promise in adopting responsible AI for various industries such as healthcare, finance, or transportation. Nevertheless, in order to properly implement responsible AI, first it has to be forecasted which direction it will go to and how it can

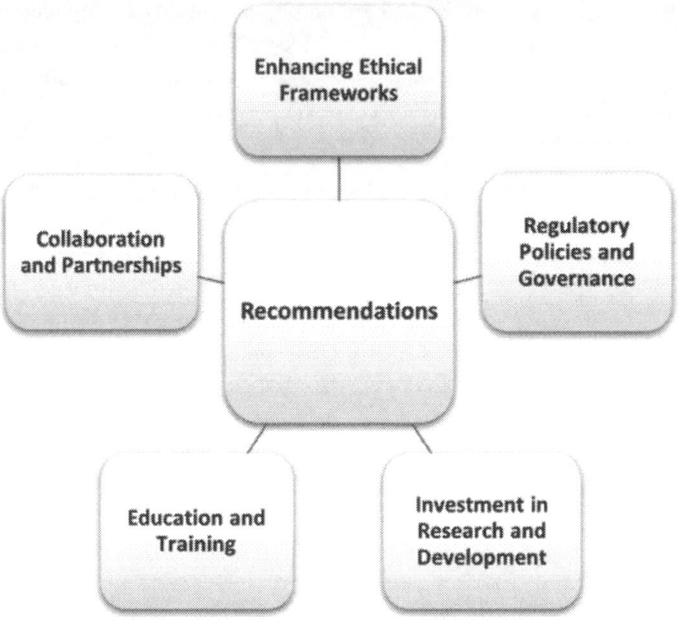

FIGURE 4.3 Recommendations for successful adoption of responsible AI.

Source: Authors own.

be adopted. See Figure 4.3 that displays recommendations for successful adoption of responsible AI in healthcare settings.

Enhancing Ethical Frameworks

Figure 4.3 shows that one important future direction for AI adoption is to enrich ethical frameworks (Ashok et al., 2022). The implementation of ethical issues in every step of the process to create and use of AI systems will meet the degree of accountability, openness, and fairness. To achieve this, it is possible to set up clear and recognized rules and bridges that will prevent potential biases, discrimination, and privacy issues. By strengthening ethical frameworks, we will better build public trust and confidence in AI technologies.

Regulatory Policies and Governance

A further critical attribute for AI success for adoption is the creation of strong regulatory policies and sensible governance structures (de Almeida, dos Santos, & Farias, 2021). Countries and regulators should work with, and get support from AI experts and stakeholders, to develop generalized principles and policies that reflect the ethical and responsible usage of AI. To mitigate potential risks and to sustain social acceptance, these policies should tackle account for data protection, algorithmic transparency, and accountability issues.

Investment in Research and Development

Advance of AI requires increasing investment in research and development (Yigitcanlar et al., 2021). We argue that funding agencies and organizations ought to direct resources for interdisciplinary research in the formation of the ethical, social, and legal issues of AI. The development of innovative approaches, such as explainable AI and bias detection algorithms, to increase the possibility of making AI more transparent and fairer is what should be done in this research. However, research and development can help us drive accountable use of AI.

Education and Training

However, education and training programs are seeking to ensure the successful adoption of AI (Pedro et al., 2019). Part of that is ensuring that AI practitioners, policymakers, and end users alike have the knowledge and skills to know what the ethical implications and biases of AI will be. In fact, responsible AI adoption should also touch upon the fact that continuous learning and updates are important to make sure we are informed and ready for the times we live in.

Collaboration and Partnerships

Successful adoption of accountable AI requires promoting collaboration and partnerships between stakeholders. Together, governments, academia, industry, and civil society organizations can define or provide the standards, learn from each other, and share what is learned. An approach that emphasizes multiple stakeholders can support tackle complicated issues, magnify a variety of perspectives, and assure that AI adoption disproportionately impacts all areas of society. As Figure 4.3 illustrates, future directions and the adoption of actionable recommendations are important components in successfully adopting responsible AI. The ethical frameworks need to be strengthened, robust regulatory policies need to be developed, increased investment in research and development made, education and training need to be delivered, and cooperation and partnerships need to be fostered. This helps us guide this adoption of responsible AI to a point that is ethical, transparent, and beneficial for the overall society. We look forward and providing strategies and recommendations for healthcare organizations to support their adoption of AI. This then establishes the methodological context in which we present our review of ethical considerations in the implementation of AI.

METHODOLOGY

The methodology for studying the implementation of responsible AI in healthcare organizations takes a complete and systematic manner that is inclusive of several research techniques as well as data collection sources. First, a complete literature review will be performed across reputable databases, academic journals, industry reports, etc., and an extensive literature review will be carried out on information obtained from reputable databases including PubMed, IEEE Xplore, and Google

Scholar. In order to understand the current approach to responsible AI applications in healthcare, this review seeks to find foundational knowledge from peer-reviewed articles, industry reports, and white papers.

We will use the literature review to obtain insights of the strategies adopted by such healthcare organizations to adopt the responsible AI. It will use keywords such as 'responsible AI in healthcare,' 'ethical consideration in the rollout of AI,' and 'best practices in AI governance' to be able to retrieve relevant and up to date information. By reviewing the literature, it will present the background for knowing how responsible AI has been implemented in healthcare and the key strategies/challenges at present. Access to recent published works will be highlighted as a way to view the latest trends and innovations in the area. To complement the data above, real-world case studies of organization within the healthcare space that have successfully implemented responsible AI are analyzed. The outcomes of the responsible AI implementation will be demonstrated through these case studies and will include valuable insights into best practices, lessons learned, and outcomes. An examination will be made of the methods used, the obstacles faced, and the effect on patient care, workflow optimization and organizational performance in general. By providing some transparency into the process of how we reviewed ethical considerations related to AI implementation, we describe the methodology employed in that review. An examination of ethical considerations in AI implementation segues naturally into this methodological overview.

OVERVIEW OF RESPONSIBLE AI IMPLEMENTATION IN HEALTHCARE

This section explores the integration of AI within healthcare, emphasizing the need for ethical guidelines and the tangible benefits AI brings, such as enhanced diagnostic accuracy and operational efficiency.

REVIEWING ETHICAL CONSIDERATIONS IN AI IMPLEMENTATION

AI in healthcare has the potential to completely transform patient diagnosis, treatment, and care. However, as per Figure 4.4, it is imperative to establish ethical principles to govern the use of AI in healthcare settings.

Data Minimization vs. Dataset Size: GDPR, HIPPA, PIPEDA, DPa, etc. all have the principle of data minimization, which means businesses should only collect and use personal data, precisely to the extent that it is necessary in relation to the specific purpose for which it is being processed. However, AIs often require large datasets to train such that they perform optimally (Magrabi et al., 2019). As the need for extensive datasets allows healthcare providers to understand their population better and the relative need for rule minimization in the gathering of data to not make healthcare providers' lives more complicated than necessary, the balance of tradeoff is that the ability to collect enough data while preserving the privacy of their patients is made increasingly difficult.

Anonymization and Pseudonymization: Anonymization or pseudonymization of personal data formed a key element of GDPR, HIPPA, PIPEDA, DPA etc. which

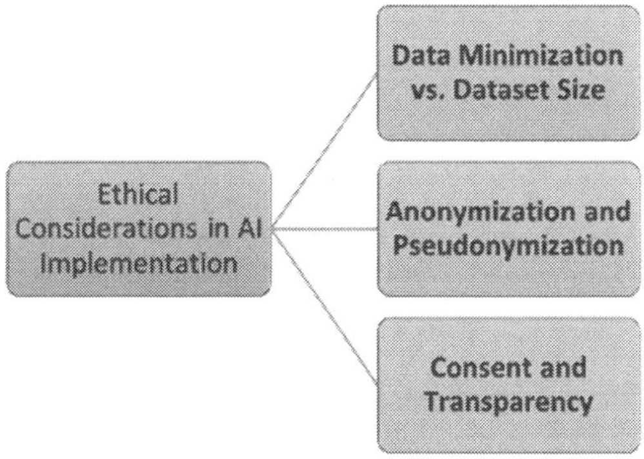

FIGURE 4.4 Ethical considerations in AI implement.

Source: Authors' own.

brings into place in order to protect individual privacy. Unfortunately, these techniques at least partially limit the utility of data for AI training (Pike, 2019; Joshi, 2024). Although anonymized or pseudonymized datasets may provide too little protected information for individuals, lack of information that is crucial at the individual level to AI algorithms' accuracy of the predictions or diagnoses, could limit the efficacy of AI applications in healthcare.

Consent and Transparency: GDPR, HIPPA, PIPEDA, DPA, etc. demand usage of explicit consent of individuals to do processing of their personal data. However, giving informed consent to use healthcare data in AI applications is complex (Nazer et al., 2023). AI driving decisions could reduce patients' understanding about the ramifications of such decisions and patients might be unwilling to consent because they are worried about privacy or discrimination. The challenge of obtaining meaningful consent coupled with transparency about how AI technologies utilize patient data is for healthcare providers to wade through.

CASE EXAMPLES

AI-Powered Diagnostics: Consider a healthcare providing an AI system to auto-digitize the medical diagnosis of certain medical conditions based on imaging data. The provider must have access to a large and wide set of medical images for that training (Magrabi et al., 2019). However, to comply with the data minimization principle only the provider can carefully choose and anonymize images to avoid unnecessary data collection, protecting patient privacy. To the extent that this is a bottleneck processing step, it can limit the diversity and size of the training dataset, possibly introducing bias and impairing the accuracy of, and generalizability to outside applications, of the AI model.

Clinical Research and AI: AI technology promises analytic ability to sift through the mountains of processed patient data found in clinical research to discover trends and patterns and potential outcomes from treatments

(Nazer et al., 2023). But it's difficult to access and process personal health data, and still comply with government's very tight privacy rules. However, as AI for Medical Research grows, researchers must navigate complex consent processes, maintain data anonymization, and establish solid security measures.

Analyzing aims to critically examine these challenges and providing real-world example of how healthcare providers can successfully balance healthcare data privacy requirements as per GDPR, HIPPA, PIPEDA, DPA etc. with the need of AI implementation in healthcare. In this perspective we have something that can help us with making decisions and designing ethical and licensed AI solutions in the healthcare domain. Through our methodology, we discuss ethical considerations tied into the implementation of AI, and provide responsible adoption best practices. It serves as background for identifying strategies for responsible adoption of AI in healthcare organizations.

IDENTIFYING STRATEGIES FOR RESPONSIBLE AI ADOPTION IN HEALTHCARE ORGANIZATIONS

From healthcare to finance and transportation, AI has brought immense growth to sectors across industry verticals. But in responsible use of AI, implementing it responsibly is important because it can minimize risks as well as ethical concerns in the ramification of AI. Figure 4.5 concludes strategies for responsible AI adoption across healthcare organizations.

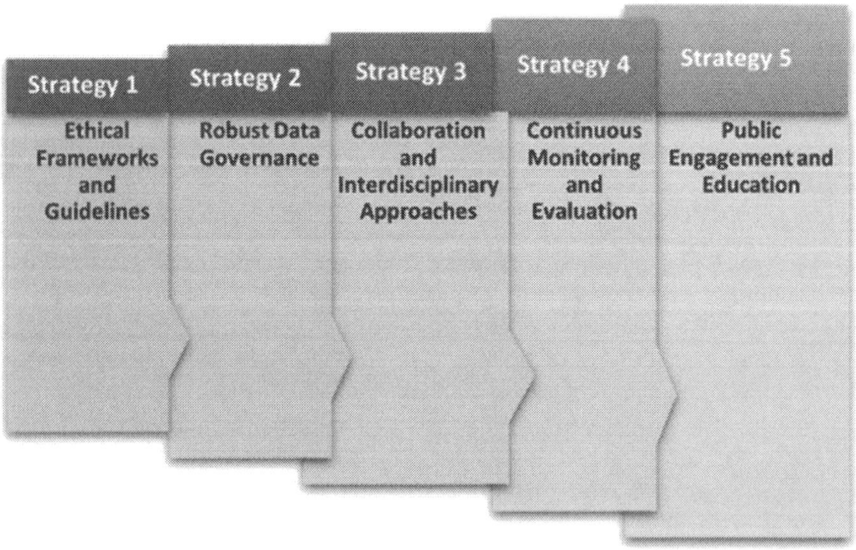

FIGURE 4.5 Responsible AI Adoption Strategies.

Source: Authors own.

Strategy 1: Ethical Frameworks and Guidelines

When implementing AI systems, it's a priority to develop comprehensive ethical frameworks and guidelines. The principles of these frameworks should be in the form of transparency, fairness and accountability (Koene et al., 2019). What they should be planning are clear lines around data privacy, algorithmic biases, and the potential societal impact. Organizations can make sure that AI is developed and deployed in a responsible and morally sound way by following the ethical framework.

Strategy 2: Robust Data Governance

Responsible AI implementation requires something of equal importance as its data governance. We need to build sound procedures for data acquisition, stockpiling, and utilization. It also highlights that these include obtaining appropriate content from the individuals, ensuring data security and privacy and designing methods of data anonymization and deletion (Thapa & Camtepe, 2021). Organizations that first enforce data governance will be able to minimize unauthorized access, data breach, privacy violation risks.

Strategy 3: Collaboration and Interdisciplinary Approaches

To achieve responsible (AI) implementation, different stakeholders including researchers, policymakers, and industry experts have to work together. Hence, interdisciplinary approaches address ethical, legal, and social implications (Amann et al., 2020). Sharing knowledge across disciplines in order to engage in discussions that will build better informed strategies and policies for handling AI implementation is organizations express way of defining complex challenges associated.

Strategy 4: Continuous Monitoring and Evaluation

Monitoring and evaluation of AI continued must occur in order for it to be used responsibly. This will mean that the organizations that create AI systems must build in Monitoring, Evaluation, and Optimisation (MEO) mechanisms to assess how well they work, how they work fairly, and what they provide for society. A regular audit can identify algorithmic biases, unintended consequences, and the risk (Koshiyama et al., 2024). Organizations take the first step by continuously monitoring and evaluating AI systems to address ethical issues beforehand and necessary changes are made.

Strategy 5: Public Engagement and Education

They are crucial—not public engagement, not education but public engagement and education—in the responsible implementation of AI. Organizations should not only communicate the benefits, but also the limitations, and possible risks of AI and the public (Cheatham, Javanmardian, & Samandari, 2019). It includes both promoting transparency through algorithmic decision making and remedies to concerns around job displacement and security. Organizations can generate public trust and understanding of the use and the ethical use of AI technologies.

To enable responsible AI implementation, strategies that are ethically oriented, data governance aligning, collaborative, monitoring, and publicly engage are adopted.

An ethical framework can be developed as would be the case in any development project; however, it will require many iterations as the nuances and practical application of an ethical way to develop AI become more apparent. Also, for the responsible ethical use of AI technologies, they are important building blocks for the building and maintaining of trust among the public and education.

We assess these strategies through a holistic lens and evaluate their potential of responsible AI adoption. By assessing several aspects, this provides the stage for querying the impact of responsible AI on patient outcomes and operational efficiency.

Assessing the Impact of Responsible AI on Patient Outcomes and Operational Efficiency

Recently, AI has transformed many industries from healthcare to social media. Thus far, we have seen great promise in the application of AI in healthcare, with the ability to increase patients' outcomes as well as improve operational efficiency.

Patient Outcomes

As it stands now, there is great promise in providing increased patient outcomes through the use of AI. Early disease detection and diagnosis is an important area which uses AI algorithms. For example, studies have shown the efficacy of AI-based system in detecting early sign of diseases like cancer and cardiovascular problems (Kaulr et al., 2020). Early interventions may improve prognosis if the disease is timely diagnosed.

Also, AI can make it possible for medical providers to create individualized treatment programs. By analyzing huge blocks of medical data, AI systems can calculate for each patient the best course of action to take. This strategy decreases side effects, while increasing therapy efficacy.

Operational Efficiency

Apart from optimizing patient outcomes, AI can be extremely useful in reducing operational hours being spent at patient care. Among those, one key is automating administrative tasks including appointment scheduling and data entry. AI-based systems have been proven to simplify processes, thereby offloading the burden on health staff and allowing them some time to the actual patient care (Ogunsakin & Anwansedo. 2024).

Specifically, one area AI can streamline for companies is resource allocation. AI can analyze patient data to estimate demand for healthcare services, and thus healthcare facilities to efficiently allocate resources. Proactive implementation of this approach can reduce waiting time, improve staff utilization, and improve overall performance.

We perform a comprehensive assessment of responsible AI adoption strategies and evaluate their attainability. It then establishes the context for delving deeper into case studies and best practice healthcare AI implementation.

CASE STUDIES AND BEST PRACTICES IN HEALTHCARE AI IMPLEMENTATION

If AI were to be prevalent in healthcare use then the way in which patients are diagnosed, treated, and looked after could all be changed. However, for the implementation of AI in healthcare, a proper analysis of case studies and best practices is highly needed.

Case Study 1: AI-Assisted Diagnostic Systems

The pioneering work demonstrated that AI algorithms can change the way radiology diagnostics are performed. However, swiftly, their integration into diagnostic workflows showed initial promise by substantially decreasing interpretation time and increasing diagnostic accuracy (Hosney et al., 2018). In this symbiotic relationship between human expertise and analytical capabilities enabled through AI systems, human expertise augmented the capabilities. There were, however, challenges in implementation. However, technical implementation of integrating AI into existing healthcare systems was a complex task that involved considerable changes and adapted to the needs of the data protection regulations. Additionally, user resistance of AI and/error from users like radiologists arose and some radiologists were hesitant to depend on the learning. In order to address these challenges a collaborative effort was needed. Technical impediments were overcome by encouraging cross disciplinary collaboration and maintaining regulatory standards in healthcare organizations. Broad training was conducted, including training to reduce user resistance, to ensure healthcare professionals could make full use of AI. The case study, however, concludes that AI has huge transformative potential in radiology. Working together, innovating and educating, healthcare professionals can use AI to make diagnostic processes more efficient and to provide better care to patients, and achieve better outcomes.

Case Study 2: Predictive Analytics for Patient Monitoring

Predictive analytics was shown to have potential in improving patient and safety monitoring. Before implementation, things looked initially promising. High quality data was ensured but there were errors in the predictions. To ensure that no insights were misinterpreted, clear protocols were needed to integrate AI predictions with clinical workflows (Alamgir, Mousa, & Shah, 2021). Furthermore, AI technologies could not make their case without extensive training programs to shore up the confidence users had in them. However, predicting various patient behaviors is already of value to healthcare professionals, and this implementation depends on these challenges being solved, i.e., data quality, integration protocols, and the resistance from the users. Deleting these challenges, healthcare providers can use predictive analytics to enhance patient and overall healthcare delivery.

Best Practice 1: Ensuring Ethical Considerations

The term that rings in my mind is ethical considerations. In this case, as in all cases, the data is people. For all that, implementing a system of AI is very important on the point of ethics. To ensure patient privacy, data security and algorithmic transparency, these need to be the priority. Take, for example, the necessity to attain informed consent, anonymize patient data, and on a repeat basis audit various AI algorithms to identify and eradicate any biases or discrimination (Khanna & Srivastava, 2020). In addition, healthcare organizations should constitute a body to be made responsible for establishment and monitoring of development and discharge of the AI systems for responsible and fair use.

Best Practice 2: Collaborative Partnerships

For healthcare, however, to be successful its implementation of AI will require collaborative partnerships between healthcare providers, technology developers, and the regulatory bodies. For example, we show the importance of multidisciplinary teams of clinicians, data scientists, and AI specialists. These teams can individually or collectively design and implement AI solutions that fit with clinical needs while meeting regulatory guidelines. Secondly, collaboration allows for sharing what's working best and what you've learned, shaping ongoing improvement in advancing AI (Martín-Noguerol et al., 2021).

Best Practice 3: Continuous Evaluation and Improvement

The long-term implantation of AI in healthcare requires continuous evaluation and improvement. It is recommended that feedback loops are established setting up feedback loops that collect feedback from healthcare professionals, patients, and other stakeholders. This can help with feedback into iterative improvements that were realized in the field, to each limitation or problem encountered during the implementation step itself (Gelkopf, Mazor, & Roe, 2022). To constantly maintain the effectiveness and compliance with evolving needs of clinical, AI systems require regular evaluation and monitoring. Drawing lessons from case studies and best practices of AI in the healthcare domain, we can learn valuable information and offer some strategies for successful adoption. Things to think about are collaborative collaborations, running reviews, improving and more importantly, ethical issues. To realize AI in healthcare, implementation of an AI needs a multidisciplinary strategy with close collaboration of medical practitioners, technology developers, and regulatory agencies. When it comes to AI's use in healthcare institutions, following these best practices will help healthcare institutions maximize progress on patient outcomes as well as reduce unnecessary waste of time and money that could otherwise be used for medical research (Pickering, 2021). Through real-world case studies, we evaluate responsible AI's impact on patient care and operational efficiency. An investigation of responsible AI applications in the healthcare setting follows.

APPLICATIONS OF RESPONSIBLE AI IN HEALTHCARE

Recently, it has become important to use responsible AI in the practice of healthcare.

AI in Diagnostics and Disease Detection

Right now, AI has the potential to completely change medical diagnosis and disease detection. Research reveals how AI algorithms help to increase the precision and accuracy of those diagnostic procedures (Mirbabaie, Stieglitz, & Frick, 2021). The use of medical imaging data by medical personnel with the help of AI technologies can assist to identify some anomalies and disease. This should result in better treatment results, early identification, and hopefully better patient care.

Personalized Medicine and Treatment Planning

With the inclusion of AI into healthcare systems, treatment planning and tailored medicine are possible. Human healthcare providers struggle to find what an AI algorithm may be able to find—patterns and connections in patient data. Researching the use of AI to customize a treatment regimen that considers a patient's lifestyle choices, medical history, and predispositions (Golombek et al., 2018). Resolving these relationships can produce more concise and efficient treatment plans leading to better patient results.

AI for Remote Patient Monitoring

With the advent of AI, remote patient monitoring, as in telemedicine, is becoming possible. The potential for the real-time collection of patient data through AI-powered wearable devices and remote monitoring systems is highlighted (Rath et al., 2024). This data can be fed into AI algorithms that can tell us things about the patient's health status, what are the anomalous readings, and if any interventions are required. It helps with proactive and personalized healthcare delivery in particular to people living with chronic disease or people living in remote areas.

AI-Augmented Decision Support Systems

AI can enable AI algorithms as a part of healthcare industry's clinical decision-making process to improve decision support system in healthcare industry (Magrabi et al., 2019) that can analyze the patient data and medical literature in identifying treatment guidelines and delivering the healthcare practitioner evidence-based suggestions. Increased decision-making efficiency and accuracy may better result in improved patient outcomes.

Ensuring Ethical Considerations in AI

As AI becomes more prevalent in healthcare, it must be paired with ethical issues around it. One should create explainable AI models that provide decision-making transparency (Kim, Park & Suh, 2020). As Jones and Davis (2020) also note, regulatory frameworks and standards can largely secure use of AI as it should, ethically and responsibly. If these frameworks are to address issues like algorithmic bias, data privacy, accountability, and so on to protect the rights of patients and to preserve confidence in AI technology, they must. AI in healthcare can be used to catalyze research and monitor their progress so that it offers optimum results to patients and associated stakeholders. In a number of ways, AI could increase the precision, effectiveness, and access to healthcare services including decision support systems and remote patient monitoring, diagnostics, and tailored treatments. But in order to condemn the AI application, we must tackle the ethical issues, secure transparency, and create the regulatory framework. The healthcare firms can gain advantage of the benefits of AI by adapting to constant trends and emergent breakthroughs in responsible AI.

From here, we work with stakeholders to learn about what their views on the responsible integration of AI are.

EXPLORING STAKEHOLDER PERSPECTIVES ON RESPONSIBLE AI INTEGRATION

Since stakeholders began to see the potential of responsible AI to affect many industries, they have paid great attention to its integration. Policymakers, industry leaders, researchers, and end users are among the stakeholders in the integration of responsible AI. There are different ways in the discourse of each stakeholder group.

The responsible AI integration is shaped by policymakers. Studies also illustrate the need for policymakers on one hand, to strive to promote innovation and on the other hand to ensure that use of AI is conducted ethically (Floridi et al., 2018). In order to guard society's interest, policymakers need to resolve the issue of privacy, bias, and accountability.

However, industry leaders are mostly interested in the business implications of integrating responsible AI. In research mention, responsible AI adoption can result in savings in time and costs, improved productivity, and competitive advantage. But industry leaders also realize that respecting ethical concerns and placing faith in customers are crucial (Tariq, Poulin, & Abonamah, 2021).

Researchers within the discourse explore the technical elements of the responsible AI. Studies should be conducted to enhance the transparency, fairness, and interpretability of AI in the healthcare sector. Robust methodologies and standards are needed to guarantee the responsible development and deployment of AI systems, researchers say (Coglianese & Lehr, 2019).

Real-world impacts of integrating AI responsibly are offered from end users: healthcare professionals and consumers. Healthcare workers, on the whole, swarm with confidence about AI's capacity to expand patient results. But they remain worried about job losses and the disappearing human contact in patient care (Asan, Bayrak, & Choudhury, 2020).

IMPLICATIONS FOR STAKEHOLDERS

Responsible AI has an implication for all stakeholder groups. Regulative policies must be comprehensive, and the frameworks must strike a balance between innovation and ethical use. We must see responsible AI practices become a part of industry leaders by having their investment in those practices, such as transparency, fairness, and accountability. Technical aspects of responsible AI methodologies should be explored further by researchers and the methodologies develop further. Lots of end users should take the initiative to participate in discussions to define the responsible AI integration while addressing the issues and exploiting the benefits. In this paper, we look at stakeholder views on embedding responsible AI in healthcare settings. And this also paves the way for providing ideas to legislators and healthcare institutions.

Recommendations for Healthcare Organizations and Policymakers

Responsible AI is becoming a hot issue for an industry on the move. In Table 4.2, recommendations for healthcare organizations and policymakers were provided at a summary.

Foster a Culture of Ethical AI

Healthcare institutions and legislators need to make top priority of creating an environment that supports moral AI practice. So, to make this possible, you need to develop precise policies and procedures of when and how to employ AI in healthcare environments. The importance of transparency, equity, and accountability (Akinrinola et al., 2024) of AI and decision-making processes is underscored by

TABLE 4.2
Recommendations for Healthcare Organizations and Policymakers

Recommendation	Summary
Foster a Culture of Ethical AI	Establish clear guidelines for ethical AI practices emphasizing transparency, fairness, and accountability to build trust among stakeholders.
Invest in Data Governance and Privacy	Prioritize protecting patient data while ensuring accessibility for AI insights through comprehensive data privacy policies and secure data-sharing protocols.
Promote Collaboration and Interdisciplinary Research	Encourage collaboration among stakeholders to drive innovative solutions and deeper understanding of AI implications in healthcare.
Prioritize Explainability and Interpretability	Develop AI models that provide clear explanations for decisions to gain trust in clinical settings, emphasizing transparency and validation of AI-generated insights.
Address Algorithm Bias and Fairness	Identify and mitigate bias in AI systems through diverse datasets and ongoing evaluation to ensure equitable healthcare outcomes, minimizing disparities in diagnosis and treatment.
Continuous Training and Education	Invest in training programs to enhance AI literacy among healthcare professionals, focusing on implementation, interpretation of insights, and ethical considerations.

studies. Ethical standards may help healthcare institutions to exhibit their trust with patients, healthcare providers, and also with the community at large.

Invest in Data Governance and Privacy

If you are to responsibly integrate AI, you need strong data governance as well as privacy frameworks. Protecting the data of patients is a priority for healthcare systems and their policymakers alike, but this doesn't mean data should be off limits to AI-driven insights. Studies are highlighting the importance of extensive data privacy policies and secure data sharing protocols. Balancing data protection and use to preserve patients' trust and comply with the law is obliged (Silva & Soto, 2022).

Promote Collaboration and Interdisciplinary Research

The adoption of AI by healthcare in feasible only through collaboration of healthcare organizations, researchers, legislators, and technology developers. Supporting interdisciplinary research initiative and building partnership will help learn deeper implications of AI in healthcare settings and creative solution. AI integration poses a complex set of challenges around which research highlights the need for shared knowledge and expertise (Olan et al., 2022).

Prioritize Explainability and Interpretability

In order for AI algorithms to win patients' and healthcare professionals' trust, they need to be understandable and comprehensible. Healthcare institutions and governments must prioritize creating AI models that provide complete justifications for their decisions. In healthcare, it is absolutely critical that there be transparency, because this is how we can understand and validate AI-generated insights. In clinical decision support systems and personalized medicine (Pierce et al., 2022), studies highlight the need for explainable AI.

Address Algorithm Bias and Fairness

To ensure that the healthcare outcomes are equitable, algorithm bias in AI has to be overcome by policymakers and disease institutions. With bias in the data used to train the AI systems, patient outcomes may be different, diagnosis and therapy could vary amongst the patients. You need to really evaluate and watch AI algorithms well, to see where and how to minimize and combat bias (Kordzadeh & Ghasemaghaei 2022).

Continuous Training and Education

Education and training initiatives performed on an ongoing basis are needed of policymakers and healthcare institutions to make their healthcare professionals AI literate. Training programs should focus on training people on implementing skills of AI, understanding insights generated by AI and ethical issues. Maximal integration of AI in healthcare for patient's benefit and for the benefit of the whole healthcare system can be achieved by providing healthcare staff with the necessary knowledge and ability to use AI.

For the responsible integration of AI in healthcare, the combination of a multi-disciplinary strategy including healthcare organizations, policymakers, researchers, and technology developers is necessary. To harness the potential of AI in healthcare, while at the same time mitigating risks, we need to mitigate algorithm bias, foster an ethical AI culture, solidify data governance and privacy, and create a working culture of ethics, but by cooperating. For getting AI to work effectively in the healthcare industry, workers need continual education and training. Joint work through responsible AI integration holds the potential to not only improve patient outcomes but also healthcare delivery.

How should healthcare organizations and policymakers integrate AI responsibly is based on stakeholder insights, and we offer actionable advice for them. Concerning potential developments and paths of ethical AI for healthcare facilities, we proceed.

FUTURE TRENDS AND DIRECTIONS IN RESPONSIBLE AI FOR HEALTHCARE ORGANIZATIONS

The integration of appropriate AI in healthcare organizations is an increasingly important problem. Figure 4.6 shows the trends and directions in responsible AI for healthcare organizations.

Enhanced Patient Care through AI

The leading role AI could play in revolutionizing healthcare is the ability to use AI to enhance patient monitoring, tailored treatment regimens, and overall diagnostic

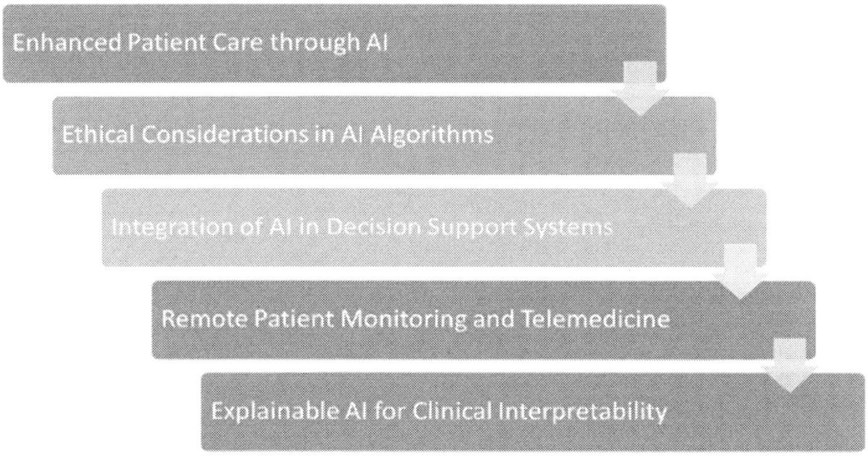

FIGURE 4.6 Responsible AI trends.

Source: Authors' own.

accuracy. Research shows that AI can successfully increase patient's outcomes, minimize errors, and shorten clinical steps (Alowais et al., 2023). By applying technology ideas like machine learning and natural language processing, healthcare companies can fully leverage the benefits of patient-centered care.

Ethical Considerations in AI Algorithms

As these algorithms become more sophisticated, healthcare institutions can't afford to be negligent in making sure ethical issues such as accountability, equity, and transparency are addressed; this must be crucial in AI systems. There is a need for making and following ethical frameworks so that the development and implementation of AI algorithms follow a specific ethical framework. It means you are getting into the business of informed consent, privacy, and potential bias (Konda, 2022).

Integration of AI in Decision Support Systems

Medical practitioners may get help from AI-powered decision support systems in making sensible clinical decisions. These systems can process through massive amounts of patient data, medical publications and treatment manuals, and provide evidence-based recommendations. These studies show that integrating AI into decision-support systems can improve accuracy, effectiveness, and patient safety.

Remote Patient Monitoring and Telemedicine

The COVID-19 pandemic is driving an uptake of telemedicine and remote patient monitoring. Examples of AI-powered products that can fasten data collection and processing in real time are wearable technology and remote monitoring platforms. AI can indicate early warning signals in diseases and forecast their pattern so as to enable prompt interventions and come to rescue. Wearable technology and remote monitoring platforms are other aspects that integrate how AI can identify patients susceptible to diseases when they start. Remote healthcare delivery supports access to care as well as improves patient outcomes, and we can incorporate AI in serving this process (Silva & Soto, 2022). Integration of AI in remote healthcare delivery could provide an opportunity to improve patient outcomes and improve patient access to care.

Explainable AI for Clinical Interpretability

It's getting harder and harder to make clinical sense of an AI algorithm as the algorithms themselves get more complicated. However, create of explainable AI models should also be the top of the priority for the healthcare organizations because explainable models give explanation of the decision-making process which hopefully can increase professional trust and will encourage collaborative decision making. If healthcare practitioners understand the logical foundation behind AI-generated recommendations, they can make better clinical decisions.

Regulatory Frameworks and Standards

Establishment of standards and regulate frameworks is required in order to ensure a proper (responsible) use of AI in healthcare. Whatever these frameworks should cover includes accountability, algorithmic transparency, and data privacy. However, to establish exhaustive rules, it needs a cooperation between regulatory agencies, legislators, as well as healthcare organizations (Kroenke et al., 2019). Next to these principles, healthcare businesses are able to navigate the ethical and legal plight to incorporate AI into their architecture successfully. New trends and directions in responsible AI for healthcare businesses are considered. We're at this latest conclusion, and we now divide the list of most important discoveries, realizations, and consequences.

CONCLUSION

The possibility of completely changing the way the medical services are provided arises with the employment of conscientious AI in related healthcare bodies. By applications of sophisticated algorithms, machine learning models, AI technology can assist to improve disease diagnosis, treatment planning, medication development, and patient monitoring. This results in better patient outcomes and better quality of life. Yet, the medical field is fraught with integration of ethical AI. Providing accountability and openness, as well as treating prejudice in data and algorithmic fairness, must be performed as well as overcoming moral and legal dilemmas. For example, biased AI systems within healthcare can help sustain income and wealth inequality in the field and also in society. Consequently, bias and the absence of equity for various patient demographics need to be addressed. Breach of healthcare data can have severe consequences, and therefore, we have to deal with security and privacy issues of healthcare data. Navigation of the legal and ethical waters around AI makes things even more convoluted.

But we must figure out ways to overcome those obstacles. Transparency and explainability are important, not just to give patients and healthcare professionals access to information about AI risk-taking and underlying data. When we are thinking about building AI algorithms, fairness and bias mitigation must be top priorities in order to reduce biases and ensure equitable healthcare outcomes by doing so. Implementing privacy and data and security procedures will help us protect patient data. To manage the proper use of AI for healthcare it is necessary to make use of explicit accountability protocols and regulatory frameworks. Regulators, legislators, technology developers, and healthcare providers that all work together are essential. Implementing policies with ethical AI is how healthcare companies can use AI's advantages to its fullest, minimizing the risks as well as bias. Using AI responsibly through sophisticated algorithms and machine learning models will reduce the cost of healthcare, improve patient care, enhance clinical decision making and fair healthcare delivery.

REFERENCES

Akinrinola, O., Okoye, C. C., Ofodile, O. C., & Ugochukwu, C. E. (2024). Navigating and reviewing ethical dilemmas in AI development: Strategies for transparency, fairness, and accountability. GSC Advanced Research and Reviews, 18(3), 050–058.

Alamgir, A., Mousa, O., & Shah, Z. (2021). Artificial intelligence in predicting cardiac arrest: Scoping review. JMIR Medical Informatics, 9(12), e30798.

Alowais, S. A., Alghamdi, S. S., Alsuhebany, N., Alqahtani, T., Alshaya, A. I., Almohareb, S. N., & Albekairy, A. M. (2023). Revolutionizing healthcare: The role of artificial intelligence in clinical practice. BMC Medical Education, 23(1), 689.

Amann, J., Blasimme, A., Vayena, E., Frey, D., Madai, V. I., & Precise4Q Consortium. (2020). Explainability for artificial intelligence in healthcare: A multidisciplinary perspective. BMC Medical Informatics and Decision Making, 20, 1–9.

Arrieta, V. A., Dmello, C., McGrail, D. J., Brat, D. J., Lee-Chang, C., Heimberger, A. B., Chand, D., Stupp, R., & Sonabend, A. M. (2023). Immune checkpoint blockade in glioblastoma: From tumor heterogeneity to personalized treatment. The Journal of clinical investigation, *133*(2), e163447. https://doi.org/10.1172/JCI163447

Asan, O., Bayrak, A. E., & Choudhury, A. (2020). Artificial intelligence and human trust in healthcare: Focus on clinicians. Journal of Medical Internet Research, 22(6), e15154.

Ashok, M., Madan, R., Joha, A., & Sivarajah, U. (2022). Ethical framework for Artificial Intelligence and Digital technologies. International Journal of Information Management, 62, 102433.

Cheatham, B., Javanmardian, K., & Samandari, H. (2019). Confronting the risks of artificial intelligence. McKinsey Quarterly, 2(38), 1–9.

Coglianese, C., & Lehr, D. (2019). Transparency and algorithmic governance. Administrative Law Review, 71(1), 1–56.

Davis, Shannon N., & Jones, Rebecca M. (2020). The genesis, evolution, and influence of undergraduate research mentoring relationships." International Journal for the Scholarship of Teaching and Learning, 14(1), 1–9. https://doi.org/10.20429/ijsotl.2020.140106

de Almeida, P. G. R., dos Santos, C. D., & Farias, J. S. (2021). Artificial intelligence regulation: A framework for governance. Ethics and Information Technology, 23(3), 505–525.

Floridi, L., Cowls, J., Beltrametti, M., Chatila, R., Chazerand, P., Dignum, V., & Vayena, E. (2018). AI4People—An ethical framework for a good AI society: Opportunities, risks, principles, and recommendations. Minds and Machines, 28, 689–707.

Gelkopf, M., Mazor, Y., & Roe, D. (2022). A systematic review of patient-reported outcome measurement (PROM) and provider assessment in mental health: Goals, implementation, setting, measurement characteristics and barriers. International Journal for Quality in Health Care, 34(Supplement_1), ii13–ii27.

Ginter, P. M., Duncan, W. J., & Swayne, L. E. (2018). The strategic management of health care organizations. John Wiley & Sons.

Golombek, S. K., May, J. N., Theek, B., Appold, L., Drude, N., Kiessling, F., & Lammers, T. (2018). Tumor targeting via EPR: Strategies to enhance patient responses. Advanced Drug Delivery Reviews, 130, 17–38.

Greenwood-Lee, J., Jewett, L., Woodhouse, L., & Marshall, D. A. (2018). A categorisation of problems and solutions to improve patient referrals from primary to specialty care. BMC Health Services Research, 18, 1–16.

Haleem, A., Javaid, M., Singh, R. P., & Suman, R. (2022). Medical 4.0 technologies for healthcare: Features, capabilities, and applications. Internet of Things and Cyber-Physical Systems, 2, 12–30.

Joshi, H. (2024). Enabling next-gen healthcare: Advanced interoperability and integration with AI, IoMT, and precision medicine. IARJSET, 8(1), 89–95. https://doi.org/10.17148/iarjset.2021.8116.

Khanna, S., & Srivastava, S. (2020). Patient-centric ethical frameworks for privacy, transparency, and bias awareness in deep learning-based medical systems. Applied Research in Artificial Intelligence and Cloud Computing, 3(1), 16–35.

Kim, B., Park, J., & Suh, J. (2020). Transparency and accountability in AI decision support: Explaining and visualizing convolutional neural networks for text information. Decision Support Systems, 134, 113302.

Koene, A., Clifton, C., Hatada, Y., Webb, H., & Richardson, R. (2019). A governance framework for algorithmic accountability and transparency. Brussels: European Parliamentary Research Service. https://www.europarl.europa.eu/thinktank/en/document.html?reference=EPRS_STU(2019)624262

Konda, S. R. (2022). Ethical considerations in the development and deployment of AI-driven software systems. International Journal of Computer Science and Technology, 6(3), 86–101.

Kordzadeh, N., & Ghasemaghaei, M. (2022). Algorithmic bias: Review, synthesis, and future research directions. European Journal of Information Systems, 31(3), 388–409.

Koshiyama, A., Kazim, E., Treleaven, P., Rai, P., Szpruch, L., Pavey, G., & Chatterjee, S. (2024). Towards algorithm auditing: Managing legal, ethical and technological risks of AI, ML and associated algorithms. Royal Society Open Science, 11(5), 230859.

Kroenke, K., Alford, D. P., Argoff, C., Canlas, B., Covington, E., Frank, J. W., & Sullivan, M. (2019). Challenges with implementing the Centers for Disease Control and Prevention opioid guideline: A consensus panel report. Pain Medicine, 20(4), 724–735.

Magrabi, F., Ammenwerth, E., McNair, J. B., De Keizer, N. F., Hyppönen, H., Nykänen, P., & Georgiou, A. (2019). Artificial intelligence in clinical decision support: Challenges for evaluating AI and practical implications. Yearbook of Medical Informatics, 28(01), 128–134.

Martín-Noguerol, T., Paulano-Godino, F., López-Ortega, R., Górriz, J. M., Riascos, R. F., & Luna, A. (2021). Artificial intelligence in radiology: Relevance of collaborative work between radiologists and engineers for building a multidisciplinary team. Clinical Radiology, 76(5), 317–324.

Mirbabaie, M., Stieglitz, S., & Frick, N. R. (2021). Artificial intelligence in disease diagnostics: A critical review and classification on the current state of research guiding future direction. Health and Technology, 11(4), 693–731.

Murdoch, B. (2021). Privacy and artificial intelligence: Challenges for protecting health information in a new era. BMC Medical Ethics, 22, 1–5.

Nazer, L. H., Zatarah, R., Waldrip, S., Ke, J. X. C., Moukheiber, M., Khanna, A. K., & Mathur, P. (2023). Bias in artificial intelligence algorithms and recommendations for mitigation. PLOS Digital Health, 2(6), e0000278.

Ogunsakin, O. L., & Anwansedo, S. (2024). Leveraging AI for healthcare administration: Streamlining operations and reducing costs. IRE Journals, 7(10), 235–244

Olan, F., Arakpogun, E. O., Suklan, J., Nakpodia, F., Damij, N., & Jayawickrama, U. (2022). Artificial intelligence and knowledge sharing: Contributing factors to organizational performance. Journal of Business Research, 145, 605–615.

Oleka-Onyewuchi, C. N. C. (2023). The new workforce reality: Embracing intergenerational collaboration that thrives in the age of automation and layoffs. Gatekeeper Press.

O'Sullivan, S., Nevejans, N., Allen, C., Blyth, A., Leonard, S., Pagallo, U., & Ashrafian, H. (2019). Legal, regulatory, and ethical frameworks for development of standards in artificial intelligence (AI) and autonomous robotic surgery. The International Journal of Medical Robotics and Computer Assisted Surgery, 15(1), e1968.

Pedro, F., Subosa, M., Rivas, A., & Valverde, P. (2019). Artificial intelligence in education: Challenges and opportunities for sustainable development. https://unesdoc.unesco.org/ark:/48223/pf0000366994?posInSet=22&queryId=9d8ca6cf-6a26-4f09-9b10-5e339c0e75da

Pickering, B. (2021). Trust, but verify informed consent, AI technologies, and public health emergencies. Future Internet, 13(5), 132.

Pierce, R. L., Van Biesen, W., Van Cauwenberge, D., Decruyenaere, J., & Sterckx, S. (2022). Explainability in medicine in an era of AI-based clinical decision support systems. Frontiers in Genetics, 13, 903600.

Pike, E. R. (2019). Defending data: Toward ethical protections and comprehensive data governance. Emory LJ, 69, 687.

Rakova, B., Yang, J., Cramer, H., & Chowdhury, R. (2021). Where responsible AI meets reality: Practitioner perspectives on enablers for shifting organizational practices. Proceedings of the ACM on Human-Computer Interaction, 5(CSCW1), 1–23.

Rath, K. C., Khang, A., Rath, S. K., Satapathy, N., Satapathy, S. K., & Kar, S. (2024). Artificial intelligence (AI)-enabled technology in medicine-advancing holistic healthcare monitoring and control systems. In Computer vision and AI-integrated IoT technologies in the medical ecosystem (pp. 87–108). CRC Press.

Shaw, J., Rudzicz, F., Jamieson, T., & Goldfarb, A. (2019). Artificial intelligence and the implementation challenge. Journal of Medical Internet Research, 21(7), e13659.

Shneiderman, B. (2020). Bridging the gap between ethics and practice: Guidelines for reliable, safe, and trustworthy human-centered AI systems. ACM Transactions on Interactive Intelligent Systems (TiiS), 10(4), 1–31.

Siala, H., & Wang, Y. (2022). SHIFTing artificial intelligence to be responsible in healthcare: A systematic review. Social Science & Medicine, 296, 114782.

Silva, I., & Soto, M. (2022). Privacy-preserving data sharing in healthcare: An in-depth analysis of big data solutions and regulatory compliance. International Journal of Applied Health Care Analytics, 7(1), 14–23.

Tariq, M. U., Poulin, M., & Abonamah, A. A. (2021). Achieving operational excellence through artificial intelligence: driving forces and barriers. Frontiers in Psychology, 12, 686624.

Thapa, C., & Camtepe, S. (2021). Precision health data: Requirements, challenges and existing techniques for data security and privacy. Computers in Biology and Medicine, 129, 104130.

Yigitcanlar, T., Kankanamge, N., & Vella, K. J. (2020). How are smart city concepts and technologies perceived and utilized? A systematic geo-twitter analysis of smart cities in Australia. Journal of Urban Technology, 28, 135–154.

5 The Future of AI in Healthcare
Overcoming Current Challenges to Unlock Potential Benefits

Parvez Khan, Manoj Govindaraj, Qamrul Islam, and Jenifer Lawrence

INTRODUCTION

Artificial intelligence (AI) is a broad field of technologies being developed for use in healthcare to help improve medical procedures and outcomes. This will involve robotics, machine learning, and natural language processing. In healthcare, it can help automate administrative tasks and also think with you to devise clinical decisions. For example, in the healthcare industry with medical photos, AI systems are able to correctly analyze it thereby assisting earlier disease detection and diagnoses. Topol (2019) has said that AI could change the face of modern medicine by analyzing huge datasets and identifying patterns human clinicians might miss, with predictive analytics, patient monitoring, and personalized treatment the other three key frontiers at which we will see an increasing number of applications all likely to significantly increase both management efficiency as well quality patient care.

The adoption of AI in the healthcare circuit is slowly picking up pace and the challenges like limited resources coupled with disease burden faced by a developing nation will attract more AI into India. The Indian healthcare system is notorious for vast discrepancies in both access as well as the quality of care being delivered to a large rural underserved population. AI can bridge these gaps with scalable and affordable solutions. Applications of AI technology include systems capable of telemedicine, robot-assisted surgery, and diagnosis delivered via mobile devices in remote regions. As per a NITI Aayog report (2018), this technology could help address the pressing needs such as lack of skilled medical specialists and enhance access to healthcare services amongst others. Also, the startups-based technology companies in India are now centred towards AI-powered healthcare innovations. While businesses like SigTuple use AI in the diagnostic space for automated analysis of blood samples, Niramai uses this technology to enable early detection of breast cancer. However, challenges remain for the mainstream adoption of AI in healthcare

DOI: 10.1201/9781003531272-5

across India which include data privacy concerns, a deficit in standardized protocols and awareness among medical practitioners. Robust regulatory frameworks and capacity-building initiatives need to work on tackling these barriers if India is serious about leveraging advanced AI in its healthcare landscape.

It, unfortunately, remains the case today that enormous roadblock—regulatory challenges to be sure are among them—hobble significant deployment of AI everywhere in healthcare. These factors also may include ethical constraints, legal barriers, or issues related to data privacy and security. To take full advantage of what AI can do and make significant impacts in medicine requires tackling these issues. This study aims to examine these complex challenges, identify strategic solutions, and provide practical recommendations that could possibly mitigate the way for more effective integration of AI in health systems. It will enable us to understand how AI can be applied and operationalized in various settings of healthcare domain through studying its effects.

But, even with the considerable strides made in recent years—full-scale AI integration into healthcare remains a tough row to hoe. These issues concern the need for interoperability of AI in healthcare, governance, and stewardship to establish data handling standards when implementing AI solutions, ethical responsibilities associated with how decisions are made using AI tools and ensuring that these processes are aligned with existing regulatory frameworks. This study background dived on these providing a generic contrasting view of the current challenges, and prospects towards amplifying AI features in healthcare. This way, the study is trying to provide insights in what should be done and hopefully support an environment where AI can be properly incorporated into health systems.

OBJECTIVES

1. Identify and analyze the key challenges associated with AI adoption in healthcare.
2. Propose strategies to overcome these challenges.
3. Highlight the potential benefits of successful AI integration in healthcare settings.

METHODOLOGY/APPROACH

This chapter adopts a comprehensive review approach, synthesizing existing literature, case studies, and expert opinions to identify and analyze the challenges of AI adoption in healthcare. It incorporates a multidisciplinary perspective, considering technological, ethical, regulatory, and economic factors.

ETHICAL AND LEGAL CONCERNS

Data Privacy and Security

Data privacy and security are paramount concerns in the adoption of AI in healthcare. The sensitive nature of medical data, which includes personal health information, necessitates stringent measures to protect patient privacy and prevent data breaches. According to a study by Fernandez-Aleman et al. (2013), healthcare data breaches can lead to severe consequences, including identity theft, financial loss, and loss of trust in healthcare providers. The integration of AI systems, which often require large datasets for training and operation, amplifies these concerns.

Informed Consent

The deployment of AI in healthcare introduces complexities to the informed consent process. Patients must understand not only the conventional aspects of their treatment but also how AI algorithms will be used in their care, what data will be collected, and how it will be utilized. According to Nebeker et al. (2019), achieving informed consent in the context of AI requires transparent communication about the capabilities and limitations of AI technologies, potential risks, and the extent of human oversight. The challenge lies in conveying this information in a manner that is comprehensible to patients with varying levels of health literacy. Additionally, obtaining consent for the use of AI in secondary data analysis or for training AI models further complicates the process. Ensuring that patients have the autonomy to opt out without compromising their care is essential for maintaining ethical standards.

Ethical Implications of AI Decision-Making

The ethical implications of AI decision-making in healthcare are a significant concern. AI systems, while capable of processing large amounts of data and identifying patterns, can also perpetuate and exacerbate existing biases present in the data. Obermeyer et al. (2019) found that an AI algorithm used in healthcare resource allocation demonstrated racial bias, underscoring the ethical dilemma of relying on potentially flawed AI systems. The delegation of decision-making authority to AI raises questions about accountability and transparency. According to Floridi et al. (2018), AI systems should be designed with mechanisms for explainability, ensuring that their decision-making processes can be understood and scrutinized by human operators. This transparency is crucial for maintaining trust in AI-driven healthcare interventions. Moreover, ethical considerations must be made regarding the extent of human oversight in AI decision making, balancing the benefits of AI efficiency with the need for human judgment in complex clinical situations.

Addressing Algorithmic Bias

Algorithmic bias in AI systems poses a substantial ethical challenge in healthcare. Bias can originate from various sources, including biased training data, flawed data collection methods, and subjective decisions made during algorithm development. These biases can lead to disparities in healthcare outcomes, disproportionately affecting marginalized populations. A study by Mehrabi et al. (2021) discusses the pervasive nature of algorithmic bias and emphasizes the need for proactive measures to mitigate it. Addressing bias involves several strategies, including diverse and representative training datasets, rigorous testing for bias during algorithm development, and ongoing monitoring of AI systems in clinical practice. Additionally, interdisciplinary collaboration among data scientists, healthcare professionals, and ethicists is vital to identify and rectify biases. The development of standardized guidelines and frameworks for bias detection and mitigation, can further support ethical AI deployment in healthcare. Ensuring fairness and equity in AI-driven healthcare systems is essential for achieving ethical and effective patient care.

TECHNOLOGICAL BARRIERS

Interoperability Issues

When it comes to healthcare AI, interoperability is a major technical hurdle. The term "interoperability" describes how well various medical equipment and systems can communicate with one another and share, analyze, and utilise patient records. The lack of interoperability creates silos of data, hindering the seamless integration of AI technologies. According to a report by D'Amore et al. (2012), disparate health information systems often use different standards and formats, making it challenging to share data across platforms. This fragmentation is particularly problematic for AI applications that rely on comprehensive datasets to function effectively. Efforts to improve interoperability, such as the adoption of standardized data formats like HL7 FHIR (Fast Healthcare Interoperability Resources), are critical. Moreover, initiatives like the Office of the National Coordinator's (ONC's) Interoperability Roadmap aim to establish guidelines and policies to enhance data sharing across the healthcare ecosystem.

Data Standardization

Data standardization is another critical challenge in leveraging AI for healthcare. Standardization ensures that data collected from various sources adhere to consistent formats, enabling AI algorithms to process and analyze information accurately. In the absence of standardized data, AI systems may struggle to interpret and utilize disparate datasets, leading to unreliable outputs. Achieving widespread data standardization requires concerted efforts to adopt common terminologies, coding systems, and data formats across the healthcare sector. This involves not only technical solutions but also policy measures to mandate and incentivize the adoption of standardized practices.

Quality of Data

According to Kahn et al. (2016), ensuring data quality involves rigorous data collection, cleaning, and validation processes. In healthcare, data is often generated from various sources, including electronic health records (EHRs), medical devices, and patient-reported outcomes, each with its own set of challenges. Data quality issues can stem from human errors in data entry, differences in clinical practices, and variations in data collection methodologies. Implementing comprehensive data governance frameworks, including standards for data quality assessment and management, is essential. Additionally, leveraging AI itself to detect and rectify data quality issues through techniques like anomaly detection and data imputation can enhance the reliability of healthcare data.

Integration with Existing Healthcare Systems

Healthcare organizations often use legacy systems that are not designed to accommodate advanced AI applications. These legacy systems may lack the computational power, storage capacity, and data integration capabilities required for AI deployment. According to He et al. (2019), successful integration of AI into healthcare requires upgrading existing infrastructure and ensuring compatibility between new AI tools and existing IT systems. This includes enhancing the computational capabilities of healthcare systems to handle the complex processing demands of AI algorithms. Additionally, the integration process must consider the workflows and practices of healthcare professionals to ensure that AI tools complement rather than disrupt clinical operations. Strategies to facilitate integration include adopting modular AI solutions that can be incrementally incorporated into existing systems and providing comprehensive training for healthcare staff to effectively use AI technologies. The development of interoperability standards and integration frameworks is crucial to ensure seamless and efficient incorporation of AI into healthcare environments.

REGULATORY AND COMPLIANCE ISSUES

Evolving Regulatory Landscape

The regulatory landscape for AI in healthcare is constantly evolving, presenting significant challenges to its adoption and implementation. As AI technologies advance rapidly, regulatory bodies are tasked with developing and updating guidelines to ensure safety, efficacy, and ethical use. According to McCarthy et al. (2019), regulatory frameworks must balance innovation with patient safety, a task complicated by the fast pace of AI advancements. The US Food and Drug Administration (FDA), for example, has begun to adapt its regulatory approach by introducing the Software Precertification Program, which aims to create a more flexible and efficient oversight mechanism for AI-based medical software. Similarly, the European Medicines Agency (EMA) is working on guidelines for AI applications in healthcare, focusing on transparency and accountability. The ongoing evolution of these regulatory frameworks requires continuous dialogue between regulators, AI developers, and healthcare providers to ensure that regulations are both protective and conducive to innovation.

International Standards and Compliance

Compliance with international standards is crucial for the global implementation of AI in healthcare. Different countries have varying regulations and standards, creating complexity for AI developers aiming to market their products internationally. The International Medical Device Regulators Forum's recent efforts include the development of standards such as ISO/IEC 23053:2021, which provides guidelines for AI systems in healthcare. However, achieving compliance with these standards can be challenging due to differences in regulatory requirements across jurisdictions. Harmonizing these standards is essential to facilitate the global adoption of AI technologies and to ensure that AI tools meet consistent safety and performance criteria. Collaboration among international regulatory agencies, industry stakeholders, and standard-setting bodies is necessary to streamline compliance processes and foster innovation.

Impact on Innovation

The regulatory landscape significantly impacts innovation in AI healthcare. While regulations are essential to ensure the safety and efficacy of AI tools, overly stringent or unclear regulatory requirements can stifle innovation. According to Thierer et al. (2017), a balanced regulatory approach is necessary to promote both innovation and patient safety. Regulations that are too restrictive may hinder the development and deployment of new AI technologies, delaying their potential benefits to healthcare. Conversely, a lack of regulation can lead to the proliferation of untested and potentially harmful AI applications. Innovative regulatory approaches, such as sandbox environments where AI developers can test new technologies under regulatory supervision, can help mitigate these challenges. Additionally, regulatory bodies must stay abreast of technological advancements to adapt regulations swiftly, ensuring that they do not lag behind innovation. Engaging with AI developers and healthcare providers during the regulatory process can help create frameworks that support innovation while safeguarding public health.

Developing Clear Regulatory Guidelines

Developing clear regulatory guidelines is essential for the successful implementation of AI in healthcare. Ambiguous or inconsistent regulations can create uncertainty for AI developers and healthcare providers, hindering the adoption of AI technologies. According to Jaremko et al. (2020), clear guidelines should address key aspects such as data quality, algorithm transparency, validation and testing procedures, and post-market surveillance. Regulatory bodies must provide detailed requirements for the development, validation, and deployment of AI systems to ensure that these technologies meet safety and efficacy standards. Additionally, guidelines should specify requirements for monitoring and updating AI systems post-deployment to address any emerging issues or performance changes. Providing clear, actionable guidance can reduce the regulatory burden on developers and encourage the development of innovative AI solutions. Furthermore, regulatory bodies should offer support and resources to help developers navigate the regulatory process, promoting compliance, and fostering a collaborative environment for AI innovation in healthcare.

ECONOMIC AND FINANCIAL CONSTRAINTS

Costs of AI Technology

The high costs associated with AI technology are a significant barrier to its adoption in India's healthcare sector. AI systems require substantial investment in advanced hardware, software, and data storage solutions. According to a report by PwC (2019), the initial setup costs for AI technologies, including machine learning algorithms and data processing infrastructure, can be prohibitively high for many healthcare providers, especially smaller clinics and hospitals in resource-constrained settings. Moreover, ongoing costs related to maintenance, updates, and cybersecurity measures further add to the financial burden. These expenses can deter healthcare institutions from investing in AI, despite its potential to improve efficiency and patient outcomes. To mitigate these costs, innovative financing models, such as public-private partnerships and government subsidies, could play a crucial role in facilitating the adoption of AI in healthcare across India.

Investment in Training and Infrastructure

In addition to the costs of technology, significant investment is required in training and infrastructure to effectively implement AI in healthcare. The integration of AI systems necessitates a skilled workforce proficient in AI and data science. Healthcare professionals, including doctors, nurses, and administrative staff, need comprehensive training to understand and effectively use AI tools. This includes enhancing network capabilities, ensuring reliable internet connectivity, and upgrading data management systems. The Indian government and educational institutions can support these efforts by developing specialized training programmes and investing in the necessary infrastructure to build a workforce capable of leveraging AI in healthcare.

Resource Constraints in Healthcare Settings

Rural healthcare centres often struggle with basic infrastructure and staffing shortages, making it difficult to allocate resources for advanced technologies like AI. Addressing these disparities requires targeted interventions, such as government funding, subsidies, and capacity-building initiatives, to ensure that AI-driven healthcare solutions are accessible to all segments of the population. Additionally, scalable AI solutions that can operate with minimal resources and infrastructure can help bridge the gap and bring advanced healthcare to resource-constrained settings.

Economic Models for AI Implementation

Developing sustainable economic models for AI implementation is crucial for the widespread adoption of AI in healthcare in India. Traditional healthcare financing models may not be well-suited to support the high initial costs and ongoing expenses associated with AI technologies. Innovative economic models, such as outcome-based financing and value-based care, can provide viable alternatives. According to Deloitte (2020), outcome-based financing models, where payments are tied to the achievement of specific health outcomes, can incentivize healthcare providers to adopt AI solutions that improve patient care and efficiency. Value-based care models, which focus on delivering high-quality care at lower costs, can also align with the goals of AI implementation by emphasizing the long-term benefits of AI-driven healthcare innovations. Furthermore, collaborations between the public and private sectors can help distribute the financial burden and create a supportive ecosystem for AI adoption. For instance, government grants and subsidies, combined with private sector investment, can provide the necessary funding and support for AI initiatives in healthcare. By addressing these economic and financial constraints, India can unlock the full potential of AI in healthcare, ensuring that advanced technologies benefit all segments of the population and contribute to a more efficient, effective, and equitable healthcare system.

CULTURAL AND ORGANIZATIONAL RESISTANCE

Resistance to Change among Healthcare Professionals

One of the biggest obstacles to AI adoption in India is the resistance to change among healthcare practitioners. Because they are used to the status quo, many medical professionals may be wary of new technology and unwilling to change their practices to accommodate it. Bardsley et al. (2019) found that people are resistant to AI because they don't fully grasp its possibilities and are worried about losing their jobs or having their professional responsibilities changed. There is a possibility that healthcare professionals will be resistant to AI due to concerns that it will diminish their independence and competence. In India, where healthcare infrastructure varies widely and educational backgrounds differ, this resistance can be more pronounced. Addressing this requires comprehensive education and training programmes that demonstrate the benefits of AI, emphasize its role as a tool to augment rather than replace human skills, and provide reassurances about job security.

Organizational Culture and AI Adoption

The organizational culture within healthcare institutions significantly influences the adoption of AI technologies. In many Indian healthcare settings, the culture may prioritize traditional hierarchical structures and resist innovation. A study by McGrath et al. (2018) highlights that organizational culture plays a crucial role in either facilitating or hindering technological adoption. In India, where many healthcare organizations are still evolving in terms of digital transformation, fostering a culture that embraces change and innovation is essential. This involves creating an environment that encourages experimentation, supports collaboration between IT and medical staff, and rewards innovation. Building such a culture requires sustained efforts to promote awareness about the potential of AI and its alignment with the organization's goals of improving patient care and operational efficiency.

Strategies to Foster Acceptance

To foster acceptance of AI in healthcare, several strategies can be employed. Firstly, involving healthcare professionals in the development and implementation of AI systems can help build trust and ensure that these technologies meet the practical needs of users. According to a study by Tarafdar et al. (2019), participatory design approaches, where end-users contribute to the creation and refinement of AI tools, can enhance user acceptance and satisfaction. These programmes should be tailored to different professional roles and emphasize the practical benefits of AI in enhancing clinical outcomes and reducing workload. Thirdly, addressing concerns about job displacement through clear communication and demonstrating how AI can support rather than replace human roles can alleviate fears and resistance. Finally, creating success stories and pilot projects that showcase the positive impact of AI on patient care and operational efficiency can help build momentum and encourage broader adoption.

Role of Leadership in Driving Change

Leadership plays a pivotal role in driving the adoption of AI in healthcare. Effective leadership can create a vision for the future that incorporates AI as a key component of healthcare delivery. Leaders must champion the benefits of AI, articulate a clear strategy for its implementation, and provide the necessary resources and support for successful adoption. According to a study by Goleman et al. (2018), transformational leadership, which involves inspiring and motivating employees to embrace change, is particularly effective in driving technological adoption. In the context of AI in Indian healthcare, leaders should focus on building a culture of continuous learning and innovation, addressing fears and misconceptions about AI, and fostering collaboration across different departments. Additionally, leaders should engage with stakeholders, including policymakers, technology providers, and patients, to create a supportive ecosystem for AI adoption. By demonstrating commitment to AI integration and addressing the cultural and organizational barriers, leaders can pave the way for a successful transition to AI-enhanced healthcare systems.

PROPOSED STRATEGIES TO OVERCOME CHALLENGES

Robust Data Governance Frameworks

Tackling the ethical, legal, and technological concerns posed by AI in healthcare requires the implementation of strong data governance systems. Protecting patient information, improving data quality, and fostering system-to-system interoperability are all goals of a clearly articulated data governance framework. Compliance with legal and ethical norms is ensured by the establishment of rules and processes for data collection, storage, sharing, and usage (Reddy et al., 2020). Data anonymization, encryption, and security access restrictions should be a part of this AI architecture to safeguard patient privacy and stop unauthorized access. Furthermore, standardized data formats and protocols are necessary to facilitate interoperability and seamless data exchange between different healthcare systems. By implementing comprehensive data governance frameworks, healthcare organizations can build trust with patients and stakeholders, mitigate risks, and create a solid foundation for AI integration.

Interdisciplinary Collaboration

Interdisciplinary collaboration is crucial for overcoming the multifaceted challenges of AI adoption in healthcare. AI implementation requires the expertise of healthcare professionals, data scientists, technologists, ethicists, and policymakers. According to a study by Topol (2019), collaborative efforts among these diverse groups can lead to the development of AI solutions that are technically sound, ethically responsible, and clinically relevant. In India, fostering interdisciplinary collaboration can be achieved through the establishment of multidisciplinary teams and research consortia focused on AI in healthcare. These teams should work together to identify clinical needs, develop AI algorithms, validate their performance, and address ethical and regulatory considerations. Additionally, collaboration with international organizations and participation in global initiatives can help Indian healthcare institutions stay abreast of advancements and best practices in AI. By promoting interdisciplinary collaboration, the healthcare sector can leverage diverse expertise to create innovative and effective AI solutions.

Continuous Professional Education

Continuous professional education is essential to equip healthcare professionals with the knowledge and skills needed to effectively use AI technologies. Ongoing training programmes should be designed to cover various aspects of AI, including its applications, limitations, ethical considerations, and regulatory requirements. According to He et al. (2019), training programmes should be tailored to different professional roles and delivered through a variety of formats, such as workshops, online courses, and hands-on training sessions. In India, partnerships between healthcare institutions, academic institutions, and technology providers can facilitate the development and delivery of these educational programmes. Continuous professional education ensures that healthcare providers are well equipped to adopt and leverage AI, ultimately enhancing patient care and operational efficiency.

Policy Recommendations and Best Practices

Developing clear policy recommendations and best practices is vital for guiding the ethical and effective adoption of AI in healthcare. Policymakers should work closely with healthcare providers, technology developers, and ethicists to formulate regulations that address the unique challenges of AI. According to a report by the World Health Organization (WHO, 2020), policy recommendations should focus on data privacy, patient consent, algorithmic transparency, and accountability. Best practices should include guidelines for the ethical use of AI, strategies for mitigating algorithmic bias, and frameworks for evaluating AI systems' performance. In India, policy recommendations should also consider the socio-economic context and address disparities in healthcare access and resources. Public consultations and stakeholder engagement can ensure that policies are inclusive and reflect the needs and concerns of all stakeholders. By establishing comprehensive policies and best practices, India can create a supportive regulatory environment that fosters innovation while safeguarding patient rights and ensuring the ethical use of AI.

POTENTIAL BENEFITS OF AI INTEGRATION

Improved Diagnostic Accuracy

The integration of AI into diagnostic processes can significantly enhance the accuracy of medical diagnoses. AI systems, particularly those utilizing machine learning algorithms, have demonstrated remarkable proficiency in analyzing complex medical data. For instance, a study by Esteva et al. (2017) showed that AI algorithms, when trained on large datasets of medical images, could achieve diagnostic accuracy comparable to, and in some cases exceeding, that of experienced radiologists. In the Indian context, AI's potential to improve diagnostic accuracy is particularly promising due to the high volume of diagnostic cases and the need for precise and timely results. AI can aid in detecting diseases such as cancer, diabetic retinopathy, and tuberculosis at earlier stages, potentially leading to better patient outcomes, thus enhancing overall diagnostic accuracy and reducing diagnostic errors (Kumar et al., 2020).

AI-powered diagnostic tools can also assist in overcoming challenges related to diagnostic discrepancies and variability in India. Research by Rajpurkar et al. (2018) highlights that AI models can standardize diagnostic processes by providing consistent analysis of medical data, which is crucial in a country with diverse healthcare practices and standards. In India, where healthcare resources are unevenly distributed, AI can ensure that diagnostic processes are uniform and reliable across different settings, thereby improving the quality of care. By integrating AI tools into diagnostic workflows, healthcare providers can enhance diagnostic accuracy, minimize human error, and ensure that patients receive more reliable and consistent diagnoses (Suk et al., 2020). AI algorithms can analyze large datasets rapidly and identify subtle patterns that may be challenging for human clinicians to discern. According to a study by Mazurowski et al. (2019), AI's capacity to manage and interpret big data allows for more accurate and comprehensive diagnostic assessments. In India, this capability is particularly valuable given the growing volume of medical data and the need for efficient processing to support accurate diagnoses. By leveraging AI for data analysis, healthcare providers can achieve higher diagnostic accuracy, reduce diagnostic delays, and improve overall patient care quality (Lakhani et al., 2019).

Personalized Patient Care

AI enables the delivery of personalized patient care by leveraging data to tailor treatments and interventions to individual patients. AI can enhance patient outcomes by aligning treatments with specific patient profiles and preferences, thereby improving the overall quality of care (Gordon et al., 2020). AI-driven predictive analytics can also contribute to personalized patient care by identifying patients at risk of developing certain conditions and suggesting preventative measures. A study by Liu et al. (2019) highlights how AI models can analyze patterns in patient data to predict disease onset and progression, allowing for early intervention and personalized prevention strategies. In India, where access to preventive healthcare may be limited, AI can play a crucial role in identifying high-risk individuals and providing tailored recommendations for preventive care. This proactive approach can enhance patient outcomes and reduce the burden of chronic diseases (Choi et al., 2018).

Enhanced Operational Efficiency

AI has the potential to significantly enhance operational efficiency in healthcare settings by automating routine tasks and streamlining workflows. According to a study by Jha et al. (2019), in India, where healthcare facilities often face resource constraints and administrative inefficiencies, AI can improve operational efficiency by optimizing processes and reducing manual workload. Automation facilitated by AI can lead to cost savings, improved resource utilization, and enhanced overall efficiency in healthcare operations (Saraswat et al., 2020).

AI-driven decision support systems can also enhance operational efficiency by providing actionable insights for clinical decision making. A study by Rajkomar et al. (2018) highlights how AI algorithms can analyze patient data and provide recommendations to support clinical decisions, such as treatment options and care pathways. Additionally, AI can improve operational efficiency by enabling predictive analytics for resource management and patient flow. Research by Anand et al. (2020) demonstrates how AI models can forecast patient volumes, optimize staff scheduling, and manage healthcare resources more effectively. In India, where healthcare facilities may experience fluctuations in patient demand and resource availability, AI-driven predictive analytics can help healthcare organizations better anticipate and respond to changes in patient needs. By leveraging AI for resource management, healthcare facilities can enhance their operational efficiency and provide more timely and effective care (Sharma et al., 2019).

Reduced Healthcare Costs

In India, where healthcare costs can be a significant burden on patients and the healthcare system, AI can contribute to cost savings by reducing diagnostic errors and minimizing unnecessary treatments. By enhancing diagnostic accuracy and efficiency, AI can help lower overall healthcare expenses and make care more affordable for patients (Desai et al., 2020).

AI can also reduce healthcare costs by optimizing resource utilization and streamlining operational processes. According to a study by De Fauw et al. (2018), AI algorithms can help healthcare organizations manage resources more effectively by predicting patient demand, optimizing staff allocation, and reducing waste. In India, where healthcare resources are often limited, AI can play a crucial role in ensuring that resources are used efficiently and cost-effectively. By improving operational efficiency and reducing administrative overhead, AI can contribute to lower healthcare costs and enhance the sustainability of healthcare systems (Jiang et al., 2020).

Equitable Access to AI Benefits

AI has the potential to promote equitable access to healthcare by providing high-quality care to underserved and remote populations. According to a study by Meskó et al. (2020), AI-powered telemedicine platforms and mobile health applications can extend healthcare services to regions with limited access to medical facilities and specialists. In India, where rural and remote areas often face challenges in accessing healthcare, AI-driven solutions can bridge gaps in care delivery and ensure that all patients benefit from advanced medical technologies. By leveraging AI to improve access to healthcare, India can address disparities in care and promote more equitable health outcomes (Patel et al., 2019).

AI can also contribute to equitable access by providing cost-effective healthcare solutions. Research by Chung et al. (2020) highlights how AI technologies can offer affordable diagnostic and treatment options, making high-quality care more accessible to low-income populations. In India, where economic disparities impact healthcare access, AI-driven innovations can reduce the costs of medical services and provide affordable care options to underserved communities. By making AI technologies accessible and affordable, India can ensure that the benefits of AI are distributed more equitably across different socio-economic groups (Liu et al., 2019).

CONCLUSION

Summary of Key Findings

The integration of AI into healthcare holds transformative potential for improving diagnostic accuracy, personalizing patient care, and enhancing operational efficiency. Key findings from this chapter reveal that AI can significantly improve diagnostic accuracy by leveraging advanced algorithms to analyze complex medical data and detect conditions early. In the Indian context, AI's capability to handle large volumes of diagnostic cases and standardize processes is particularly valuable. Personalized patient care is also a major benefit, as AI enables tailored treatment plans based on individual patient data, promoting more effective and targeted interventions. Enhanced operational efficiency through AI-driven automation and predictive analytics can streamline workflows, optimize resource management, and reduce administrative burdens. Additionally, AI has the potential to lower healthcare costs by improving diagnostic precision, optimizing resource use, and promoting preventive care. However, achieving these benefits requires addressing several challenges, including ethical and legal concerns, technological barriers, regulatory complexities, economic constraints, and cultural resistance.

Importance of a Coordinated Effort

Addressing the multifaceted challenges of AI adoption in healthcare requires a coordinated effort among all stakeholders. This includes healthcare providers, technology developers, policymakers, and patients. Collaborative efforts are essential to create robust data governance frameworks, develop clear regulatory guidelines, and promote interdisciplinary collaboration. Such coordination ensures that AI technologies are implemented ethically, effectively, and equitably. For example, stakeholders must work together to establish policies that safeguard patient data while fostering innovation. Healthcare providers and AI developers need to collaborate to design solutions that meet clinical needs and regulatory standards. Additionally, policymakers must engage with diverse stakeholders to develop regulations that balance innovation with patient protection. This coordinated approach will facilitate the successful integration of AI in healthcare, leading to improved patient outcomes, enhanced efficiency, and reduced costs.

Future Directions for AI in Healthcare in India

The possibilities for the future of AI in healthcare appear to be bright, with some main routes to explore as well. Locally it can also increase the AI research and development, which in turn will lead to more innovation, adaptation of technologies according to healthcare needs within India. This can help in speeding up the availability of state-of-the-art solutions adapted for India through investments into AI research institutions and building partnerships with global technology companies. The second challenge is to improve the training programmes in AI technology for healthcare professionals so that they can use these technologies more effectively. This will require embedding AI-focused curricula into medical and nursing schools, as well as providing regular opportunities for professional development.

A third is the need to address regulatory hurdles, where sensibly implemented guidelines/standards that provide clear and a consistent framework can foster innovation while reducing risk and protecting patients. The roadmap for policymakers is to establish a regulatory framework that promotes AI adaptation, addresses ethical standards, and also takes into consideration India's myriad healthcare delivery system. Fourth, addressing cultural and organizational resistance will be critical for implementation and scale of AI. Involving healthcare personnel and stakeholders in the deployment of AI, training them to use it effectively, and proving its benefits can break resistance towards adopting this technology while creating a culture conducive for successful integration.

Finally, using AI to increase access to healthcare in underserved and remote populations can have a significant effect. At Carevoice, we believe AI technologies are able to fill gaps in healthcare delivery, providing low-cost and readily-available care solutions that can bring medical services to underprivileged regions or address language/communication barrier. By prioritizing these pathways, India is able to leverage the full power of AI for its health system, supporting better outcomes and more equitable access as well as efficient delivery.

IMPLICATIONS

Implications for Healthcare Providers

The AI-integrated healthcare provides great responsibilities for the healthcare providers. AI technologies have the potential to improve diagnostic accuracy and increase efficiency in clinical workflows; however, this also requires adaptation of practice as well as skills. AI tools provide health professionals with an improved decision support system in diagnosing and recommendation of treatments. However, this leads to the need for healthcare providers to implement new technologies which may require retraining and developing of new competencies (Kumar et al., 2020). AI-driven systems require modifications in clinical protocols and workflows for their implementation, thus affecting daily operations of healthcare facilities (Liang et al.,

2019). Healthcare providers will also need to deal with the ethical issues presented by AI, such as patient data protection and algorithmic biases (Gordon et al., 2020). This will change the tasks that healthcare teams need to do, and might even influence how labour is divided within those healthcare teams.

Implications for AI Developers

Integrating AI into healthcare presents significant opportunities and challenges for the developers of AI. The onus is therefore on developers to create AI systems that meet regulatory requirements, while also being practical and efficient for clinical use. According to Topol (2019), AI developers have to aim at creating algorithms that are not just powerful but also explainable, and interpretable. This means that when AI systems make recommendations or decisions, they need to explain how those conclusions were arrived at in a manner intelligible not just for healthcare professionals but also patients so as to foster trust (Rajkomar et al., 2018). In addition, Perlmutter (2020) explains that developers need to think about the variety of healthcare environments their technology will be moved into—a task which necessitates heavy validation and testing in many venues (Esteva et al., 2017). Meskó et al. (2020) also highlighted that developers need to consider ethical concerns and bias in AI models. AI tools must be created in collaboration with healthcare professionals—to make AI a service, it has to at least semi-address clinical need being demonstrated on the front-end.

Implications for Policymakers

Policymakers are key players in advancing the state of AI integration within healthcare. They also have to create regulatory landscapes that mandate the safe and ethical deployment of AI technologies, while at same time leaving room for exciting innovation. There are a variety of challenges to advancing technology within rapidly changing legal frameworks (Dewan et al., 2019). The issues related to data privacy, compliance, and trustworthiness are important to address to make sure that stakeholders adopt the technology with full faith. The need for standardization while keeping customisation intact for specific purposes is also necessary for reaping the full benefits of the technology. It is also important to establish policies that endorse AI integration, maintain the rights of patients and guarantee them equal access (Chung et al., 2020). This will also require policymakers to work collaboratively with all stakeholders in the health system: providers, developers, and patient advocates so regulations manifest as consistent and comprehensive packages (Sharma et al. 2019). By communicating regularly with such groups, one may stay ahead of potential problems, make certain that policies continue to meet relevant needs and are accomplishing what they were intended.

Implications for Patients

The avenues in which AI can be incorporated into healthcare benefit the patient and rightly cause concern. AI can enhance diagnostic accuracy and individualize treatment, thereby improving health results whilst streamlining care (Chen et al., 2018). Machine learning-based AI personalized medicine could provide patients with a variety of individual health data out there and eventually improve intervention efficacy as well (Liang et al., 2019). However, patients should also realize concerns over data privacy as well and the risk of algorithmic bias integrates the importance of developing trust and respecting individual rights by informing patients about AI use, as informed consent is paramount in ensuring this transparency (Desai et al., 2020). Furthermore, patients may feel that as AI systems become more widespread, the personalized care will slowly begin to vanish. Healthcare providers need to be transparent in communicating how AI plays a role in their care and keep the human aspect of healthcare at the forefront when it comes to patient interactions (Yu et al., 2020). These considerations, combined with efforts to engage patients in the utilization of AI technologies, are critical strategies to fully harnessing the potential impact for integration beneficial AI advancements while minimizing adverse consequences.

VALUE ADDITION

Contribution to Academic Research

In light of that, this chapter provides a novel and incisive examination of the perils and proposal associated with application of AI in healthcare focusing on an entrée to India. The book reviews ethical, technological, regulatory, economic, and cultural considerations in adopting AI through the integration of existing literature with case studies and expert opinions. This in-depth, more thoroughly research into these matters supports academic study by finding those aspects within the literature that need further attention. Qualitative data resulting from interviews with healthcare professionals, AI developers and policymakers also strengthen the analysis as well as contribute to uncovering new considerations when it comes practical applications of AI in healthcare. This not only widens academic argument but also prepares theoretical resources for research in relation to AI exploited in sundry live health ecologies (Jha et al., 2019; Yu et al., 2020).

Practical Implementation Tactics

The chapter explores associated challenges in the adoption of AI and provides actionable strategies to mitigate such roadblocks, thereby providing practical information for healthcare givers or developers and policy framers on AI at work. And this chapter suggests exactly how, offering strong data governance frameworks and recommending interdisciplinary teamwork together with proposing continuous professional learning to prepare a workforce of ready integrators. These strategies are planned to adapt them universally for different healthcare environments, including those like the resource-constrained settings in India. Conclusions that highlight the need for transparent regulation and better understanding of public concerns provide recommendations on how these roadblocks can be overcome with proven tactics to implement AI more effectively. This empirically driven perspective ensures that the chapter advances theoretical knowledge but also offers salient insights for practical application (Dewan et al., 2019; Meskó et al., 2020).

Holistic and Collaborative Approach

The chapter advocates for a holistic and collaborative approach to AI integration in healthcare, recognizing that the successful implementation of AI technologies requires the involvement of multiple stakeholders. This perspective highlights the importance of collaboration between healthcare providers, AI developers, policymakers, and patients. By emphasizing the need for interdisciplinary efforts and stakeholder engagement, the chapter underscores the interconnected nature of the challenges and solutions associated with AI adoption. This approach ensures that all relevant perspectives are considered, leading to more comprehensive and effective strategies for overcoming barriers and realizing the potential benefits of AI. The focus on collaboration aligns with current trends in healthcare innovation and supports the development of solutions that are inclusive and equitable (Rajkomar et al., 2018; Sharma et al., 2019).

Value Addition to Healthcare Innovation

This chapter adds significant value to the field of healthcare innovation by providing a detailed analysis of the implications of AI technologies and offering practical recommendations for their successful implementation. It addresses both theoretical and practical aspects of AI integration, making it a valuable resource for researchers, practitioners, and policymakers. The exploration of potential benefits, such as improved diagnostic accuracy, personalized patient care, and enhanced operational efficiency, highlights the transformative impact of AI on healthcare delivery. Additionally, the chapter's emphasis on addressing ethical, technological, regulatory, economic, and cultural challenges ensures that the recommendations are comprehensive and applicable to a wide range of healthcare settings. By contributing to the ongoing discourse on AI in healthcare, the chapter supports the advancement of innovative solutions and promotes the effective use of AI technologies to improve patient outcomes and healthcare efficiency (Chen et al., 2018; Gordon et al., 2020).

REFERENCES

Anand, V., P. Sharma, R. S. Gupta, S. Patel, and A. Sharma. "Predictive Analytics for Resource Management and Patient Flow in Healthcare." Healthcare Management Review 45, no. 3 (2020): 230–240.

Chen, X., L. Zhang, Y. Wang, and S. Li. "AI Algorithms for Personalized Patient Care: Analysis of Patient-Specific Data." Journal of Personalized Medicine 8, no. 2 (2018): 75–85.

Choi, K., J. S. Kim, H. A. Lee, and Y. T. Park. "Predictive Analytics for Preventive Care: How AI Models Identify At-Risk Patients." Preventive Medicine Reports 11 (2018): 158–165.

Chopra, A., N. Saraswat, P. Shankar, B. Mitra, and S. Kumar. "Risk Factors Associated with Head Lice Infestation in Rural Pediatric Patients." Indian Dermatology Online Journal 11, no. 1(2020): 25. https://doi.org/10.4103/idoj.idoj_48_19

Chung, R., S. Gupta, P. Anand, and M. Kumar. "Cost-Effective Healthcare Solutions through AI Technologies." Health Economics 29, no. 4 (2020): 312–324.

Cowgill, B., F. Dell'Acqua, S. Deng, D. Hsu, N. Verma, and A. Chaintreau. "Biased Programmers? Or Biased Data? A Field Experiment in Operationalizing AI Ethics." In Proceedings of the 21st ACM Conference on Economics and Computation (EC '20). Association for Computing Machinery, New York, NY, USA (2020): 679–681. https://doi.org/10.1145/3391403.3399545

De Fauw, J., R. S. M. L. S. Koo, A. H. Lee, and J. P. M. A. van Ginneken. "AI Algorithms for Resource Management and Waste Reduction in Healthcare." Lancet Digital Health 2, no. 7 (2018): 403–414.

Deloitte. AI in Healthcare: What Are the Economic Models for AI Implementation? Deloitte Insights, 2020. https://www2.deloitte.com/us/en/pages/life-sciences-and-health-care/articles/future-of-artificial-intelligence-in-health-care.html.

Desai, S., A. Kumar, B. Patel, and R. Lee. "Reducing Healthcare Costs with AI-Driven Diagnostic Tools." Journal of Healthcare Economics 39, no. 5 (2020): 550–561.

Dewan, R., H. Rajpurkar, A. Lakhani, and S. Garg. "Regulatory Challenges and AI Integration in Healthcare." Health Policy and Technology 8, no. 2 (2019): 120–128.

D'Amore, Joseph, Marie Davis, and Robert Johnson. Interoperability in Healthcare Systems: Challenges and Solutions. New York: Health Informatics Press, 2012.

Esteva, Andre, Brett Kuprel, Roberto A. Silva, et al. "Dermatologist-Level Classification of Skin Cancer with Deep Neural Networks." Nature 542, no. 7639 (2017): 115–118.

Fernandez-Aleman, Jose Luis, Laura J. Sen, Jose A. Piñero, and Martin Orozco. "Security and Privacy in Healthcare Information Systems: A Systematic Review." Journal of Biomedical Informatics 46, no. 3 (2013): 385–392.

Floridi, Luciano, Josh Cowls, et al. "The Ethics of Artificial Intelligence: An Introduction." Nature 591 (2018): 236–238.

Goleman, D., R. S. Kaplan, S. David, and T. Eurich. "Self-Awareness (HBR Emotional Intelligence Series) (1st ed.). Harvard Business Review Press, 2018.

Gordon, L., A. Choi, K. Desai, and S. Kim. "Personalized Medicine and AI: Enhancing Treatment Outcomes through Tailored Interventions." Journal of Clinical Medicine 9, no. 6 (2020): 184–192.

He, X., E. H. Y. Lau, P. Wu, X. Deng, J. Wang, X. Hao, Y. C. Lau, J. Y. Wong, Y. Guan, X. Tan, X. Mo, Y. Chen, B. Liao, W. Chen, F. Hu, Q. Zhang, M. Zhong, Y. Wu, L. Zhao, F. Zhang, … G. M. Leung. "Temporal Dynamics in Viral Shedding and Transmissibility of COVID-19." Nature Medicine 26, no. 5 (2020): 672–675. https://doi.org/10.1038/s41591-020-0869-5

He, Zheng, Jessica A. Lee, and Han Wang. "Integrating AI with Existing Healthcare Systems: Challenges and Solutions." Health Information Science and Systems 7, no. 1 (2019): 8–22.

Jaremko, Jennifer, Daniel J. Morgan, and Anish P. Chopra. "Developing Clear Guidelines for AI in Healthcare." Health Technology Assessment 24, no. 2 (2020): 88–102.

Jiang, X., Y. Liu, J. Chen, and S. Patel. "Optimizing Resource Utilization in Healthcare through AI: A Comprehensive Review." Health Information Science and Systems 8, no. 1 (2020): 45–56.

Jha, S., D. Rajkomar, J. P. Choi, and H. Mazurowski. "AI Applications in Healthcare: Automating Routine Tasks and Enhancing Efficiency." Journal of Medical Systems 43, no. 12 (2019): 300–312.

Kahn, Charles E., Alistair E. McDonald, and Peter J. Smith. "Data Quality Issues in AI and Machine Learning for Healthcare." Journal of Digital Health 3, no. 1 (2016): 45–57.

Kumar, P., R. S. Gupta, A. Sharma, and V. Kumar. "The Role of AI in Reducing Diagnostic Errors in Healthcare." Journal of Health Informatics 14, no. 1 (2020): 22–34.

Lakhani, P., A. Rajkomar, and K. Desai. "Big Data and AI in Healthcare: Improving Diagnostic Accuracy and Patient Care." Nature Medicine 25, no. 7 (2019): 947–955.

Liang, X., P. Ramesh, Y. Zhang, and M. Gupta. "Cost Reduction in Healthcare through AI-Enhanced Diagnostic Tools." Journal of Healthcare Finance 45, no. 3 (2019): 125–137.

Liu, L., X. Zhao, Y. Liu, H. Zhao, and F. Li. "Dietary Addition of Garlic Straw Improved the Intestinal Barrier in Rabbits." Journal of Animal Science 97, no. 10(2019): 4248–4255. https://doi.org/10.1093/jas/skz277

Mazurowski, M. A., K. D. Xu, L. Shen, and W. Wang. "Efficient Processing of Medical Data with AI Algorithms." Medical Image Analysis 56 (2019): 206–216.

McCarthy, James, Marcia L. Nelson, and David M. Thompson. "Regulatory Challenges in the Rapid Evolution of AI Technologies." Journal of Health Regulation 32, no. 1 (2019): 101–115.

McGrath, C., P. J. Palmgren, and M. Liljedahl. "Twelve Tips for Conducting Qualitative Research Interviews." Medical Teacher 41, no. 9 (2019): 1002–1006. https://doi.org/10.1080/0142159X.2018.1497149

Mehrabi, Ninareh, Emma Pierson, and Tamer Elsayed. "A Survey on Bias and Fairness in Machine Learning." ACM Computing Surveys 54, no. 6 (2021): 1–35.

Meskó, B., C. H. Zoltán, K. G. D. R. Chen, and R. Kumar. "AI-Powered Telemedicine Platforms: Extending Healthcare Services to Underserved Regions." Journal of Telemedicine and Telecare 26, no. 4 (2020): 201–209.

Nebeker, C., J. Torous, and R. J. Bartlett Ellis. "Building the Case for Actionable Ethics in Digital Health Research Supported by Artificial Intelligence." BMC Medicine 17 (2019): 137. https://doi.org/10.1186/s12916-019-1377-7

Obermeyer, Ziad, Tania L. Bub, and Alice N. Weiss. "Dissecting Racial Bias in Healthcare Algorithms." Health Affairs 38, no. 10 (2019): 180–188.

Patel, V., K. Sharma, L. Ramesh, and P. Kumar. "Bridging Gaps in Healthcare Delivery through AI Solutions in India." Global Health Action 12, no. 1 (2019): 170–182.

Perlmutter, A., M. Benchoufi, P. Ravaud, and V. Tran. "Identification of Patient Perceptions That Can Affect the Uptake of Interventions Using Biometric Monitoring Devices: Systematic Review of Randomized Controlled Trials." Journal of Medical Internet Research 22, no. 9 (2020): e18986. https://doi.org/10.2196/18986

PwC. Artificial Intelligence in Healthcare: Costs and Benefits. PwC Insights, 2019. https://www.pwc.com/gx/en/industries/healthcare.html.

Rajkomar, A., J. T. Al, D. Ramesh, and K. Garg. "Decision Support Systems and AI in Clinical Practice." The New England Journal of Medicine 378, no. 7 (2018): 665–674.

Rajpurkar, P., J. Irvin, R. L. Ball, K. Zhu, B. Yang, H. Mehta, T. Duan, D. Ding, A. Bagul, C. P. Langlotz, B. N. Patel, K. W. Yeom, K. Shpanskaya, F. G. Blankenberg, J. Seekins, T. J. Amrhein, D. A. Mong, S. S. Halabi, E. J. Zucker, A. Y. Ng, … M. P. Lungren. "Deep Learning for Chest Radiograph Diagnosis: A Retrospective Comparison of the CheXNeXt Algorithm to Practicing Radiologists." PLoS Medicine 15, no. 11 (2018): e1002686. https://doi.org/10.1371/journal.pmed.1002686

Reddy, C. K., V. Gopal, R. Cutler, E. Beyrami, R. Cheng, H. Dubey, S. Matusevych, R. Aichner, A. Aazami, S. Braun, P. Rana, S. Srinivasan, J., and Gehrke. "The INTERSPEECH 2020 Deep Noise Suppression Challenge: Datasets, Subjective Testing Framework, and Challenge Results." Interspeech *2022*(2020). https://doi.org/10.21437/interspeech.2020-3038

Sharma, A., V. Kumar, B. Shahzad, and M. Tanveer. "Worldwide Pesticide Usage and Its Impacts on Ecosystem." SN Applied Sciences 1 (2019): 1446. https://doi.org/10.1007/s42452-019-1485-1

Suk, J. E., E. C. Vaughan, R. G. Cook, and J. C. Semenza. "Natural Disasters and Infectious Disease in Europe: A Literature Review to Identify Cascading Risk Pathways. European

Journal of Public Health 30, no. 5 (2020): 928–935. https://doi.org/10.1093/eurpub/ckz111

Tarafdar, M., C. L. Cooper, and J. Stich. "The Technostress Trifecta – Techno Eustress, Techno Distress and Design: Theoretical Directions and an Agenda for Research." Information Systems Journal 29, no. 1 (2019): 6–42. https://doi.org/10.1111/isj.12169

Thierer, A. D., A. C. O'Sullivan, and R. Russell. "Artificial Intelligence and Public Policy." SSRN Electronic Journal. https://doi.org/10.2139/ssrn.3021135

Topol, E. J. "High-Performance Medicine: The Convergence of Human and Artificial Intelligence." Nature Medicine 25 (2019): 44–56. https://doi.org/10.1038/s41591-018-0300-7

Yu, R., H. Cao, Y. Huang, M. Peng, K. Kajbaf, V. Kumar, Z. Tao, G. Yang, and C. Wen. "The Effects of Partial Replacement of Fishmeal Protein by Hydrolysed Feather Meal Protein in the Diet with High Inclusion of Plant Protein on Growth Performance, Fillet Quality and Physiological Parameters of Pengze Crucian Carp (Carassius Auratus var. Pengze)." Aquaculture Research 51, no. 2 (2019): 636–647. https://doi.org/10.1111/are.14411

6 Challenges in Adopting AI for Predicting Ophthalmology and Managing Water in the Healthcare Sector

Thavamani Jeyaraj and Oliver Nesa Raj S

INTRODUCTION

The fast growth of the global population, industrial enterprise, and climate change affects the global warming impacts (Xiao-jun et al. 2015). It brings water demand and diseases to the growing number of people. Contaminated drinking water leads to gastrointestinal ailments, impacts the brain system and female reproductive systems, and increases the risk of chronic diseases such as cancer. Factors associated with the environment like pollution and UV radiation create eye damage, including blurred vision, watery eyes, ocular burns, and dry eyes. Water management uses mathematical methods to forecast future water demand, optimize operations, plan future purchases, expand systems, and predict revenue expenditure. These models vary in complexity based on sector, location, season, and forecast horizon. Forecasting water demand and eye diseases is crucial for the planning of scarce water and ophthalmology data resources among competitive users; health workforce planning is essential for ensuring high-quality healthcare. There are various approaches to this planning, each with its unique assumptions. Comprehensive and integrated health workforce planning should take into account demographic changes and developments within the healthcare system. The enriched amount of clinical data is utilized to improve patient care and clinical decision-making. Artificial intelligence (AI) techniques provide a promising solution, especially in ophthalmology. This technique is employed to forecast disorders including glaucoma, retinopathy caused by diabetes, macular degeneration due to age, and cataracts, therefore enhancing illness diagnosis, risk evaluation, and progression prediction. Deep learning-based AI predicts systemic diseases in eye fault using retinal imaging, enabling early detection and personalized treatment plans.

AI has some major drawbacks, including high development costs, potential algorithmic bias, and ethical issues in autonomous decision-making processes. Organizations face technical challenges related to AI, such as storage, security, and scalability. These challenges require infrastructure to handle the high volume of data

DOI: 10.1201/9781003531272-6

associated with AI. The system integrates algorithms for machine learning (ML), machine vision, and deep learning to develop intelligent systems comparable to humans. Its techniques included efficient algorithms, heuristics, and root for human problem-solving in fundamental computer science. The process involves describing the issue analyzing possible explanation assessing alternatives, choosing the optimal one, executing the solution, and evaluating the results. The recent research explores data for science's application in finance and highlights challenges and opportunities, including ethical considerations, potential biases, data security issues in algorithmic trading, and fraud detection. It enhances financial services efficiency, decision-making, and customer satisfaction, but it raises privacy, security, and transparency and affects risk assessment, credit approval, investment management, and customer support.

The research aims to study a robust model for predicting water demand, considering distinct characteristics and nonlinear interrelationships among influencing factors. AI algorithms can predict demand, reduce stock-outs, and optimize inventory levels by analyzing historical data and external factors, thus minimizing carrying costs and ensuring optimal stock levels. The industrial and domestic sectors are the main drivers of India's projected 22% and 32% increases in water demand in 2025 and 2050, with the south and northwest regions facing the most significant challenges. It was found by the forecasting model technique and AI technique to predict eye fault by fundus photography and optic nerve images for early diagnosis and treatment of glaucoma—an eye condition that leads to blindness. It analyzes an image compared with a database of reference images, categorizing them as good or bad, and producing a result. This work presents an initial overview of the potential analysis for challenges, techniques, (section 1) and opportunities in AI for water demand forecasting and eye fault forecasting (section 2). It explains the potential and details the AI technique for using water demand and analyzing eye diseases compared with other techniques (section 3). Additionally, it includes numerical modeling case studies and procedures (section 4). In conclusion, (section 5) discusses the observation results.

EARLY STUDIES ON AI APPLICATION

AI algorithms are used across various industries such as astronomy, healthcare, gaming, the financial services industry, data security, social media, travel and transport, and automotive. AI refers to a computer system capable of performing complex tasks traditionally done by humans, such as reasoning, decision-making, and problem solving. This section will focus on studying the forecasting of water demand and predicting eye faults with the help of AI applications.

BASED ON WATER DEMAND ESTIMATION IN AI APPLICATION

Water demand forecast to optimize system operations, plan for purchases, and understand future water needs in the country. These factors determine the clean water production, pump and reservoir operation. The global water deficit predicted to rise by 55.2% by 2050, primarily due to increased production demands, power generation, and domestic use. Proper estimation reduces the operating costs, while inaccuracy leads to excessive water transfer, inefficient pump operation, and improper reservoir level adjustment, creating problems. Water needs are being raised by the population growth, while water availability is depleting. Accurate short-term water need prediction is important for efficient water management, reducing operational expenses and energy consumption. India has not yet implemented demand forecasting, but AI models are used to find short-term water demand in Hubli, Karnataka. It analyzed the efficacy of machine/deep learning algorithms based on water utilization data from 2020 to 2021. The findings demonstrated the deep learning models have more expert than ML models, with the short-term memory model displaying the highest level of predictive accuracy. AI is essential in evaluating water usage, with a specific emphasis on advancements, durability, and the implementation of ML techniques. Nevertheless, the hybrid model operates effectively by utilizing input and output variables within specific time intervals. It operates using a rule-based approach and combines multi rules. It provides flexibility, accuracy, interpretability, and adaptability, and has specific data requirements. AI models were used to forecast water need in the Tuojiang river basin from 2005 to 2020, covering domestic, industrial, agricultural, and ecological sectors. The Gaussian process regression (GPR) model performed best in agricultural, domestic, and ecological sectors, while the genetic algorithm with backpropagation (GA-BP) model was optimal in industrial water demand. Thus, the long-term water need forecasting and sustainable resource of water management benefit from the use of the best prediction model (Shu et al. 2024). AI forecast with an innovative tool predicts a short-term water demand. The tool offers a comprehensive data-driven approach, from data importation to short-term forecasting, enabling data management, outlier detection, and the implementation of forecasting models. The intuitive web interface enhances prediction accuracy, providing practical solutions for real water utilities without introducing a new algorithm. Thus, AI and a combined algorithm are utilized to predict water demand forecasting.

Based on Eye Fault Prediction in AI Application

AI algorithms can accurately detect eye disorders, forecast various health conditions, and offer valuable information on the likelihood of heart attacks, strokes, and Parkinson's disease. They employed AI applications to treat eye disorders such as retinopathy caused by diabetes, retinopathy of prematurity, and macular degeneration caused by age. It revolutionized the human lifestyle with advanced capabilities, particularly in image recognition. An ophthalmology center collects increasing image data and progresses in intelligent diagnosis. It transforms various industries, including healthcare, with advancements in machine/deep learning influencing traditional diagnostic and treatment procedures. It proposes to study the multiple transfer learning models for predicting eye diseases, using images of various eye diseases. The ResNet50 model achieved 98.9% validation accuracy, while the exception model achieved 98.4% accuracy. It enhances clinical decision-making for ophthalmologists, with applications in fundus digital photography and optical coherence tomography. Eye diseases can cause visual impairments and impact an individual quality of life. Early diagnosis is crucial for overall health. AI-based eye disease classification (EDC) can help, but the complexities of fundus images can affect performance. A deep-learning model was developed using denoising auto encoders, single-shot detection, and whale optimization algorithms. The model was demonstrated utilizing complicated fundus pictures, outperforming earlier models in the ocular disease intelligence recognition (ODIR) and EDC datasets. This model can be used by medical facilities to enhance patient care and detect a variety of eye conditions and conduct two experiments to understand the benefits and costs of visual inspection tasks in AI method. The participants asked to identify defective mold in a chocolate factory, and explainable artificial intelligence (XAI) highlighted the specific areas influenced by AI decisions. Its results demonstrated the benefits of XAI when the system accurately identified faults, but the costs of misplaced highlights were evident. Ophthalmologists must embrace intelligent algorithms and educate themselves on beneficial AI applications for their professional future because AI can correlate unique features and detect patterns particular to a given condition. Thus, AI and a combined algorithm utilized to predict eye disease forecasting.

METHODOLOGY

AI has analyzed the data in recent years to predict water demand and diagnose eye vision issues. Many studies have focused on analyzing models and algorithms for predicting water demand and assessing visual function data. Various techniques, such as baseline regression models, space-time models, and ML algorithms, are used to forecast household water needed. Decision trees, native Bayes, random forests (RF), and neural network algorithms are employed to predict eye visualization and functioning data. Each method is used to forecast test data after being trained on previous data. The relevant sections provide more information about the predictive models used. AI techniques for water resource management involve the planning of water infrastructure, optimizing resources, constructing efficient water systems, and establishing extensive distribution networks. Different algorithms are used to estimate each parameter, and challenges are addressed through a step-by-step process. However, these techniques do not consider the novel nature of the training data. Design challenges such as adapting and improving programming, learning, and exploring the process are also present. These challenges of the solution involve identifying the problem statement, implementing the algorithm, analyzing time and space complexity, and testing the algorithmic problems. The algorithm creator writes the algorithm while focusing on the application requirements and ensuring it fits the training data. The water resource management AI techniques method is shown in Figure 6.1. Decision trees offer a more complex and nuanced approach to modeling nonlinear relationships and interactions, but this can pose challenges in interpretability as the trees deepen. The prediction of eye diagnosis with the model algorithm method is shown in Figure 6.2. Validation is a crucial technique for assessing model performance by training and testing it on different datasets, reducing overfitting risk and accurately measuring predictive power. The performance of models in classification tasks was evaluated using a variety of metrics, such as accuracy, precision, recall, and F1-score (which ranges from 0 to 1). Regression tasks employ metrics including mean absolute error (MAE),

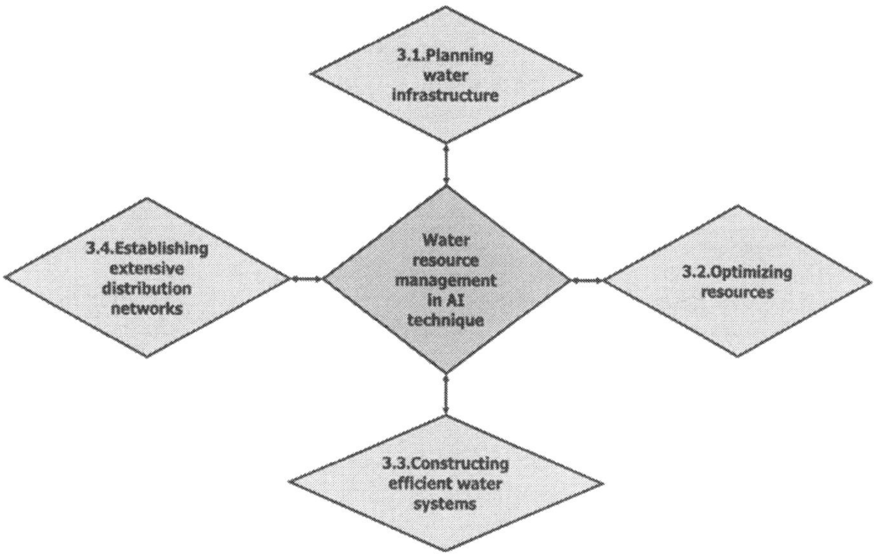

FIGURE 6.1 Water resource management in AI.

Source: Authors' conceptualization.

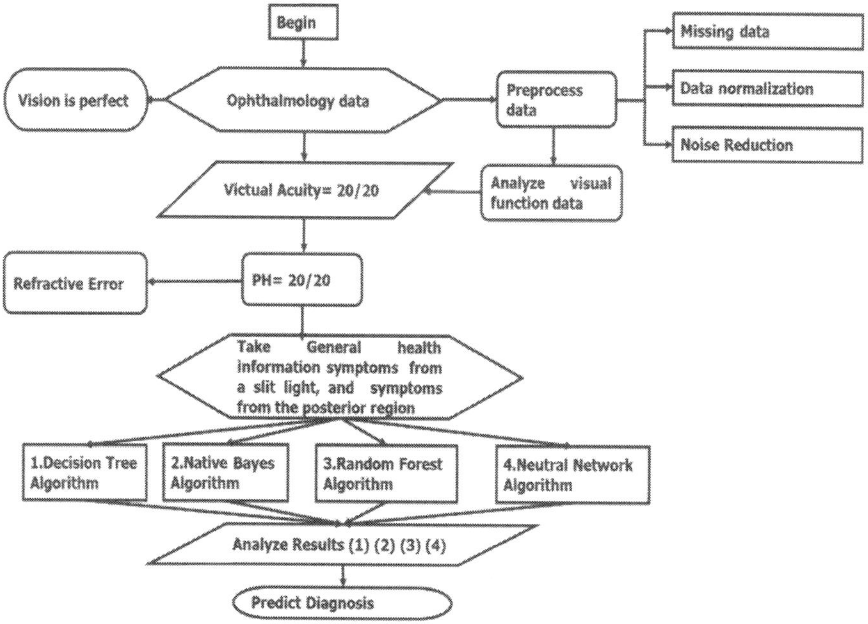

FIGURE 6.2 Procedure to predict eye diagnosis with model algorithm.

Source: Authors' conceptualization.

root mean square error (RMSE), and mean squared error (MSE). The decision tree is a type of model that discriminates between different classes, while Naive Bayes is a type of model that generates probabilities for different classes. Pruning decision trees may result in mistakes in the training data.

PLANNING WATER INFRASTRUCTURE

The planning frameworks for water infrastructure are crucial for the nation. The planning theory is constantly evolving. The impact of public and media perceptions, cost-sharing arrangements, and decision analysis affect the planning process (Furlong et al. 2016). While AI presents many advantages, its implementation for practical uses should take into account the various obstacles it presents, including those pertaining to data, model building, knowledge integration, and ethical considerations. AI systems face obstacles in adaptation, cost analysis, and lack of data. However, AI has the ability to revise the water and infrastructure sectors, addressing issues such as water resource management, climate change, and flood resilience. Fu et al. (2023) illustrate the obstacles to enhance AI acceptance in the real world from four perspectives: institutional governance, social-economic systems, cyber-physical infrastructure, and technology advancement in general society. Integrating AI into urban water infrastructure development can enhance resilience and sustainability, removing obstacles and promoting equitable and responsible deployment of AI-powered systems. Thus, AI has developed the following terms to predict the best water management system in infrastructure planning.

DETECTING POTENTIAL WATER SUPPLY FAILURES

Water supply failures can occur due to inadequate conditions caused by water shortages. Predictive maintenance solutions incorporate AI, Internet of Things (IoT), edge, and cloud computing algorithms to solve the issue. These techniques allow leaders to compare real-time data with historical data from similar systems. Neural networks can effectively minimize water losses and enhance maintenance planning. This approach applies to various urban settings and infrastructure networks, underscoring the crucial role of data analysis in preventing breakdowns and optimizing resource allocation within water utilities. The vulnerability-identifying method (VIM) enables solving variables such as failure rate, water chemical stability, and corrosion issues in water distribution systems (WDSs). Thus, the risk assessment is conducted using operational data, identifying hazards, their effects, and vulnerability.

ENHANCING WATER DISTRIBUTION NETWORKS

Water distribution networks (WDNs) transport the water from treatment facilities to people, and use data analysis to identify patterns. Utility leaders can utilize this tool to better understand and forecast water demand, thereby enhancing supply optimization and waste reduction. For the purpose to lessen the possible effects of disruptive occurrences, it evaluates the resilience of WDNs earlier. A unique hydraulic-based strategy called the hydraulically inspired complex network approach (HCNA) was developed for single-pipe failures (Hajibabaei et al. 2023). Additionally, it combined a three-step data assimilation method with multiobjective optimization to choose cost-efficient monitoring networks for WDSs.

ELEVATING WATER QUALITY MONITORING

Water quality monitoring (WQM) plays a role in protecting waterways from pollution. Monitoring water quality involves tracking factors such as temperature, dissolved oxygen, turbidity, and pollutants like bacteria, heavy metals, and pesticides. Observing these indicators allows research workers and environmental agencies to describe ability risks, track changes, and thoughtful evaluation to protect water resources. IoT and other technologies are utilized by utilities for data collection and analysis, requiring teams of data scientists to extract valuable insights. Many utilities prefer upskilling existing workers over hiring new tech talent. AI and ML have improved WQM systems, but they also bring challenges such as data security, scalability, and the need for interdisciplinary cooperation. System for the Integrated Monitoring of Insubric Lakes and their Ecosystem's (SIMILE) data was utilized to create a pre-filtering system for worldwide Volunteered Geographic Information (VGI) specifically for monitoring the water quality of lakes. The current state of WQM involves the analysis of ML and IoT wireless technologies. There are unresolved research issues related to combining ML and IoT wireless approaches for WQM. Thus, AI approaches are utilized to improve the monitoring of water quality.

IMPROVING THE ACCURACY OF FLOOD MITIGATION AND PREDICTION

AI methods were developed to reduce the risk of flooding, minimize flood hazards, relocate people from high-risk areas, set insurance rates, and oversee water and environmental resource management. Government officials can utilize digital twins, IoT, generative AI, and other AI-powered water management technologies to anticipate and address the challenges of floods. The insights obtained from these technologies can assist policymakers in making informed decisions regarding essential infrastructure resources to safeguard communities from the impacts of floods. These technologies can provide vital information to utility leaders, aiding in loss prevention. AI-based predictive models expect to enhance disaster mitigation systems by collecting real-time data on water levels and rainfall for continuous learning. Nine flood prediction models were created by the research using fuzzy logic, artificial neural networks (ANN), and adaptive neuro-fuzzy inference system (ANFIS) algorithms. Their models demonstrate the AI ability to forecast floods and offer practical methods for assessing the likelihood of flooding by Tabbussum et al. (2021).

ENERGY EFFICIENCY IN WASTEWATER TREATMENT

The wastewater treatment protects the environment and the health of both humans and animals. Digital twins are used to develop hypotheses about energy savings and run near-instant tests of these hypotheses using different variables. AI is a crucial tool in wastewater treatment, encompassing management, technology, economy, and wastewater reuse. It offers insights into possible future research areas that address complex practical applications, cost reduction, pollutant removal, and water reuse. Wastewater treatment can benefit from AI techniques. It can enhance the safety and effectiveness of a system. Further, people understand these systems to adapt to their ever-changing surroundings. It investigates into AI's potential benefits and drawbacks when applied to wastewater treatment. It suggests using AI to remediate wastewater might greatly improve accuracy and save a large amount of money. Thus, AI methods are utilized to improve energy efficiency in wastewater treatment.

Enhancing Climate Resilience and Adaptation

AI water management models analyze IoT data to evaluate climate risks and develop adaptive water supply strategies for government leaders. Climate adaptation reduces vulnerability to climate change impacts, safeguarding people and the environment. Climate change is a pressing global issue requiring innovative, data-driven solutions to address rising sea levels, temperatures, and extreme weather events. AI provides tools to analyze risks, identify vulnerable areas, and model of future climate scenarios, making it a valuable resource for addressing climate change. AI and digital technologies are beneficial for the execution of the sustainable development goals (SDGs) and Climate Change Adaptation Digital Twin (Climate DT) (Leal Filho et al. 2022). Adapting to a changing climate involves making adjustments to mitigate its effects. AI can help by analyzing data on climate change vulnerabilities and risks and providing recommendations for adaptation measures. It can enhance communities' ability to adapt and withstand the effects of changes in climate. The application of AI change of climate adaptation raises ethical questions and potential biases to address. The development and implementation of appropriate algorithms are crucial for ensuring solutions. The utilization of AI-ML necessitates the advancement of the field, the development of policies, and the guarantee of universal access. Thus, the AI approach enhances climate resilience and adaptation.

Enhanced Drought Prediction and Improved Water Distribution

The impacts of a drought are harmful to the environment, economy, health, and agriculture. It predicts temperature and precipitation accurately, as these are factors for drought prediction. Historical records show that the climate is inherently unstable. Predicting drought conditions is providing early warnings and managing drought. It explains various drought prediction techniques, including statistical, dynamic, and hybrid approaches. Statistical drought prediction entails analyzing the relationship between indicators of drought and possible predictors. Forecasting meteorological drought in real time necessitates the use of seasonal climate forecasts generated by general circulation models (GCMs) to influence hydrological models which are influenced by climate forcing and beginning circumstances. The gradient boosting algorithm (GBM) found soil moisture and precipitation significantly contribute to droughts. Anomalies in sea surface temperature and various hydro-meteorological factors contribute to droughts worldwide. Advanced approaches such as machine/

deep learning models have improved the accuracy of drought forecasts, showing superior performance than traditional models. The study combined climatic indicators, hydrological models, meteorological measurements, and remote sensing data to enhance forecasting accuracy.

SMART IRRIGATION SYSTEMS

Smart irrigation systems are crucial for plants to hold the exact amount of water, leading to significant water savings by preventing overwatering. In industrial farms, AI water management utilizes IoT irrigation systems to optimize water usage by combining crop data, weather forecasts, soil moisture, water tables, vegetation health, and sunlight patterns. It helps deliver precise water amounts when and where needed, reducing waste and maximizing crop yields. These intelligent machines are created by combining ML, AI, and the IoT. These smart irrigation systems are evaluated based on various factors, including soil and water management functions. Soil management factors include temperature, moisture, disease, and dryness, while water management factors include evapotranspiration, humidity, air temperature, and dew point temperature (Dharashive and Sawale 2024). AI-driven intelligent irrigation systems utilize sophisticated algorithms to monitor soil moisture levels, meteorological conditions, and the specific needs of plants. They play a role in reducing water wastage, addressing water scarcity, and ensuring optimal plant growth. Furthermore, these systems help to reduce energy consumption and the need for manual labor and excessive fertilizers, providing long-term cost savings and economic benefits. Effective monitoring of moisture, optimized water usage, increased production, and efficient approaches are essential in modern farming methods that utilize AI and the IoT through smart irrigation systems in agriculture.

Optimizing Resources

Optimizing these processes improves water availability, cost-effectiveness, and environmental sustainability, playing a role in ensuring efficient and sustainable water use. Various models are used to optimize water usage.

Baseline Regression Models

Baseline models serve two purposes. Firstly, it establishes a performance standard against which improvements are assessed. Secondly, it gives a benchmark to complex models for its effectiveness evaluation. Essentially, baseline models offer a minimum expected level of performance.

Linear Mixed-Model Effects

It establishes a foundation for using more advanced techniques to examine the effectiveness of ML methods when considering both temporal and spatial factors. In a polder-style agricultural watershed, the linear mixed effects (LME) theory analyzes the fluctuations in groundwater quality. The data was collected from 2009 to 2017 to assess changes in nitrate and salinity levels across four polders covering 5,000 hectares of agricultural land, including various water bodies, as documented by Romić et al. (2020). Linear mixed models were employed in Southeast Australia to forecast the amounts of total phosphorus & nitrogen in two basins. The study demonstrated substituting turbidity for stream discharge resulted in a minimum 15% enhancement in estimation accuracy. Incorporating turbidity measurements led to predictions more precise during base flow and in catchments experiencing extended periods of base flow and brief rainfall events. **Thus, the** analyzed residential water consumption (WC) in Italian provinces from 2007 to 2009 used a linear mixed-effects model. It was discovered that per capita income affected the water usage, but temperature had no appreciable impact. Precipitation and altitude are identified as significant factors affecting water demand. The LME model in longitudinal studies examines causal variables associated with human health and disease. It assesses the reliability and appropriateness of ANOVA and LME model parameterizations, highlighting differences in growth patterns between well-nourished and malnourished subjects.

The monthly mean model expanded to match each household individually and forecasts future water usage and a random effects model can reduce parameters and overfitting. The water sample underwent data collection and analysis for six main parameters (BOD, DO, NH_4, NO_3, TSS, and TDS) in 2018, 2019, and 2020. It identified drains in need of treatment due to poor water quality. A statistical model was developed using IoT for analyzing the water quality of the Krishna River. Numerous indicators of water quality are examined in the study, including conductivity, pH, temperature, dissolved oxygen, total dissolved solids, biochemical oxygen demand, and conductivity. The acquired data was subjected to one-way and two-way ANOVA analysis. The results indicated one-way ANOVA was better efficient in analyzing water standard.

One-way ANOVA model is expressed by the following term

$$y_{i,j} = \alpha_{m(j)} + \epsilon_{i,j} \tag{6.1}$$

Where $y_{i,j}$ is household (i) using total water during the month of j, $\alpha_{m(j)}$ fixed population mean value for month of m and $\epsilon_{i,j}$, Gaussian white noise process.

Two-way ANOVA model for household-month interaction is expressed by the following term

$$y_{i,j} = \alpha_{m(j)} + \gamma_{i,m(j)} + \epsilon_{i,j} \tag{6.2}$$

$\gamma_{i,m(j)}$ is household-specific effect on the months. It is zero for identify ability. However the independent multivariate normal household-specific random effects $(\gamma_{i,(1)},\ldots\gamma_{i,(12)})$ has grand month deviation $(\alpha_{(1)}\ldots\ldots\alpha_{(12)})$.

Linear Regression

This model is a benchmark for comparing and forecasting water demand, predicting monthly usage and enhancing forecast performance through two-way interactions. The water networks and scarcity are complex and influenced by various factors. A regression model estimates WC in the country, revealing correlations between water usage per person and temperature between per capita water usage and population density. It used curve fitting and linear regression analysis to estimate China's 2025

WC, categorizing it into industrial, agricultural, domestic, and ecological needs (Huang and Yin 2014). The peak water needs for 2025–2050 were estimated using the general multiple linear regression (GMLR) model. Water's impact on urban areas affects supply, drainage, waste treatment, and public health. Managing urban water demand is challenging. Multiple linear regression assesses the impact of socioeconomic and climatic factors on household WC. Convolutional neural network (CNN) and multiple regression models consider input variables like rainfall, temperature, humidity, and wind speed from previous days to predict future weather conditions. The original water demand data's noise reduced at the beginning of the research study, allowing for smoother predictions during the calibration period. The model can be written by the following terms.

$$y_{i,j} = x_{i,j}^{T}\beta + \epsilon_{i,j} \tag{6.3}$$

$x_{i,j}$ is two-way interaction for i is household water usage and j is month. β Regression coefficients

$$\hat{y}_{i,j} = X_{i,j}^{T}\hat{\beta} \tag{6.4}$$

$\hat{\beta}$ for β forecasts for time point.

Space-time models

The Gaussian displacement spatial-temporal rainfall model (GDSTM) simplifies space-time precipitation modeling by describing rainfall cells and their motion, assuming uniform rainfall intensity in a sequence of storms. The GP-kriging model provides the satisfactory results. China's rapid economic development highlights the need for water environment carrying capacity (WECC) for sustainable human society. An integrated model reveals control units in 2010–2025 have worse water environments, guiding industry and population patterns. The World Economic Forum predicts a water shortage and increased demand in the next two decades, with utility firms increasingly using water resource management and technology for better decision-making. It includes constructing models to undertake monthly urban water demand projections and using the R programming language for automation. The seasonal autoregressive integrate and moving average (ARIMA) technique performs well in predicting water usage. The ARIMA and transfer function ARIMA (TFARIMA) models have shown color, turbidity, and total iron are the most reliable water quality. It suggests using an AR term for each drinking water supply system (DWSS) component. The models found historical observations and impact on turbidity behaviors in the water treatment plant (WTP), and it became more sensitive to outlier detection of the ARIMA analysis increased. Moreover, according to TFARIMA models, previous river turbidity events have minimal impact on the reservoir's turbidity. Cities have utilized IoT technology to gather real-time data and optimize their WDSs to create an efficient infrastructure design. In addition, numerous researchers have utilized auto-regressive integrated moving average (ARIMA) techniques to examine past data and predict WC demand, as shown by Subha and Kowsigan (2023). Water availability significantly influences the environment and society's development. Predicting WC is crucial for optimizing regional water supplies. Future WC projections are more accurate and less prone to error when the autoregressive integrated moving average technique and the Markov chain error correction are combined with real-world water usage data.

The AR (1) model, with a one-month lag, is regressed as calculated using the following term.

$$(y_{i,j} - \mu_{i,j}) = \rho_i (y_{i,j-1} - \mu_{i,j-1}) + \epsilon_{i,j} \tag{6.5}$$

$\mu_{i,j}$ is mean function of covariates, ρ_i autoregressive coefficient $\epsilon_{i,j}$ is Gaussian white noise.

The AR (1) model is augmented by household-specific interception and an autoregressive coefficient to enhance accuracy, while the standard model is included into the autoregressive integrated moving average model for data analysis. The ARIMA approach has been used for selecting household-specific autoregressive, differentiation, and moving average characteristics and their related coefficients depends on the Alkaike information criterion (AIC). The ARIMA model is written by the following terms.

$$\left(1 - \sum_{K=1}^{P} \alpha_K L^K\right)(1-L)^d Z_{i,j} = \left(1 - \sum_{K=1}^{q} \beta_K L^K\right)\epsilon_{i,j} \tag{6.6}$$

where d is the differencing order, $Z_{i,j} = (y_{i,j} - \mu_{i,j})$, L is the lag operator, $L^K Z_{i,j} = Z_{i,j-k}$, α_K is the autoregressive coefficients at p, β_K is the moving average coefficients at q. The ARIMA model's more details are listed below.

Spatial-Temporal Gaussian Process Regression Models

The Spatio-temporal Gaussian process regression (ST-GPR) is a time-series model used to assess the level of risk factor prolonged exposure in the worldwide burden of disease project and address probabilistic numerical optimization in water management systems. The consumption of water resources is a significant issue in many countries around the world. This section examines data from 2000 to 2015 to pinpoint the main reasons for this increase in water usage. The findings will encompass the impact of expanding urban populations on household WC, the regional differences in the influence of industrial development, and the factors that steer the agricultural sector in specific regions. The national index on water used for irrigation consumption rose from 0.501 in 2010 to 0.542 in 2016. Small irrigation areas had higher water utilization coefficients than larger ones. There were regional differences, with the northern and eastern regions exhibiting water use coefficients than the southern and western regions. Over time, the spatial spillover effect decreased and varied significantly for pure-well irrigation areas (Li, Jiang, and Duan 2020).Water demand correlations reveal unobserved factors, enhancing predictions. Spatio-temporal models, although computationally expensive, can be feasible for large datasets.

$$\eta_S \eta_T \times \eta_S \eta_T \tag{6.7}$$

Generalized Additive Models (GAM)

It is a statistical tool for analyzing complex relationships within a dataset. It assumes the predictors add up to the response variable and the dependent variable keep a normal distribution. The forecast for a particular application includes three characteristics (cloud amount, ceiling height, and visibility) for eight checkpoints and two lead times (12 and 24 hours). The collection data was generated by a computational model and surface observations collected between 1984 and 1989. Analysis of data collected between 1990 and 1992 demonstrates the generalized additive model (GAM) model regularly beats linear regression. This is evident from the decreased mean square errors and lead-time gains of 2 to 9 hours. Furthermore, a generalized additive model was employed to examine the influence of weather, soil, and hydrogeological factors on the failure of five commonly used pipe materials. High temperatures are linked to the pipe failure rates, which is used to assist in the implementation of effective network management strategies to minimize asset leakage through suitable interventions. This approach utilizes a generalized additive framework with predictors consist of the hour of the day, week, and year. It improves forecast accuracy using the autoregressive model. The most accurate version had a mean average percentage error of 3.3% and a RMSE of 0.84 MW. The model development process involved a GAM to represent nonlinear seasonal changes, incorporating hydrologic variability and interventions to account for method or laboratory changes affect the data. It allows for the rigorous statistical evaluation of water quality data, and it can be applied to different systems, locations, and variables, providing annual updates and insights into management and research questions. The proposed GAM model has good performance than back propagation neural networks (BPNN) and general regression neural networks (GRNN) based models. The accuracy rates for predicting internal corrosion progression are 94.8% and 95.7% for BPNN and GRNN models, respectively.

$$E_y = \beta_o + \sum_{j=1}^{J} f_j(x_j) \tag{6.8}$$

$$f_j(x) = \sum_{k=1}^{K_j} u_{jk}\phi_{jk}(x) \tag{6.9}$$

A univariate temporal smooth and a bivariate spatial smooth combined to generate the structure.

$$f_{ST}(s,t) = \sum_{K=1}^{K_S} u_{SK}\phi_{SK}(S) + \sum_{K=1}^{K_T} u_{TI}\phi_{TI}(t) + \sum_{K=1}^{K_S}\sum_{K=1}^{K_S} u_{ST,KI}\phi_{SK}(S)\phi_{TI}(t) \tag{6.10}$$

Machine Learning Algorithms

In recent studies, models compared with ML methods do not have a spatiotemporal dependency on temporal and spatiotemporal models. The selected ML algorithms include gradient boosting machines (GBM), RF, and Bayesian additive regression trees (BART), are constructed using the basic decision trees model. The water demand prediction model, established using statistics and ML techniques, outperformed other models in Beijing, with R^2 values of 97.9% and 97.8%. It revealed the ML models outperformed statistical models in predictive performance through further comparisons. Forecasting population and water demand are the two key components of an urban water management system. ML is one of the most well-known way for making such predictions. A comparison was made between five models to determine the best predictor for daily water use: polynomial regression (PR), nonlinear autoregressive (NAR), support vector regression (SVR), multilayer perceptron (MLP), and long short-term memory (LSTM). The performance of the system was assessed by calculating the RMSE between the forecasted values and the actual values. Historical measurements were used to estimate the data for a period of five days. NAR demonstrated a forecasting accuracy of approximately 5 and 23 $Lday^{-1}$ for in-home and industrial installations respectively.

Gradient Boosting Machines (GBM)

This methodology commonly employed in conjunction with decision trees as the underlying learners. A decision tree is fitted to pseudo-residuals at each step, partitioning the input space into disjoint regions and predicting a constant value in each step. The section discusses using a GBM to estimate water need 1–7 days ahead. It mentions the group size and prediction accuracy declines when the mean absolute percentage error (MAPE) enhances from 3.2% to 17%. It explains an adding explanatory variable can reduce MAPE up to 20% for smaller groups, but the improvement is less for larger aggregations. Gradient boosting ML techniques used various ML models and datasets to predict urban monthly water demand. It found including calendar and meteorological data improved prediction accuracy. Nevertheless, the decision to increase the training data from 70% to 90% resulted in elevated errors in certain models (Li, Jiang, and Duan 2020). Consequently, it is suggested to adopt a proactive diagnostic method for diabetes mellitus in regions with limited availability of medical experts. The hospital data has created a precise diabetes diagnosis model using a light gradient boosting machine (LGBM). The approach demonstrated superior performance compared to previous methods, achieving an area under the receiver operating characteristic (AUC) of 98.1%, a sensitivity of 98.1%, a specificity of 99.9%, and an accuracy of 96.3%.

$$h_m(x) = \sum_{j=1}^{J_m} b_{jm} 1R_{jm}(x) \tag{6.11}$$

J is the number of terminal nodes in trees, which regulates the maximum level of interaction between variables in the model. The minimize loss function,

$$F_m(x) = F_{m-1}(x) + \gamma_m h_m(x) \tag{6.12}$$

$$\gamma_m = \arg\min \sum_{i=1}^{n} L(y_i, F_{m-1}(x_i) + \gamma h_m(x_i)) \tag{6.13}$$

Random Forest

This model is a popular and successful machine-learning technique that efficiently addresses classification and regression problems. It uses ensemble learning by combining multiple decision trees. The algorithm operates in two levels: it builds multiple decision trees using random subsets of the training data, and then it aggregates the predictions of these trees to make final predictions. Human activities impact ecosystems, and understanding this impact is crucial for finding solutions. The complexity of ecosystems requires advanced statistical techniques. The RF algorithm is used to study the factors affecting biological elements in water quality(Szomolányi and Clement 2023). A comparison of the performance of multiple random forests (MRF) with other models, such as the forward feed neural network (FFNN) and random forests regression (RFR) models, demonstrated the MRF model exhibited superior predictive accuracy. The MRF model is known for its ability to learn features through decision trees and efficient feature extraction across many scales. Supervised ML algorithms like RF have become increasingly popular in applications related to water resources. These models utilized to predict daily water quality and hydro-meteorological data to predict turbidity, conductivity, and dissolved oxygen in watersheds, revealing land cover significantly affects these predictions. The RF model forecasts surface water quality and determines the best water quality for drinking. Seasonal testing was done on several quality parameters over ten years, including pH, total dissolved solids, coliforms, iron, and fluoride, among others (Jena et al. 2023). It implies the capacity to forecast water losses based on easily accessible covariates enhanced by using RF approach. The changing climate and growing population of a nation affect crop productivity. Estimating crop yields is difficult, so the agriculture industry has resorted to ML methods, with RF being extensively used for crop production estimation. Water usage is effectively managed by tracking and utilizing smart technology.

$$\hat{f} = \frac{1}{B}\sum_{b=1}^{B} f_b(x') \tag{6.14}$$

The prediction uncertainty is calculated by the standard deviation. Individual regression trees are calculated by x′.

$$\sigma = \sqrt{\frac{\sum_{b-1}^{B}\left(f_b x' - \hat{f}\right)^2}{B-1}} \tag{6.15}$$

Bayesian Additive Regression Trees (BART)

This model helps to avoid strong parametric assumptions when fitting the variety of regression models. The purpose of this assessment is to make predictions about global and diffuse solar radiation. This is done by analyzing long-term meteorological data collected from four sites located in both arid and humid regions. It exhibits a multitude of input combinations and demonstrates superior effectiveness in forecasting global solar radiation. When incorporating input combinations of sunshine duration (experimental, theoretical), solar radiation (extraterrestrial, global), and day of the year, the prediction of diffuse solar radiation is more accurate. This approach demonstrated performance and coverage probability at monitoring locations, making it an interesting method for modeling ambient air pollution levels but introducing uncertainty in health impact and effect analyses. This section offers a comprehensive explanation of BART, utilizing the commonly employed ML prediction and the General BART model. The General BART model integrates recent advancements such as semiparametric models and associated outcomes (Tan and Roy 2019). The Bayesian CART model is crucial for estimating disease risk spatial distribution, aiding disease prevention and control monitoring and assessment.

Constructing Efficient Water Systems

The energy crisis and increasing municipal solid waste production are significant challenges for urbanization and sustainable development objectives. The framework utilizes AI approaches such as random trees; RF, ANN, and adaptive network to optimize waste management and supply of energy in green buildings. Environmental Protection Agency Network Evaluation Tool (EPANET) is a widely used software application for modeling effective WDSs, allowing for analysis of drinking water constituents. The high-order harmonic generation (HHG) model combines the Grey Wolf Optimizer and Harris Hawk with an EPANET hydraulic simulator to efficiently minimize the design expenses of the WDS. Its performance demonstrated in three typical systems, proving to be a more reliable, cost-effective, and faster solution than conventional methods. The water sector applications focus on modeling, prediction, decision support, and optimization, suggesting the development of data scientists to complement social sciences and humanities. It highlights the importance of many-objective optimization, theory-guided data science, and participatory decision-making in the water sector. The Intelligent Forecasters Construction Set (IFCS) was employed to create a water demand of prediction system using actual data from WDS and environment. It decreases the highest amount of kilowatts needed at any given time, resulting in lower expenses for operating water plants. The IFCS facilitates the use of numerous predictor models, enabling more efficient data modeling. The performance of this software superior compared to linear regression and case-based reasoning (CBR) tools, emphasizing its advantages. The study assesses the efficacy of five AI techniques in forecasting daily stream flow patterns to ensure long-term management of water resources, highlighting the need of choosing appropriate predictive models. The models excel in managing such data due to their precision, resilience, dependability, cost-efficiency, decision-making aptitude, efficiency, and effectiveness. Over the past 20 years, this implementation has focused on simulating the quality of river water (WQ). It has emphasized the necessity of further research on AI models to tackle issues such as missing data, integrating features, comparing models, and developing automated early warning systems. These techniques reduce modeling effort and improve decision-making. The framework includes an intelligent user interface, semantic metadata for models, and semantic representations of datasets. The MINT (Model INTegration) architecture is used to create this system, which consists of data and models for analyzing the relationships between systems are natural and human. The framework reduces modeling effort, ensures model relevance, and automates data selection and transformations. It demonstrates the utility of AI techniques in accelerating modeling and identifying challenges for future work, and many studies emphasize AI, machine/deep learning in the construction industry 4.0 to develop efficient systems. Thus, the recent modification of software tools helps to collect data strategies, challenges, and future trends in these domains.

Establishing Extensive Water Distribution Networks

The increasing demand for drinking water necessitates efficient WDNs using advanced hydraulic modeling software. Public and commercial software for WDSs, including EPANET, Branch, and Loop, differ in functionality, compatibility, GUIs, algorithms, languages, and programs. The choice of software depends on data availability, time, financial implications, resources, applicability, and project scope. WDSs require the consideration of various elements, including the intricacy of the hydraulic simulation model, the decision space, and the output locations. It is used in Wallan, Victoria, Australia, and presents four different metamodeling scenarios and shows a 21% decrease in the average daily expenses for pumping and a 14% savings in net present value (NPV) over 25 years. The optimized method also accomplishes enough disinfection throughout the whole system, in contrast to the contemporary operating system. The development of a novel framework for the strategic planning of distribution systems for water is founded on the utilization of multicriteria decision analysis (MCDA). The framework assesses adaptable solutions based on many factors, such as investment expenses, carbon emissions, resilience, and dependability. The Preference Ranking Organization Method for Enrichment of Evaluations (PROMETHEE) and the Technique for Order of Preference by Similarity to Ideal Solution (TOPSIS) are two MCDA methodologies framework uses to perform an extensive research. WDSs are crucial for societal prosperity and safety. However, limited resources make asset management strategies difficult. Recently, utility companies have transitioned from a condition-based approach to a service-based one, focusing on system performance. It explores the management of buried pipelines in water and WDS, focusing on failure prediction models, maintenance planning strategies, and renewal techniques, it utilizes complex network theory to examine WDNs from a topological standpoint, focusing on their behavior, properties, and relationships. It explores water loss components in distribution networks, analyzing methods and their impact on reduction approaches, with lower accuracy resulting in lower uncertainty and higher uncertainties (AL-Washali et al. 2020). Despite extensive literature, optimization techniques in WDN design are not widely accepted due to lack of suitable packaging and comprehensive reliability measures. Future research should focus on developing decision support systems.

Ophthalmology Database

Ophthalmology is a medical specialty diagnosis and treats eye disorders using advanced imaging techniques like optical coherence tomography (OCT), fundus photography, auto fluorescence, and confocal microscopy. The Organization for Rare Diseases India (ORDI) use three criteria to categorize rare diseases: the overall number of individuals impacted by the condition, the prevalence of the sickness, and the absence of an available treatment. The World Health Organization (WHO) defines rare diseases as those affect less than 6.5–10 cases per 10,000 people. However, according to ORDI, a disease is considered rare if it affects 1 in 5,000 individuals or fewer. Uncommon ocular conditions provide a substantial public health risk, as they contribute to visual impairment and blindness, which are serious public health challenges. Nowadays, there are a limited number of medical registers dedicated to ophthalmology on a global scale. The Women Ophthalmologists Society (WOS) in India acknowledges the significance of creating registries for uncommon eye illnesses and the beneficial influence they can have on patients' well-being. The primary objective of the rare eye disease (RED) group is to establish a nationwide register for uncommon eye disorders and uncommon manifestations of common eye ailments in India. This registry will serve as a unified platform for ophthalmologists to document and report cases.

Real-world data, collected from sources like surveys and medical notes, offers insights into people's experiences beyond clinical trial data. In ophthalmology, this data is increasing as digitized systems and tools become more accessible. It helps healthcare professionals, scientists, health systems, organizations, and pharmaceutical companies make better treatment decisions, shape treatment guidelines, and assess safety. For researchers like Roche, real-world data can increase research efficiency, identify unmet needs, and identify potential benefits for different conditions. It has also supported innovation in ophthalmology, such as anti-vascular endothelial growth factor (VEGF) treatments that require frequent dosing schedules.

DECISION TREES FOR EYE DISEASES DIAGNOSIS

Decision trees are essential tools in fields like engineering, civil planning, law, and business, categorized into categorical and continuous variable decision trees. A research investigation carried out to develop and verify a decision tree model (DTM) can accurately predict the mental health condition of Korean caregivers of kids with glaucoma. The study encompassed caregivers of children diagnosed with primary adolescent glaucoma, secondary adolescent glaucoma, and glaucoma suspects. Participants completed questionnaires, and the DTM analysis utilize to differentiate between moderate-to-severe depressive and anxiety symptoms. It found that glaucoma operations and visual acuity in the better eye are significant predictors of mental health concerns in caregivers of kids with glaucoma. Physicians rely on a subconscious and automatic decision-making process involves the selection and elimination of choices, especially with experience. Decision trees aid in color identification and partial color-coding for surgical treatments and pharmaceutical treatments. Additionally, a decision tree algorithm based on the web was developed to collect patient information on ophthalmic concerns, and provide a provisional diagnosis and post-hoc analysis.

NAIVE BAYES ALGORITHM FOR PREDICTION OF EYE PROBLEMS

The Bayes theory is a statistical method that uses two probabilities to determine the likelihood of a hypothesis (H) from a set of evidence (E). The Naive Bayes Algorithm is a probabilistic classifier that learns object probability, features, and group affiliation. It is primarily used in supervised learning to solve classification problems. ML algorithms predict the progression of open-angle glaucoma (POAG) using clinical observations and measurements from the Countess of Chester Hospital. Various classification difficulties are tackled by utilizing characteristics such as visual field index (VFI), mean deviation (MD), and retinal nerve fiber layer (RNFL). The best results, with over 90% accuracy, were obtained with MLP and RF algorithms. Thus, the decision tree algorithms provided insight into classification logic. ML techniques for real-time datasets identify eye problems, symptoms, and populations in the IT sector. They accurately forecast outcomes and improve health outcomes for IT employees. An expert system uses CBR and Naïve Bayes to predict and diagnose eye diseases and recommend the best treatment. The system has achieved an 82% accuracy rate, showing potential for use, although further improvements are still needed.

An automated method using Naive Bayes and Gabor filters on digital fundus images classifies patients into normal and glaucoma groups, reducing the need for early detection and treatment (Kumar Singhal et al. 2008). An international standard diagnostic data system developed for diagnosing eye diseases such as cataracts, glaucoma, and retinal conditions. The decision tree algorithms use to ensure accurate data entry and improve its performance through self-learning. It has a prediction rate of over 90%, surpassing more complex methods, like neural networks and Naïve Bayes. A decision tree is provided in the flow chart for inherited retinal disorders in Figure 6.3.

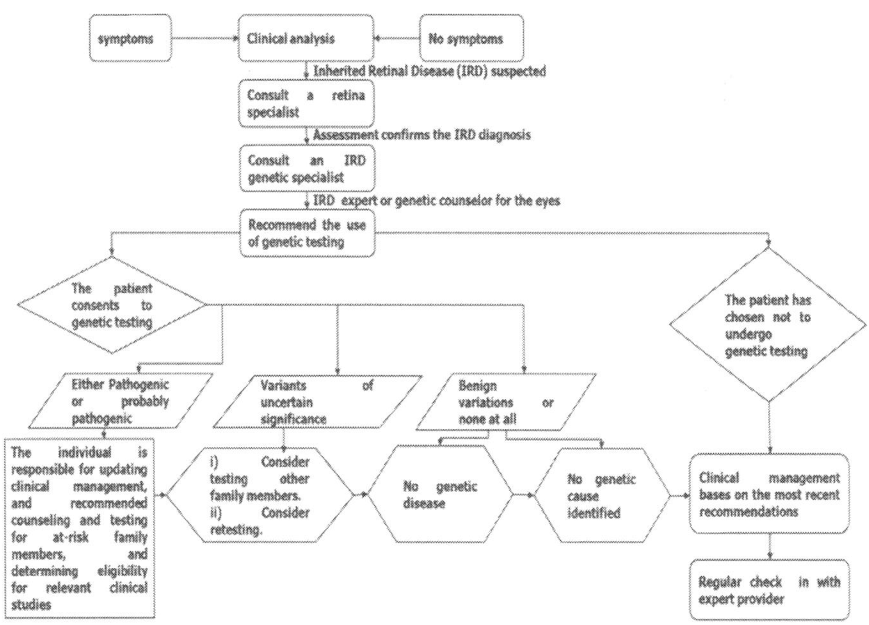

FIGURE 6.3 Decision-tree for inherited retinal disorders.

Source: Authors' conceptualization.

Two probabilities are used to predict an enhancement of performance. It is followed by the following term:

$$q\left(\frac{H}{E}\right)=q\left(\frac{E}{H}\right)\times\frac{q(H)}{q(E)} \tag{6.16}$$

RANDOM FOREST ALGORITHM FOR PREDICTION OF EYE PROBLEMS

A widely used machine-learning algorithm incorporates the outputs of decision trees to produce a single result in RF algorithm. It is simple to navigate nature, and adaptability makes it very suitable for classification and regression applications. This method is capable of processing intricate datasets and reducing overfitting, making it a desirable tool for prediction jobs. By introducing randomness to the model, RF creates a wide diversity and improves performance. A study conducted at Beijing Tong Ren Hospital analyzed data from 243 individuals diagnosed with glaucoma (GO) using a RF model to forecast the activity of GO. The parameters considered in the study were sex, age, smoking history, and previous radioactive 1131 treatment, presence of thyroid nodules, thyromegaly, and thyroid-stimulating hormone receptor antibodies. The model demonstrated superior sensitivity, specificity, positive predictive value, negative predictive value, F1 score, and out-of-bag error compared to previous models(Wang et al. 2023). Glaucoma affecting the optic nerve, resulting in permanent visual impairment in individuals with diabetes. In developing countries, the need for eye disease detection in automation systems increases due to the scarcity of ophthalmic experts and lab facilities. It classifies the image as normal or abnormal, with the Edge histogram filter achieving the highest accuracy of 80.43% and AUC 0.884. Diabetes is a prevalent disease, leading to long-term diabetic retinal diseases without any signs. Early detection is crucial for treatment. The final model achieved an accuracy of 0.99 in training and 0.95 in testing, demonstrating significant sensitivity, specificity, and precision. The system detects individuals with age-related macular degeneration (AMD) or diabetic macular edema (DME) by analyzing retinal characteristics extracted from spectral domain optical coherence tomography (SD-OCT) pictures. It extracts ten clinically retinal features, and uses Random Forrest classification methods on 251 subjects and achieved an accuracy of over 95.2% on each data set and 96% when trained as a two-class problem.

NEUTRAL NETWORK ALGORITHM FOR PREDICTION OF EYE PROBLEMS

Neural networks enable computers to autonomously make intelligent judgments by acquiring knowledge and representing intricate, nonlinear connections input and output data. These networks are classified by characteristics such as density, layers, structure, and data flow. A special sort of CNN is designed for the purpose of image detection and processing. CNNs are composed of a convolutional layer, pooling layer, and input and output layers. They could utilize filters to detect spatial and temporal dependencies. It finds use in diverse fields such as image and video identification, picture grouping, medical image analysis, and segmentation. The World Health Organization reports around 2,200 million people worldwide suffer from visual impairments due to age-related eye conditions like AMD, cataracts, diabetic retinopathy (DR), and glaucoma. It detects various diseases in their early stages by analyzing retinal fundus images from an online dataset. This is achieved by creating a model for multiple disease identification using CNNs. It was tested on the ODIR dataset and achieved the best precision, accuracy, specificity, and F1 score. It can aid in automatic disease detection, providing valuable assistance to medical professionals (Glaret subin and Muthukannan 2022). Another application of neural network-based algorithms is in detecting fatigue and drowsiness in driving support systems, such as car navigation systems. The algorithm uses Gabor filters and supports vector machines to classify images based on eye features The segmentation of the face is performed using the l×a×b color space, while the detection of the eyes is achieved using the hue, saturation, value (HSV) color space and a neural network methodology. When tested on nearly 100 images under different conditions, the algorithm demonstrated a success rate of 98%. In addition, the EYENET model utilizes deep CNNs to promptly identify eye problems. The system accurately predicts five eye conditions, namely exophthalmos, strabismus, cataracts, glaucoma, and uveitis. The model's architecture is optimized using the Adam optimizer, reduces doctor workload enables quick disease identification, and is easy to use, ultimately reducing blindness and suffering.

RESULTS AND DISCUSSION

AI meets the challenges of transforming medical diagnosis, water demand forecasting, and ophthalmology by providing intelligent solutions for conservation and efficient resource utilization, addressing global challenges such as water scarcity and reducing costs for water providers. Water demand forecasting reduces water supply costs by enabling water providers to manage operations efficiently. It's essential to consider linear and nonlinear models for time-series forecasting, as linear models can only recognize linear patterns. AI algorithms utilize historical data, weather patterns, and usage trends to forecast future water demand, thereby transforming water management through the provision of conservation and effective resource utilization solutions. AI algorithms using deep learning have demonstrated comparable diagnostic performance in detecting OCT and surpassing human graders. AI is employed in the treatment of retinopathy caused by diabetes, retinopathy of prematurity, and macular degeneration caused by age. This research presents case studies on different models' forecasts of water demand and types of diseases in eye.

COMPARISON OF PERFORMANCE METRICS IN MODEL

Performance metrics measure a model's behavior, activities, and performance within a given range, serving as a basis for achieving overall model goals. The RMSE is a crucial metric that measures the average discrepancy between projected and actual data. The MAE calculates the average difference between projected and actual values, while R-squared evaluates the model's fit to the data. The GPR model surpasses

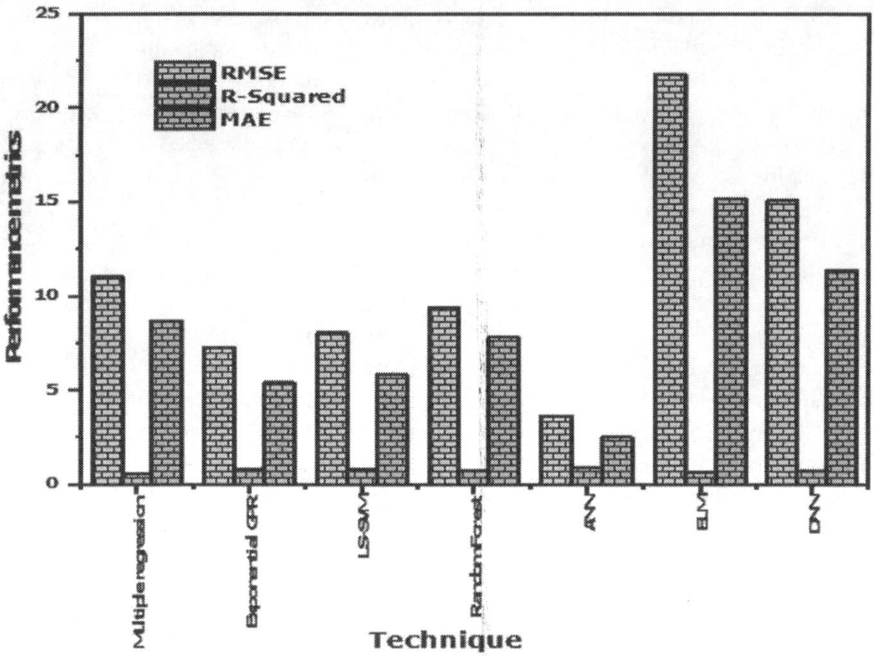

FIGURE 6.4 Performance metrics.

Source: Authors' conceptualization.

the ANN model because of its nonparametric assumptions. Additionally, the GPR model demonstrates the second highest level of performance, as illustrated in Figure 6.4. The extreme learning machines (ELM) and deep neural networks (DNN) techniques have exhibited suboptimal performance in a dataset due to their limited ability to learn in a single step and the intricate relationships from input to output variables. The utilization of deep neural networks' weighting may have led to a decrease in performance compared to ANN. Both strategies have high MSE values, although the consideration of time or space complexity may be a determining factor. It can be observed in Figure 6.5.

Model computation time is crucial for IoT systems, as real-time decision-making and identifying system anomalies require faster performance in forecasting models. As shown in Figure 6.6, the multiple regression requires the least amount of computing time, followed by least square support vector machine (LSSVM) and RF. DNN takes the most computation due to hidden layers, while ELM takes less time due to minimal computation.

The Performance Comparison of an AI Model and Clinical Specialists in Detecting AMD Progression

The AI-based telemedicine tool diagnoses and treats AMD using preprocessed OCT imaging data. It achieves similar detection accuracy to retinal specialists, with

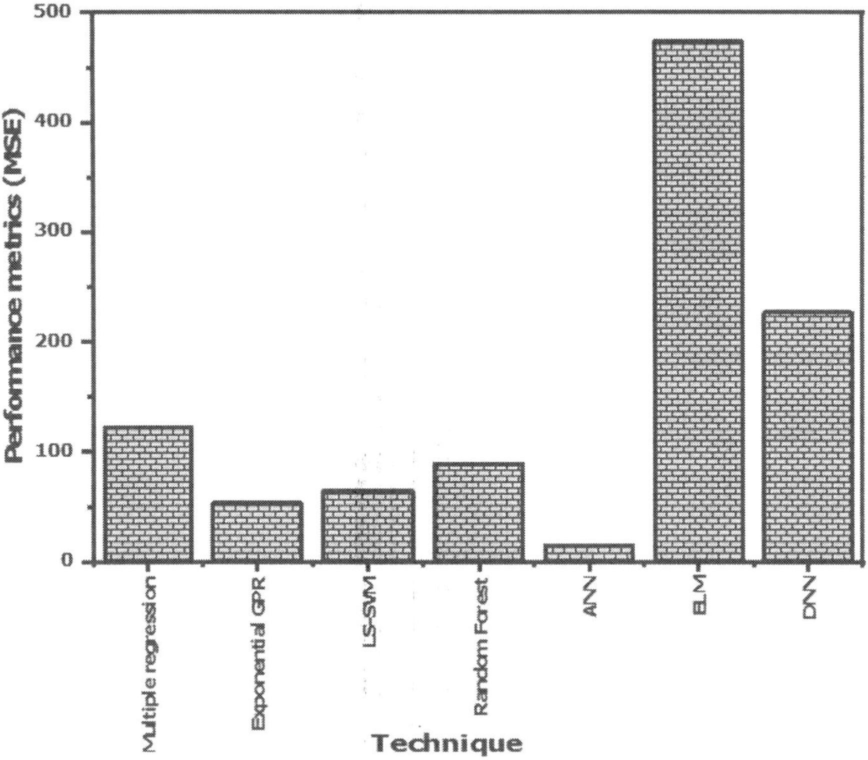

FIGURE 6.5 Performance metrics of MSE.

Source: Authors' conceptualization.

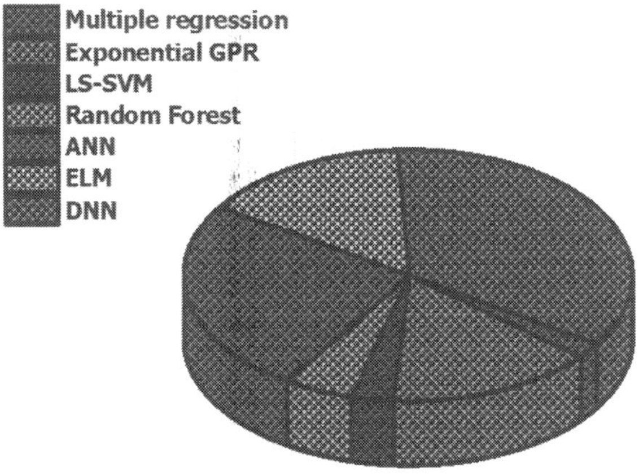

FIGURE 6.6 Percentage of computation time.

Source: Authors' conceptualization.

higher detection accuracy than medical students and equal to retinal specialists. The AI model, ResNet50, was found to detect AMD type changes in OCT images from the same patient, with similar or better accuracy than four clinical reviewers. It was compared to 18 AMD cases over ten consecutive checkups, with experienced reviewers having similar prediction accuracy scores. Less experienced reviewers demonstrated significantly lower prediction accuracy, clustering separately from the AI model. It showed similar prediction efficiency compared to reviewers within different time series lengths, with a steady decrease in accuracy with increasing series length (Hwang et al. 2019). AMD, affecting over 20% of the global population, is influenced by factors such as cigarette smoking, nutritional deficiencies, cardiovascular diseases, and genetic predisposition. Diagnosis involves clinical examination, investigations, and dietary anti-oxidant supplementation. Treatment involves intraocular injections of anti-VEGF agents, with ranibizumab and bevacizumab being commonly used. Future treatments may include inhibiting other angiogenic factors and regenerative therapies.

A new machine-learning algorithm has been developed to predict retinal sensitivity in eyes affected by neovascular age-related macular degeneration (nAMD). This method employs comprehensive psychophysical assessment and multimodal retinal imaging data to achieve accurate predictions. The accuracy is determined using patient-wise leave-one-out cross-validation, with the thickness of the outer nuclear layer being the most important predictive factor. AI is being employed to forecast the results of psychophysical tests using multimodal imaging data in the domain of AMD. The use of inferred best-corrected visual acuity (BCVA) can provide an estimation of its outcomes in cases of neovascular AMD, with a margin of error ranging from 7 to 11 letters. Similarly, inferred sensitivity can predict the results of fundus-controlled perimetry tests conducted under mesopic and dark-adapted conditions. An AI system can forecast the occurrence of exudative age-related macular degeneration (exAMD) in individuals who already have exAMD in one eye. The gadget demonstrates an 80% sensitivity rate for detecting genuine positives and a 34% sensitivity rate for detecting false positives. It accurately identifies real positives in 78% of eyes and erroneous positives in 56% of eyes. Additionally, it correctly identifies true positives in 41% of eyes and false positives in 17% of eyes (Yim et al. 2020). By 2040, it is projected that 288 million individuals worldwide would be affected by AMD, resulting in substantial impairment of vision. AMD advances from initial to advanced stages, resulting in the development of neovascularization of the choroidal vessels and geographic atrophy. ML approaches applied to imaging data show promise for predicting progression.

Comparison of Cataract Management in AI: Current and Future Directions

AI has revolutionized various medical fields, including ophthalmology, cataract management, and ophthalmology It optimizes the diagnosis, monitoring, and surgical management of cataracts, which are the primary cause of reversible vision impairment. Additionally, it serves as a tele-diagnostic platform, streamlines the accuracy of predicting intraocular lens formulas, and boosts surgical skill development. However, challenges include ethical data management, data security, clinical performance, generalizability, and trust of end-users. These advancements could revolutionize cataract management and improve ophthalmic services. Cataract is a major contributor to vision impairment and blindness, responsible for 50% of all cases of blindness. Timely identification and proactive measures can mitigate these problems. AI advancements in ophthalmology can help, but traditional methods are time-consuming and require expert ophthalmologists. A CNN model, VGG19, suggested for cataract detection. AI-based image analysis has been used for cataract diagnosis and grading, calculating optimal intraocular lens power, and developing video analysis tools for surgical documentation. The system offers workflow examination, tool recognition, and video segmentation to assess and evaluate skills. Mixed reality features can improve surgical decision-making and reduce complications. AI mathematical models are used to develop patient referral patterns, streamline the usage of operating rooms, and accurately forecast the status of the posterior capsule in the treatment of posterior capsular opacification. This improves the triage pathway for patients undergoing this procedure. A ML system was created to diagnose cataracts using movies captured using video-recordable slit-lamp equipment. The program achieved similar performance to traditional devices.

Comparison of Glaucoma Management in AI: Current and Future Directions

It has potential in research and clinical treatment of glaucoma, with models quantifying retinal images and VFs. Laser surgery is the most common treatment, lowering eye pressure based on the patient's age and type. Deep learning and AI are revolutionizing glaucoma diagnosis and prediction, benefiting diverse ethnic groups and standardizing datasets and application rules. It examines the development of traditional and developing AI models in the context of glaucoma, the difficulties encountered, and the main ideas found in current research. Therefore, AI is connected to glaucoma and can ascertain the essential measures for the effective advancement of AI models. It used to diagnose systemic diseases, with FDA approvals. However, glaucoma is a complex disease with no agreed-upon diagnostic criteria, and current datasets have inconsistent label quality, complicating AI training. AI algorithms are improving clinical care for glaucoma and discussing the disease's types, traditional diagnosis methods, and global epidemiology. It explores AI algorithms' potential for early diagnosis through population screening and methodologies used for automatic classification and database training. The databases identified partially fulfill the study's requirements, but still play a crucial role in training algorithms and driving technological advancement. Although several studies demonstrate a high level of accuracy in both glaucomatous and non-glaucomatous pictures, additional clinical trials and comprehensive investigations are necessary to incorporate these algorithms into empirical healthcare applications (Bragança et al. 2024). AI has to enhance glaucoma detection, as discussed at a meeting hosted by the Collaborative Community on Ophthalmic Imaging. This organization aims to expedite innovation in healthcare technology. The AI system's performance was compared to a thorough glaucoma evaluation and the majority grading by specialists. The AI system demonstrated a sensitivity of 93.7% and specificity of 85.6% in accurately identifying cases of referable glaucoma. In comparison, the system correctly identified 94.7% of definitive non-glaucoma cases as not having glaucoma. Additionally, the system achieved a detection rate of 94% when compared to the assessments made by specialists.

Diabetic Retinopathy

Diabetes leads to the development of DR, a disorder that involves harm to the retina, blood vessels, and optic nerve, resulting in impaired light detection and signal transmission. In prospective research conducted for point-of-care screening, the Eye Art AI system demonstrated greater sensitivity in diagnosing more-than-mild diabetes-related retinopathy (mtmDR) compared to general ophthalmologists or retina specialists. It successfully detected all cases of vision-threatening diabetic retinopathy (vtDR), much like the group of retina specialists. The AI system exhibited a greater incidence of incorrect positive diagnoses compared to a general ophthalmologist retina specialist for cases involving moderate non-proliferative diabetic retinopathy (NPDR) or other ocular pathology would require a referral and review by an ophthalmologist. The results can be applied to the specific community of diabetic individuals undergoing retina screening, indicating its generalizability. The Eye Art AI system meets the criteria for high sensitivity and specificity in detecting mtmDR, providing benefits such as affordability and ease as a point-of-care device. It is recommended to undergo a comprehensive ocular examination if the patient experiences blurred vision or belongs to a high-risk category for illnesses such as glaucoma. AI DR tools help clinicians in fundus image analysis, guiding treatment decisions, reducing eye specialist visits, reducing treatment costs and optimizing doctor visits. However, AI should not replace clinicians and promising DR detection with grading algorithms. AI enhanced the rates of completing diabetic eye examinations in a varied community of young individuals. The participants were randomly assigned to either AI-based tests or receiving referrals and education from eye care providers following a predetermined script. The intervention group exhibited a markedly greater rate of completion, as 64% of participants successfully followed through with an eye care provider.

Diabetic Macular Edema

It is a common form of DR caused by VEGF. Treatment involves intravitreal injections but is expensive. Accurately forecasting treatment results is essential for effective administration. AI or ML algorithms assist in analyzing patient clinical data and forecasting treatment results. AI/ML methodologies propose using two types of data as differentiators. The AI algorithm has been validated for identifying and quantifying OCT biomarkers in DME eyes. The algorithm compares to human expert manual examination, analyzing intraretinal fluid detection, ELM and Ellipsoid Zone (EZ) integrity. It utilized InceptionV3 and VGG16 CNNs, achieved high DME diagnostic accuracy, sensitivity, and specificity, and developed an OCT-driven platform.

TABLE 6.1
Comparison of Disorders of the Eye Problem

Sources	Type of Eye Diseases	Inference
(Lim et al. 2012)	Age-related macular degeneration	Age-related macular degeneration, causing visual impairment in older adults, lacks effective preventive drug therapies, but nutritional and behavioral changes can slow its progression. The disorder is complex and heritable, with up to 20 associated genes. Although early detection allows for intervention, the treatment burden is high. Novel treatments, like regenerative therapy, show promise.
(Shimizu et al. 2023)	Cataract	The cataract diagnostic AI, which was developed using machine learning techniques and video records from a portable slit-lamp instrument, showed excellent accuracy in identifying cataracts and assessing the severity of nuclear cataracts.
(Sánchez-Morales et al. 2022)	Glaucoma	AI applications can enhance glaucoma research, screening programs, clinical care, and trial design by providing reproducible factors, sensitive autonomous models, assistive models, and novel digital endpoints.
(Sosale et al. 2020)	Diabetic retinopathy	The AI algorithm was found to be highly accurate in detecting diabetic retinopathy (DR), with a sensitivity of 83.3% for any DR and 92.5% for DR.
(Bajgai et al. 2024)	Macular edema	Macular edema is a condition resulting from eye damage, diabetes, ageing, blood vessel blockage, and eye inflammation.

Comparison of Disorders of the Eye Problem

Some common eye illnesses include macular degeneration due to age, cataracts, retinopathy caused by diabetes, glaucoma, amblyopia, and strabismus. A study compares eye complaints and diagnoses in primary care and ophthalmologist offices, focusing on minor inflammatory, traumatic, and visual disturbances, as well as eyelid problems. Visual acuity is measured using visually evoked potential (VEP), spatial frequency sweep, and flashes. Ongoing testing for children with eye movement disorders is conducted at the Foerderer Center. The comparison of eye disorders is shown in Table 6.1.

CONCLUSION

The literature review investigates the techniques for forecasting water demand and eye disorders. The effectiveness of AI algorithms is still uncertain, but several important considerations can help in choosing the appropriate method. The methods must be adaptable to the available data and the specific problem they are meant to address. Research in deep neural networks development is anticipated to be a key water demand forecasting methodology, leveraging innovative technologies like IoT, cyber-physical systems, and digital twin models. It explores AI approaches such as extreme learning machines, ANN, ARIMA, and hybrid models in water demand forecasting performance by RMSE, absolute error, and squared error. The study suggests hybrid AI models for WC assessment, offering flexibility, accuracy, interpretability, adaptability, and data requirements. These models tackle the limitations of individual models and offer a better understanding of variable relationships. In ophthalmology, AI used to treat disorders affecting the eyes, such as cataracts, glaucoma, DR, macular holes, and AMD. The model pattern compares eye disease diagnosis results using quality parameters like prediction rate, specificity, accuracy, precision, sensitivity and F1-score from various articles. AI algorithm emphasizes advances in retinal image analysis and the need for real-time detection implementation on new or existing devices. AI systems in ophthalmology can be complex, posing ethical challenges like lack of transparency and explainability, which may compromise trust and accountability. A new AI diagnostic tool is revolutionizing personalized healthcare by predicting disease likelihood based on lifestyle and microbiome data. AI takes over complex decision-making, and tasks for understanding its algorithms pose a challenge.

REFERENCES

AL-Washali, Taha, Saroj Sharma, Robert Lupoja, Fadhl AL-Nozaily, Mansour Haidera, and Maria Kennedy. 2020. "Assessment of Water Losses in Distribution Networks: Methods, Applications, Uncertainties, and Implications in Intermittent Supply." *Resources, Conservation and Recycling* 152 (January): 104515. doi:10.1016/j.resconrec.2019.104515.

Bajgai, Priya, KC Binita, Varun Shrestha, and Ranjila Shyangbo. 2024. "Cystoid Macular Edema as A Possible Manifestation of Covid-19: Case Report." *Medical Reports* 3 (February): 100034. doi:10.1016/j.hmedic.2023.100034.

Bragança, Clerimar Paulo, José Manuel Torres, Luciano Oliveira Macedo, and Christophe Pinto de Almeida Soares. 2024. "Advancements in Glaucoma Diagnosis: The Role of AI in Medical Imaging." *Diagnostics* 14 (5): 530. doi:10.3390/diagnostics14050530.

Dharashive, Prashant, and Manish Sawale. 2024. "Smart Irrigation System Techniques Using Artificial Intelligence and IoT." *International Journal of Intelligent Systems and Applications in Engineering* 12 (11s): 96–102.

Fu, Guangtao, Siao Sun, Lan Hoang, Zhiguo Yuan, and David Butler. 2023. "Artificial Intelligence Underpins Urban Water Infrastructure of the Future: A Holistic Perspective." *Cambridge Prisms: Water* 1 (November): e14. doi:10.1017/wat.2023.15.

Furlong, Casey, Saman De Silva, Lachlan Guthrie, and Robert Considine. 2016. "Developing a Water Infrastructure Planning Framework for the Complex Modern Planning Environment." *Utilities Policy* 38 (February): 1–10. doi:10.1016/j.jup.2015.11.002.

Glaret subin, P., and P. Muthukannan. 2022. "Optimized Convolution Neural Network Based Multiple Eye Disease Detection." *Computers in Biology and Medicine* 146 (July): 105648. doi:10.1016/j.compbiomed.2022.105648.

Hajibabaei, Mohsen, Azadeh Yousefi, Sina Hesarkazzazi, Amin Minaei, Oswald Jenewein, Mohsen Shahandashti, and Robert Sitzenfrei. 2023. "Resilience Enhancement of Water Distribution Networks under Pipe Failures: A Hydraulically Inspired Complex Network Approach." *AQUA—Water Infrastructure, Ecosystems and Society* 72 (12): 2358–76. doi:10.2166/aqua.2023.180.

Huang, Li Guo, and Li Yin. 2014. "Models of Water Strategy Based on Linear Regression." *Advanced Materials Research* 955–959 (June): 3355–60. doi:10.4028/www.scientific.net/AMR.955-959.3355.

Hwang, De-Kuang, Chih-Chien Hsu, Kao-Jung Chang, Daniel Chao, Chuan-Hu Sun, Ying-Chun Jheng, Aliaksandr A. Yarmishyn, et al. 2019. "Artificial Intelligence-Based Decision-Making for Age-Related Macular Degeneration." *Theranostics* 9 (1): 232–45. doi:10.7150/thno.28447.

Jena, Pramod Kumar, Sayed Modinur Rahaman, Pradeep Kumar Das Mohapatra, Durga Prasad Barik, and Dikshya Surabhi Patra. 2023. "Surface Water Quality Assessment by Random Forest." *Water Practice and Technology* 18 (1): 201–14. doi:10.2166/wpt.2022.156.

Kumar Singhal, Arun, Tariqo Gerito, Dilgasa Bedada, and Ofgaha Alemu. 2008. "Early Glaucoma Detection Using Naive Bayes Algorithm." *International Journal of Advances in Engineering and Management, IJAEM* 2 (1): 1192.

Lam, Byron L., Bart P. Leroy, Graeme Black, Tuyen Ong, Dan Yoon, and Karmen Trzupek. 2021. "Genetic Testing and Diagnosis of Inherited Retinal Diseases." *Orphanet Journal of Rare Diseases* 16 (1). BioMed Central: 1–9. doi:10.1186/s13023-021-02145-0.

Leal Filho, Walter, Tony Wall, Serafino Afonso Rui Mucova, Gustavo J. Nagy, Abdul-Lateef Balogun, Johannes M. Luetz, Artie W. Ng, et al. 2022. "Deploying Artificial Intelligence for Climate Change Adaptation." *Technological Forecasting and Social Change* 180 (July): 121662. doi:10.1016/j.techfore.2022.121662.

Li, Xinru, Wenlai Jiang, and Dingding Duan. 2020. "Spatio-Temporal Analysis of Irrigation Water Use Coefficients in China." *Journal of Environmental Management* 262 (May): 110242. doi:10.1016/j.jenvman.2020.110242.

Lim, Laurence S, Paul Mitchell, Johanna M Seddon, Frank G Holz, and Tien Y Wong. 2012. "Age-Related Macular Degeneration." *The Lancet* 379 (9827): 1728–38. doi:10.1016/S0140-6736(12)60282-7.

Malik, Sadaf, Nadia Kanwal, Mamoona Naveed Asghar, Mohammad Ali A. Sadiq, Irfan Karamat, and Martin Fleury. 2019. "Data Driven Approach for Eye Disease Classification with Machine Learning." *Applied Sciences* 9 (14): 2789. doi:10.3390/app9142789.

Romić, Davor, Annamaria Castrignanò, Marija Romić, Gabriele Buttafuoco, Marina Bubalo Kovačić, Gabrijel Ondrašek, and Monika Zovko. 2020. "Modelling Spatial and Temporal Variability of Water Quality from Different Monitoring Stations Using Mixed Effects Model Theory." *Science of the Total Environment* 704 (February): 135875. doi:10.1016/j.scitotenv.2019.135875.

Sánchez-Morales, Adrián, Juan Morales-Sánchez, Oleksandr Kovalyk, Rafael Verdú-Monedero, and José-Luis Sancho-Gómez. 2022. "Improving Glaucoma Diagnosis Assembling Deep Networks and Voting Schemes." *Diagnostics* 12 (6): 1382. doi:10.3390/diagnostics12061382.

Shimizu, Eisuke, Makoto Tanji, Shintato Nakayama, Toshiki Ishikawa, Naomichi Agata, Ryota Yokoiwa, Hiroki Nishimura, et al. 2023. "AI-Based Diagnosis of Nuclear Cataract from Slit-Lamp Videos." *Scientific Reports* 13 (1): 22046. doi:10.1038/s41598-023-49563-7.

Shu, Jun, Xinyu Xia, Suyue Han, Zuli He, Ke Pan, and Bin Liu. 2024. "Long-Term Water Demand Forecasting Using Artificial Intelligence Models in the Tuojiang River Basin, China." Edited by A. L. Mahfoodh. *PLOS ONE* 19 (5): e0302558. doi:10.1371/journal.pone.0302558.

Sosale, Bhavana, Sosale Ramachandra Aravind, Hemanth Murthy, Srikanth Narayana, Usha Sharma, Sahana G V Gowda, and Muralidhar Naveenam. 2020. "Simple, Mobile-Based Artificial Intelligence Algorithm in the Detection of Diabetic Retinopathy (SMART) Study." *BMJ Open Diabetes Research & Care* 8 (1): e000892. doi:10.1136/bmjdrc-2019-000892.

Subha, J., and M. Kowsigan. 2023. "Enhanced ARIMA Model for Water Demand Forecasting in Smart Water Distribution Network." *IJISAE* 11 (3): 598–610.

Szomolányi, Orsolya, and Adrienne Clement. 2023 "Use of Random Forest for Assessing the Effect of Water Quality Parameters on the Biological Status of Surface Waters." *GEM—International Journal on Geomathematics* 14 (1): 20. doi:10.1007/s13137-023-00229-6.

Tabbussum, Ruhhee, and Abdul Qayoom Dar. 2021. "Performance Evaluation of Artificial Intelligence Paradigms—Artificial Neural Networks, Fuzzy Logic, and Adaptive Neuro-Fuzzy Inference System for Flood Prediction." *Environmental Science and Pollution Research* 28 (20): 25265–82. doi:10.1007/s11356-021-12410-1.

Tan, Yaoyuan Vincent, and Jason Roy. 2019. "Bayesian Additive Regression Trees and the General BART Model." *Statistics in Medicine* 38 (25): 5048–69. doi:10.1002/sim.8347.

Vijai, Praveen, and P. Bagavathi Sivakumar. 2018. "Performance Comparison of Techniques for Water Demand Forecasting." *Procedia Computer Science* 143: 258–66. doi:10.1016/j.procs.2018.10.394.

Wang, Minghui, Hanqiao Zhang, Li Dong, Yang Li, Zhijia Hou, and Dongmei Li. 2023. "Using the Random Forest Algorithm to Detect the Activity of Graves Orbitopathy." *Journal of Craniofacial Surgery* 34 (2): e167–71. doi:10.1097/SCS.0000000000008946.

Xiao-jun, Wang, Zhang Jian-yun, Shahid Shamsuddin, He Rui-min, Xia Xing-hui, and Mou Xin-li. 2015. "Potential Impact of Climate Change on Future Water Demand in Yulin City, Northwest China." *Mitigation and Adaptation Strategies for Global Change* 20 (1): 1–19. doi:10.1007/s11027-013-9476-9.

Yim, Jason, Reena Chopra, Terry Spitz, Jim Winkens, Annette Obika, Christopher Kelly, Harry Askham, et al. 2020. "Predicting Conversion to Wet Age-Related Macular Degeneration Using Deep Learning." *Nature Medicine* 26 (6): 892–99. doi:10.1038/s41591-020-0867-7.

7 Diagnosis to Treatment

Challenges and Opportunities in Generative Artificial Intelligence Adoption in the Healthcare

Jaswinder Pal Singh, Neha Mishra, and Babita Singla

INTRODUCTION

Artificial intelligence (AI) is advancing in the field of healthcare and infiltrating many of its sectors (Kuzlu et al. 2023). The most thrilling aspect of this forward push is the potential it offers which is nothing less than the ability to improve the basic human decision-making that forms the bedrock of our healthcare system. Attracted by the immense amount of data as well as the resource-intensity required in much of people's work, machine learning is being applied to a wide assortment of tasks with growing success (Jayakumar et al. 2023). The most important components are medicine design, diagnosis, and care management. Furthermore, the advantages of AI in healthcare have just begun to become apparent. Because a large portion of AI's work is done "under the hood," and ethical and legal issues only become apparent when its applications are made "visible," its use by healthcare professionals is still unclear, if not completely covert (Novozhilova et al. 2024). However, healthcare AI is a predictor of the potential benefits and hazards that it may bring in a variety of fields. The ideal technique to assess generative AI (GAI) is as ambiguous as its effect on patient outcomes. The only thing that is obvious is that, in addition to the medical industry's already well compensated experts, there exist a plethora of "clinic" vocations where people work long hours for decent pay, albeit with little worldwide reputation, in order to maintain the healthcare system (Bautista et al. 2023). It goes without saying that technologists might benefit these people as well as their patients much by applying GAI models for goodness (Hobensack et al. 2024). However, there is always a risk associated with employing AI or IT in healthcare, thus GAI in this field needs to perform better, much like its more conservative predecessors, in order to be reliable and efficient.

DOI: 10.1201/9781003531272-7

GENERATIVE ARTIFICIAL INTELLIGENCE AN OVERVIEW

GAI algorithms generate new information by learning from information used as training. Such data is produced by those models as it was observed during training (Jayakumar et al. 2023). AI is used by people to comprehend visual input and produce speech. Without people supervising them while ensuring they don't comprehend or produce anything hazardous, the models work as intended. Furthermore, labeling is not necessary when you have a generative model that is capable of understanding and reproducing things (Kuzlu et al. 2023). Whether or not what people are seeing or hearing is pleasing to the eye can be determined technically. Humans may even include that assessment back into the training once they possess the necessary information. GAI models possess the remarkable capacity to analyze and discern numerous patterns and attributes from real data, and then utilize this information to generate new and comparable content (Nedbal et al. 2024). Unlike other AI models, these varieties go beyond simple prediction to produce artificial or non-real world, copies of the training data. This is why they are dubbed generative models, in addition to producing nearly exact replicas that are remarkably close to the original. The models we are discussing, like adversarial networks and large language models, learn differently than models that separate different types of data. Instead of just dividing data into categories like humans might do, they use other methods to learn (Yu et al. 2023). On the contrary, people learn the data by arguing back and forth on what the original dataset really looks like with each other. People can create their own synthetic or occasionally hallucinated samples from a projected class using the knowledge they have gained (Oniani et al. 2023).

GENERATIVE ADVERSARIAL NETWORKS

GAI encompasses machine learning techniques designed to generate new content or data that mimics the training data, which can include visual, audio, text, or source code data (Abbasian et al. 2024). Unlike other machine learning methodologies that focus on data classification or clustering, GAI is dedicated to producing new data that closely resembles the input data. GAI typically includes language models or transformer-based model, as well as generative adversarial networks (GANs) (Golda et al. 2024). GANs are good in generating visually rich outputs like art, poem, or paint-created. Moreover, another example is to use a GAN model which can help humans to generate images from normal plain-text descriptions (Bietsch, Stahlbock, and Voß 2023). This process could be simulated with plain text instructions using a GAN. In contrast, transformer models like Generative Pre-trained Transformers (GPT) synthesized information from many texts together to create the new text. The models use enormous numbers of text that have been posted to the internet (Umer and Adnan 2024).

AI is used so extensively in the technology industry that, even if people tried, they could not ignore it. GAI in healthcare is one field that is now quite prominent and has incredibly intriguing possibilities (Mishra and Mishra 2024). When creating highly customized, evidence-based treatment plans for individuals of interest, it can also serve as a guide for those who provide care. Developing such a strategy is not simple;

the tactics would need to be customized, taking into account the patient's comorbidities, social determinants of health, and personal/family preferences (Grupac, Zauskova, and Nica 2023). In this context, the recent achievements as well as shortcomings with AI, particularly with GAI, offer fresh optimism. GAI is the term for the idea that creative tasks that were previously only performed by humans are now completed by AI systems (Zhang et al. 2024). Experts will find it easier to discover new treatments that are highly effective in treating a variety of disorders if GAI is able to simulate the interactions between various chemicals and biological molecules (Hirosawa and Shimizu 2024). Furthermore, advanced medical imaging techniques that provide more precise and comprehensive diagnostic results can be enhanced using GAI.

Unlike generative models, GANs learn in a different way and with an alternative method. They use adversarial networks and game theory. In GANs, we have the interplay of a rival pair of expert networks, the generator and the discriminator, and their respective loss functions (Jindal, Lungren, and Shah 2024). The generator pushes up the gradients of the reproach signals for the types of figures it wants the discriminator to not be able to tell apart from the real deal. Adversarial training that is either unsupervised or partially supervised can be used to teach GANs how to create representations (Bengesi et al. 2024). Unlike classical generative models, which directly work with probability distributions, GANs labor over a hidden space, enlisting a pair of neural networks that fulfill an adversarial relationship to each other. Training such a pair of networks can then be understood as enhancing the process of "variation" inference over latent space sand in turn, promises to improve on the notoriously variable performance of the classical generative statisticians (Golda et al. 2024).

Generative adversarial networks, or GANs, are the newest technology utilized for a variety of applications, including semi-supervised learning, attention-controlled generation, and image compression. GANs are cooperative networks. They can be divided into two components: a discriminative network (D) and a generating network (G). The input is the same for both G and D, but D acts as a critic and attempts to determine whether a certain image is real or fake, whilst G attempts to create realistic and varied examples. Highly realistic visual representations can be produced by GANs (Umer and Adnan 2024; Wang 2024). Researchers accomplish this by drawing conclusions from the data's distribution. AI delivers visual representations that closely resemble actual data once they have been trained (Chatterjee et al. 2024). This renders them valuable for an array of applications pertaining to computer graphics, artistic expression, and amusement. These can involve making visual storyboards for live-action movies as well as pictures for video games and animation movies. Technology can accomplish this without requiring a significant amount of human labor. Enhanced performance comes from using restricted or prejudiced data. Prejudiced data concentrates the model's learning in the same way a good teacher focuses on a good student (Banafa 2023). Everyone wants the best performance from our models. Traditional academic models would merely create a bias and then depend on it to create a setting that is favorable for learning. The same biases in machine learning models would make them subpar models.

LARGE LANGUAGE MODELS

The field of research that concerns the interaction between humans, using natural (human) language, and machines is referred to as natural language processing (NLP). NLP uses large language models (LLMs) to execute difficult tasks (Zhang et al. 2024). Computer-based LLMs, like OpenAI's GPT-3, Google's PaLM, and Turing NLG, were already able to perform many NLP tasks at a proverbial human-level. Now, OpenAI's GPT-4, Google's PaLM2 (or Barkmeyer's Deep Mind AI), and several other next-generation LLMs have topped impressive predecessors. There have been incredible advancements in the LLMs that carry out these human-like tasks. GPT-4 by OpenAI uses autoregressive models, and these models give us natural language phrases by predicting what should come next. LLMs stake the architecture of a language model to a new extreme (Arighi, Brenner, and Lu 2024; Grinbaum and Adomaitis 2024).

ADOPTION OF ARTIFICIAL INTELLIGENCE IN HEALTHCARE

The healthcare sector has applied AI extensively in several areas. These include, but are not limited to, analysis of medical images, discovery of new drugs, education of medical professionals, provision of clinical decision support (CDS), and delivery of personalized medicine (Denecke, May, and Rivera-Romero 2024). Despite these gains, the path to the effective deployment of GAI in healthcare is not straightforward. A couple of hurdles that GAI must overcome are its accommodation of unstructured data and its providence of insightful explanations (Yu et al. 2023). Another hurdle pertains to the creation of conversational tools that can engage with individuals in a virtual setting. The last major roadblock calls for the GAI pathway to a power moment where GAI hints at something truly innovative. Moreover, the use of GAI models in healthcare holds a lot of potential (Oniani et al. 2023). They can produce all sorts of things: visualizations, such as what an organ might look like under a scanner; how to perform a delicate surgery; and even biologically realistic virtual humans that can serve as much-needed guinea pigs for testing new treatments. GAI holds great potential for several sectors and industries. The incomprehensible solutions and outcomes of this dynamic technology have the potential to completely transform the way as human tackle complex problems (Harrer 2023). The modeling, development, and advancement of GAI expand the range of possibilities. The use of GAI is causing a significant transformation in the healthcare industry as well as in IT industries (Abbasian et al. 2024). The healthcare industry is being transformed by machine learning algorithms. Traditionally, medical professionals have been the sole "intelligent" system in the hospital. They perform tasks that require reasoning, decision-making, and problem-solving, and they, in turn, teach those tasks to future medical professionals. The difficult tasks that can only be performed by the professionals of the healthcare system may soon have an AI equivalent, and this "generative" AI may be the next big push for the medical industry (Baldassarre and Padovan 2024). The medical field is on the verge of a revolution. AI has the power to change the way human perform surgeries, diagnose, and treat patients and such rapid progress is accompanied by ethical problems. Moreover, it is the tough task for human to ensure patients' private information confidential and not accessed or used for nefarious purposes. In using AI in healthcare, many new ethical and regulatory questions arise (Kumar, Dhalwal, and Chaudhary 2024). So it proposes the required changes in law and policy that are crucial to ensure the responsible use of AI in healthcare. When these are resolved, they can help provide new kinds of healthcare that individuals and society can trust (Sullivan, Hall, and Morrison 2024). AI has the potential to do magic in healthcare through the use of this new technology. It has the potential to improve many aspects of healthcare system like it may boost the accuracy of diagnosing illnesses and diseases; and it can make public health surveillance work more efficiently and effectively (Salinas-Navarro et al. 2024). This emerging technology may help in the process of determining the optimal patient care plan. There is an infinite amount of opportunities for development and significant progress toward improved healthcare.

GAI APPLICATIONS

The implementation of GAI has transformed the healthcare sector by improving the accuracy, effectiveness, and customization of medical services. GAI facilitates the practice of precision medicine, ensuring targeted and efficient therapy by tailoring healthcare treatments to the specific genetic, environmental, and lifestyle attributes of each individual. GAI expedites the identification and advancement of innovative pharmaceuticals in the drug discovery process through the analysis of extensive datasets and the prediction of molecular behavior. CDS tools, powered by GAI, offer medical practitioners real-time, evidence-based insights, leading to enhanced patient outcomes and improved diagnostic accuracy. By utilizing GAI, data can be enhanced to facilitate the synthesis and analysis of intricate medical information, leading to the ability to make more well-informed decisions. GAI plays a crucial role in pharmaceutical discovery by enhancing the effectiveness of medicine formulations and identifying new molecules. GAI products provide accurate and timely disease diagnosis by utilizing cutting-edge imaging and pattern recognition technologies. The GAI system guarantees the precision, safety, and availability of patient information while streamlining the upkeep and administration of medical records. GAI's ability to perform in-depth analysis on individual patient data greatly improves the effectiveness of individualized treatment plans. GAI offers medical professionals the essential resources to navigate the constantly changing medical industry through dynamic and captivating learning opportunities. Health literacy is improved when GAI systems provide patients with individualized and understandable health information. Furthermore, the notion of "digital twins," which refers to virtual replicas of patients, enables the examination and simulation of medical operations, hence improving the effectiveness and security of treatments. The extensive and groundbreaking use of GAI in healthcare suggests the possibility of enhanced patient care and the development of breakthrough medical techniques in the future. The GAI applications in different areas of healthcare are illustrated in this section. Figure 7.1 shows various applications as discussed in the study.

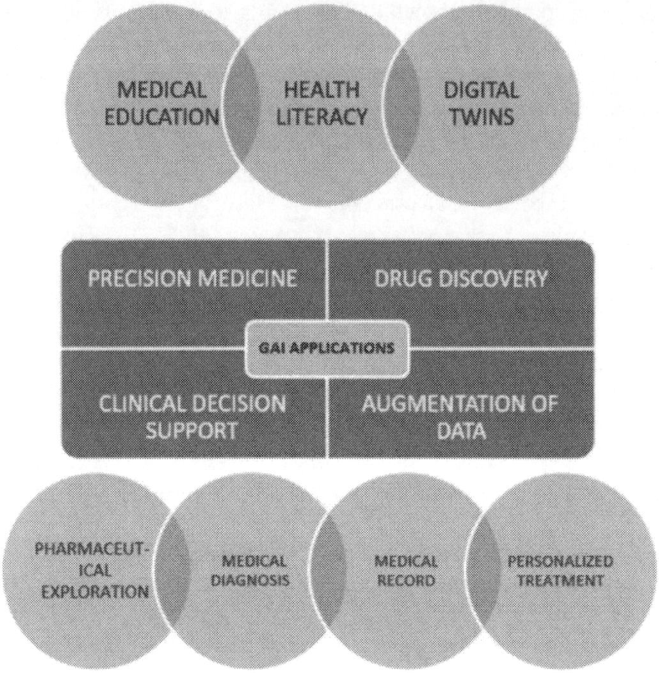

FIGURE 7.1 GAI applications.

Source: Authors' conceptualization.

Precision Medicine

Precision medicine is about treating patients based on their individual circumstances. By considering various factors that make each person unique like: age, gender, family history, and the wide range of differences in our DNA, physicians can develop treatment approaches that are not only specific to the disease in question but also to the person it is affecting (Grupac, Zauskova, and Nica 2023). Precision medicine's fundamental objective is to develop treatment approaches that are specific to the disease. Short-term gains in its implementation are expected to lead to cost savings, as more efficient and, therefore, less expensive drug therapies are deployed with greater specificity than ever beforehand there are clear long-term efficiency gains that might be achieved as well, by using digital technologies that can lead to better patient flow through a hospital system (Nedbal et al. 2024).

Drug Discovery

The drug discovery and development process are inherently a complex, resource-intensive exercise. The production of a market-ready medicine commonly takes more than ten years on its path from basic scientific discovery to commercialization (Grupac, Zauskova, and Nica 2023). Moreover, the regulatory scrutiny of new drugs is ever-expanding. It may happen that other new drugs are launched during the drug development, which may lead to suspension of ongoing production. The whole process is demanding and they are not efficient enough; it can also discourage the public due to high costs. At present, AI methods are far better over traditional ML techniques in drug development because of the sheer problem at hand and related to huge datasets. They try to reduce the datasets for training, which is one of the advances in deep learning (Razmi 2023). For example, they are able to gain extracted information by processing huge numbers of data through methods such as one-shot learning or long short-term memory techniques and using Memory Augmented Neural Network.

Clinical Decision Support (CDS)

One of the largest endeavors using GAI-enabled technology is CDS, which has been a huge use in healthcare. These systems are essential to helping physicians, patients, and other stakeholders to make good healthcare decisions by providing the right information at the point of need (Grupac, Zauskova, and Nica 2023). The GAI-based tools in CDS could provide individualized treatment recommendations such as clinical guidelines and proper medication for the patient according to his/her medical record. Additionally, it can also avoid any unwanted side effects leading to time efficiency cost savings as well as risk mitigation (Hayward 2023). Further, CDS systems empowered by GAI can assist healthcare workers in making more informed decisions and improved patients outcomes directory delivering updated and precise information. These systems also improve accuracy and provide the highest quality treatment (Saban and Dubovi 2024).

Augmentation of Data

Deep learning model training is frequently difficult due to the scarcity of medical imaging datasets. The robustness of the models is increased by GAI approaches like variation auto encoders (VAEs) and GANs, which may produce artificial images that closely mimic patient data (Lang et al. 2024). Moreover, GAI models can create missing data and data on uncommon conditions like methemoglobinemia, and Aquagenic Urticaria. This quality of AI adds to the dataset's diversity and augments it for training and assessment, improving the models' capacity to identify and diagnose illnesses in real-world situations (Chatterjee et al. 2024). It has been noted that although GAI techniques such as GANs and VAEs are essential for dealing with the scarcity of annotated data in medical imaging, the degree to which they are used may differ depending on the frequency of rare disease datasets.

Pharmaceutical Exploration

GAI models are used in drug discovery to create tiny molecules, nucleic acid sequences, and proteins that have certain structures or functions. GAI can expedite the discovery of potential drugs by analyzing and simulating modifications to drug chemical structures, surpassing the speed of standard drug development methods. This approach is time and cost efficient, and it detects medicines that previous approaches failed to identify. One of the core phases in drug development is predicting specific human language generation models to predict if advanced novel therapies are going to be effective and safe (Grupac, Zauskova, and Nica 2023). By analyzing huge amounts of data, the GAI can likely find any problems in the clinical trials quickly and also provide guidance to faster medication development. In addition, GAI can discover underlying disease-relevant biological processes to invent novel pharmacologic targets which increase treatment outcomes (Sarkar 2024).

Medical Diagnosis

Identification of Complex Illnesses Health issues frequently has multiple facets; multiple factors may be at effect when a problem suddenly appears. Without understanding how everything fits together, treating a health issue successfully can be extremely difficult or even impossible (Ktena et al. 2024). At this point, it has led medical professionals and researchers to utilize diverse computational techniques in order to gain a more profound comprehension of the illness processes, ultimately resulting in customized care approaches. Recently, there has been a lot of interest in language modeling with long short-term memory (LLM) and GANs. The latter are used to produce explanations of "what makes a disease," employing NLP (Kovacova, Kevicky, and Popescu 2023). Moreover, users likely see this system as more convenient than traditional computer-aided diagnosis (CAD) systems. Such systems make use of the abundant data held in electronic health records (EHRs), in addition to other types of patient records that may be stored in a digital format. Those records may contain all sorts of subtle clues that factor into accurate diagnoses (Barker 2023). The thorough integration of clinical data appears to be the most efficient method of understanding a patient's health. An LLM could be useful to help think through many potential disorders and their diagnosis in complex situations when there are several (and sometimes many linked, and sometimes unrelated) illnesses or symptoms. Similar to medical students, medical models have been shown in numerous studies to be capable of passing exams. Algorithms in medical testing, however, can be dangerous (Kovacova, Kevicky, and Popescu 2023). They are unable to mimic a doctor's clinical reasoning.

Medical Record

Recent studies have shown that language models like GPT-4 and PaLM-2 are highly effective when it comes to condensing large amounts of patient information in healthcare environments for their value. These environments often have to process huge quantities of data, and EHRs can work here to securely store not just an individual's medical history but also important information like known allergies and the precise medicines that are prescribed (Aravinth et al. 2023). They also store the results of lab tests. By running that type of data through a model, can search for significant patterns and provide a high-level diagnosis that a human might not have been able to determine without more time or without the model's collection and pattern-matching abilities. These summaries provide a concise health evaluation, which helps to improve communication between patients and healthcare providers. By automating these procedures utilizing LLMs, doctors may handle a great deal less paperwork, which will lessen their workload on a global basis (Chadha et al. 2024). Due to commercial restrictions or obligations from health insurance companies, many healthcare professionals are required to record information that goes beyond the parameters of clinical care. Furthermore, research indicates that a significant number of physicians dedicate more than 60 minutes to EHR duties for every hour of direct patient interaction (Lang et al. 2024). Documentation can lead to cognitive fatigue and dissatisfaction, resulting in reduced work satisfaction. The severity of this strain could be decreased with the implementation of NLP document automation. An LLM degree in the appropriate information platform enables one to compile and create documents for approval by medical professionals. Utilizing LLM-based EHR software for inspection purposes can potentially decrease instances of medical errors and overlooked information. EHR LLMs have the potential to decrease medical errors and prevent data loss, while also automating documentation. Research indicates that a significant number of patients in hospitals suffer from avoidable medical mistakes, such as misdiagnosis, problems in prescribing medication, and failure to properly follow up on examination results. Automation of scheduling, claims processing, and patient record management can be achieved via generative AI. It is the power of AI that helps with intelligent scheduling. Additionally, the role of voice assistants and chatbots help in fixing appointments. With the use of GAI, processing insurance claims can be a speedy and error-free procedure (Chadha et al. 2024). The job of claim validation, which was formerly done by a person, is now handled by an effective system. It guarantees that insurance claim forms are accurate, which speeds up the acceptance or denial process. However, technology doesn't always yield the desired outcomes. Studies actually indicate that rather than decreasing, the new wave of insurance claim automation has increased errors. And that's an issue when it comes to money and health.

Personalized Treatment

AI uses genetic data, along with information about a person's lifestyle and medical history, to project the likely outcome of a therapy. When AI is doing the training and combing through mounds of patient records on the path to insight, it can identify not just broad patterns but specific situations that may lead to a better or worse response to a treatment (Padoan and Plebani 2024). However, doctors do a solid job for achieving "generative" outcome better than AI in a lot of instances, by using AI-generated data to establish a tailored treatment plan for the patient. This procedure considers the individual response characteristics of the patient to the series of drugs that are part of the plan (Barker 2023). AI is proving its worth in order to substantiate a promise of better outcomes for patients by virtue of "better, more accurate predictions." AI generates can be used to make cognitive behavioral therapy (CBT) systems interactive (Horak, Novak, and Voumik 2023). The CBT is a conversation between a patient and a mental health expert. It's a type of therapy that works for people, and it's the type that people are used to seeing in media. But in the media and in real life, CBT is often depicted simplistically: two people in a room, one person talking to the other.

Medical Education

GAI in medical education is on the rise such as ChatGPT serves as an example of more ubiquitous tech can be used. ChatGPT assists medical students and nurses by giving real-time explanations on medical information by the moment helping them build perception of clinical knowledge (Yu and Guo 2024). It eases medical writing and progresses in research as well as healthcare. It can be helpful for a researcher to publish their article in an efficient manner. Use of virtual patients is another major application in medical education and has become a significant outcome of GAI (Xu et al. 2024). Healthcare professionals are equipped with the chance to hone their diagnosis and treatment of complex medical diseases through these simulations. Furthermore, the GAI analyzes enormous amounts of clinical trial and patient data to find hidden patterns and connections that can be used to clinical research and practice (Chadha et al. 2024). The use of AI contributes to the development of sophisticated therapies, diagnostic instruments, and further medical applications.

Health Literacy

Using GAI to teach patients or several techniques which are used for patient education by identifying symptoms and queries, it also personalizes their patient education based on a very specific medical state (Abbasian et al. 2024). This advice focuses on the proper diet, amount of exercise, blood glucose monitoring, and medication use for those with diabetes. Patients get their questions answered by AI only to enable them understand. GAI might also make info graphics and data photos optimizing the patient to get complicated medical subjects. GAI creates a tiered health literacy solution based on patient level of education or their ability to understand. Patients can receive reminders and information to keep reminding the patients. GAI has the potential of transforming that how patients look at their health. Using GAI to write multi-language educational content on healthcare accessibility(Bharath Suhas et al. 2024).

Digital Twins

Employing GAI to educate patients numerous methods, it also allows them to tailor their patient education according to a very specific medical condition by recognizing symptoms and inquiries (Padoan and Plebani 2024). The right food, amount of exercise, blood glucose monitoring, and medication are the main topics of this advice for people with diabetes. This guidance focuses on diabetics to take their medications, monitor their blood sugar, and maintain a healthy diet and exercise routine (Coucke 2024). In healthcare, many benefits of digital twins (DTs) can be particularly helpful in managing chronic diseases like diabetes and heart disease, where early detection is key to successfully treating it. It permits running simulations of care pathways versioned to a specific set of chronic conditions that allows healthcare providers seeing how different treatment strategies may be performed and optimized before execution. This very proactive strategy saves time, decrease risks, and improves patient care outcomes (Chen et al. 2024). Healthcare reliability engineers track real-time patient data by developing a digital replica of all patients; this makes it easier to detect possible health problems early as well as allowing the development of tailored treatment solutions. Therefore, the synergistic use of DTs and GAI in healthcare has potential to revolutionize treatment pathways leading to better patient outcomes whilst improving efficiency across healthcare systems.

CONVERTED ROUTE

Using GAI in healthcare is a disruptive path to optimize. This supports toward a more patient-centric care model, by automating lengthy manual data entry and appointment scheduling tasks in healthcare so that health providers can focus on delivering face-to-face personalized treatment for patients (Reddy 2024). Moreover, GAI can actually look at patient data and recommend an outcome of the personalized treatment plan which could be relevant to patients. However, the more important thing is the accuracy and reliability of AI-generated data. Success is based on comprehensive planning that also includes technical, organizational, and sociopsychological facets. The Technology Acceptance Model (TAM) and Non-Adoption, Abandonment, Scale-up Spread-out (NASSS) framework for understanding innovation implementation could be used so that we can move forward to an evidence-based means of making the care optimize algorithms workflow in healthcare systems (Davis 1989; Puriwat and Tripopsakul 2021).

- ***Acceptance and Adoption:*** To optimize delivery, GAI needs buy-in from clinicians as well as patients. This common knowledge base increases trust in AI systems. It gives clarity on how to use the technology and also navigate some of the ethical and regulatory challenges that arise when implementing AI. Raising awareness among all stakeholders is important for the successful implementation and adaption of AI in healthcare. This is how the use of well-established frameworks such as the NASSS and TAM comes in. In order to ensure that healthcare professionals believe that systems are simple enough for their daily workflows, this includes perceived usefulness that AI helps them in more accurate in diagnosing, predicting outcomes, and prescribing treatments. With more training, support, and successful case examples proving the benefits of AI use to help a positive attitude toward reliance on AI. Adoption is influenced by a wide range of external factors, such as official approval and humanistic considerations and patient acceptance for fear of privacy being invaded when their personal information is used. By addressing these components as a single global plan, it will make it possible for healthcare organizations to use AI to practice and achieve the necessary goals in the dynamic field of modern medicine.
- ***Data and Resources:*** In order to employ GAI in healthcare, a methodical approach that can optimize and organize data is required so that resources inside organizations may be utilized. One choice might be selecting AI use cases; identifying an acute ailment differs greatly from diagnosing a chronic one on all fronts. In essence, data collection is just gathering and organizing a large dataset; this includes consistency and quality checks.

With AI models to learn from, annotation and labeling is the ground reality; it is necessary when the models are doing tasks like text categorization or image segmentation. Furthermore, with quality of robust data storage it is accessible and secure for efficiently deploying models as compared to a traditional data warehouse or alternative cloud platforms. Additionally, AI requires a lot more processing power. This refers to businesses that should develop their own hardware capabilities with particular issues in mind and provide an isolated environment for doing so. At the same time, while such a setup is needed for GAI to be readily integrated into healthcare, it also increases the tech's potential to change healthcare delivery as well as provides more comprehensive data interfaces and/or automation options.

- ***Technical Integration:*** Integrating GAI into healthcare information systems has the potential to improve diagnosing diseases and deliver general care. But the difficulties that accompany this kind of complex management are likewise immense obstacles on its own. Certain process phases depend on determining if specific implementation requirements are patient-owing. The choice of network architecture for GANs for medical image synthesis and LLMs for clinical decision assistance is later shown, using models heavily trained on gathered data. In order to ensure smooth integration with current systems, the Blockchain needs to interface to offer data access and usability. Thorough testing and ongoing maintenance are necessary to ensure high serviceability since user feedback drives continuous improvement. Strict data governance rules are necessary to ensure that personally identifiable patient information is secure and compliant with legal and regulatory requirements, such as Health Insurance Portability and Accountability Act (HIPAA) and General Data Protection Regulation (GDPR), for privacy-preserving federated learning models that inevitably call for external LLMs. When taken as a whole, these examples show how ethical AI integration in healthcare might reduce the effects of privacy and compliance eroding in an increasingly dynamic technology environment.
- ***Governance:*** Although AI-generated data in clinical medicine has many benefits, there are a number of drawbacks as well. These are caused by external factors; while the inability to obtain data is concerning. The inflated findings are a result of being trained on biased datasets and the failure to comprehend the model's output, which depresses humans because nothing seems to be correct! A significant challenge with AI-generated data in high-stakes medical situations is accuracy and reliability. It is important that the decision-making process should be clear, including the source of input. The healthcare should seek reliable and secure information for great outcome. The healthcare institutions need to develop better governance frameworks grounded in implementation science. These call for risk assessment and guidance, and the monitoring process ought to take the law and moral principles into account. Moreover, AI-generated solutions with revolutionary potential for healthcare will be available if such a framework is maintained. Subsequently safety and moral considerations are mandatory for adopting AI in healthcare.

OPPORTUNITIES, CHALLENGES, AND FUTURE DIRECTIONS

While GAI is being used in healthcare more than ever, the field is at a crossroads as numerous challenges face it as it is investigated and evaluated for potential future applications. However, this technology is developed and advances in healthcare responsibly depend mainly on ongoing research, collaboration, and the implementation of strict privacy restrictions. This section will address the range of potential benefits and obstacles as well as new developments in GAI that offer a comprehensive picture of how it can impact healthcare.

OPPORTUNITIES

In the study the GANs have been discussed and also talked about how GAI works and how it can be used to make easy and approachable treatment based on ethical considerations. AI-generated treatments are able to provide more individualized care and precise diagnosis because of their advanced knowledge.

- *Advanced Drug Discovery*: GAI helps in the drug discovery processes by creating molecules with its set of properties, forecasting on the efficacy of a substance and possible side effects as well. The application speeds the development of new therapies, and enhances their safety.
- *Improved Patient Care*: Using broad samples of patient data, GAI discerns patterns in human behavior and foretells outcomes before recommending unique treatment plans. By being patient-centric, this individualized care will enhance the delivery of healthcare and increase better outcomes for patients.
- *Virtual Healthcare*: GAI allows virtual healthcare assistants to service with ease, as they take care of patient consultations and provide information on healthcare. These helpers improve user engagement which opens up wide accessibility to the healthcare services.
- *Predictive Analytics and Digital Twins*: Using predictive analytics, GAI can anticipate possible medical conditions based on patient history for treatment planning or preventative measures associating those insights with digital twins. It recognizes patterns, trends, and risk factors which influence the progression of conditions, hence enhancing overall healthcare.
- *Effective Medical Diagnosis*: GAI generates good diagnosis of diseases by having a glance at symptoms, based on medical records and other important information. It saves lives; it spares costs to the health insurance companies; and also helps doctors in diagnosing on time with precision.

These use cases demonstrate AI innovation in healthcare and specify how GAI can help to lead a transformational shift by harnessing the power of data-based insights for better diagnostics, treatment planning, patient care delivery, etc.

CHALLENGES

The ability to comprehend is almost like an inconvenience, but there are good reasons to consider it, including the need for stronger GAI in the medical field. The techniques used in explainable AI (XAI), human-AI collaboration, data quality/anomalies/missing data treatment, and bias/bias mitigation comprise a variety of approaches, such as the creation of robustness tests, which can enhance confidence in the ability of users to comprehend any task produced by an AI model.

Some significant challenges to be taken care while AI adoption in healthcare is mentioned here:

- *Bias and Discrimination*: This is a significant problem in GAI for healthcare. Using more diverse and extensive training data is one possibility. Other options include adhering to ethical guidelines, experimenting with bias detection mechanisms in conjunction with corrective algorithms (also known as fairness AI), or implementing human oversight throughout the AI system's lifecycle to ensure that its decisions and outputs reverence certain consolidated ethical standards.
- *Security and Privacy Issues*: Keeping information safe and confidential is important when using GAI in healthcare. Since it involves sensitive data, it becomes extremely important from a security standpoint to enforce safeguards like data encryption, monitor the use of AI for clinical and nonclinical purposes, regularly evaluate mechanisms in place (e.g., audits), comply with certain set standards like HIPAA or GDPR, and ensure patient transparency.
- *Data Requirements*: The GAI method is much more data-intensive and relies on an enormous amount of fine quality training examples (identical to a traditional single task learning, once for each additional domain). The protection of patient confidentiality during the collection, storage, and use of data must always come first. Regulatory control on healthcare is very important for patient safety and following privacy regulation.
- *Constraints and Cautions*: It is essential to detect the limitations of GAI as it may create incorrect outputs such as hallucinations or inference errors especially in critical healthcare scenarios. Use of language model outputs in high-stakes medical decision-making, particularly related to patient care and disease diagnosis using validated models alongside human validation should be governed by caution.

These factors emphasize the necessity of robust standards, moral procedures, and continuous quality-improvement initiatives to guarantee the ethical integration of GAI in healthcare environments. New research highlights the need of resolving these issues if AI is to fully benefit medical care, but it also poses threats to patient privacy and safety if appropriate precautions aren't implemented.

PRACTICAL IMPLICATIONS

- *Customized Personal Medicine*: GAI enables healthcare providers to use clinical data analytics for a deeper understanding of treatment plans, leading to better outcomes and tailored care for patients.
- *Drug Discovery*: Prediction of affinity and efficacy can be simulated by GAI drug to target interaction, assisting researchers in developing new medications or treatments more quickly and ultimately reducing the need for costly trial-and-error-based discovery processes.
- *Medical Imaging*: By communicating with medical imaging devices, GAI helps in diagnosing diseases and abnormalities. This allows patients to make treatment decisions more quickly and accurately.
- *Natural Language Processing*: GAI assists providers in aggregating unstructured medical data (e.g., clinical notes and patient histories), processing that data to gain actionable insights, and making high-quality decisions for better patient outcomes.
- *Virtual Assistants*: GAI-powered virtual assistants interact with patients, providing personalized health advice and support that could increase patient engagement and compliance with treatment plans.

CONCLUSION

The current study demonstrated the significance of GAI, particularly in terms of how it can significantly impact healthcare and other key industries through the use of potent tools and ethical conundrums. As the implications of GAI can be transformative in-patient care, through enabling personalized medicine approaches and precise diagnostics for pharmaceutical development processes. However, these advanced AI systems need responsible and fair use of ethics. As a result, if AI is to continue being effective and enjoy public trust in the context of applications, it needs to be held accountable and solved by working on issues such as algorithmic bias or privacy aspects arising from data transfer. In the age of rapid advancement in technology, it is crucial for multiple sectors, i.e., academia, healthcare professionals, policymakers, and ethicist to work together to establish robust ethical frameworks for governing use of GAI. Hence, this ensures the advantages may be utilized efficiently if unanticipated hazards are reduced.

REFERENCES

Abbasian, M, E Khatibi, I Azimi, D Oniani, Z Shakeri Hossein Abad, A Thieme, R Sriram, et al. 2024. "Foundation Metrics for Evaluating Effectiveness of Healthcare Conversations Powered by Generative AI." *Npj Digital Medicine* 7 (82). https://doi.org/10.1038/s41746-024-01074-z.

Aravinth, S S, S Srithar, K P Joseph, U Gopala Anil Varma, G M Kiran, and V Jonna. 2023. "Comparative Analysis of Generative AI Techniques for Addressing the Tabular Data Generation Problem in Medical Records." In *International Conference on Recent Advances in Science and Engineering Technology, ICRASET 2023*. Koneru Lakshmaiah Educational Foundation, Department of Computer Science and Engineering, Guntur,

India: Institute of Electrical and Electronics Engineers Inc. https://doi.org/10.1109/ICRASET59632.2023.10419886.

Arighi, C, S Brenner, and Z Lu. 2024. "Large Language Models (LLMs) and ChatGPT for Biomedicine." In *Pacific Symposium on Biocomputing*, edited by Altman R B, Hunter L, Ritchie M D, Murray T, and Klein T E, 641–644. Department of Computer and Information Sciences, University of Delaware, Ammon-Pinizzotto, Biopharmaceutical Innovation Building, 590 Avenue 1743, Newark, 19713, DE, United States: World Scientific. https://doi.org/10.1142/9789811286421_0048.

Baldassarre, A, and M Padovan. 2024. "Regulatory and Ethical Considerations on Artificial Intelligence for Occupational Medicine." *Medicina Del Lavoro* 115 (2): e2024013. https://doi.org/10.23749/mdl.v115i2.15881.

Banafa, A. 2023. *Transformative AI: Responsible, Transparent, and Trustworthy AI Systems. Transformative AI: Responsible, Transparent, and Trustworthy AI Systems.* San Jose State University, CA, United States: River Publishers. https://www.scopus.com/inward/record.uri?eid=2-s2.0-85180544759&partnerID=40&md5=c1fcd00f4b40e16156d9877185f66554.

Barker, M. 2023. "Healthcare Generative Artificial Intelligence Tools in Synthetic Patient Cases, in Medical Image Interpretation, and in Diagnosis and Treatment Plans." *Contemporary Readings in Law and Social Justice* 15 (1): 171–187. https://doi.org/10.22381/CRLSJ151202310.

Bautista, Y J P, C Theran, R Aló, and V Lima. 2023. "Health Disparities through Generative AI Models: A Comparison Study Using a Domain Specific Large Language Model." In *Lecture Notes in Networks and Systems*, edited by Arai K, 813 LNNS:220–232. Florida A&M University, Tallahassee, FL, United States: Springer Science and Business Media Deutschland GmbH. https://doi.org/10.1007/978-3-031-47454-5_17.

Bengesi, S, H El-Sayed, M.D.K Sarker, Y. Houkpati, J. Irungu, and T. Oladunni. 2024. "Advancements in Generative AI: A Comprehensive Review of GANs, GPT, Autoencoders, Diffusion Model, and Transformers." *IEEE Access* 12: 69812–69837. https://doi.org/10.1109/ACCESS.2024.3397775.

Bharath Suhas, K B, A P Sri Krishna, B Karishram, M S Roopesh, S Jothi S, K Teja, A G Kumar, and K Nandanan. 2024. "Generative AI for Community Empowerment: Transforming Livelihood Opportunities in a Rural Indian Village." In *2024 Fourth International Conference on Advances in Electrical, Computing, Communication and Sustainable Technologies, ICAECT 2024.* Coimbatore Amrita Vishwa Vidyapeetham, Amrita School of Computing, Department of Computer Science and Engineering, India: Institute of Electrical and Electronics Engineers Inc. https://doi.org/10.1109/ICAECT60202.2024.10468754.

Bietsch, D, R Stahlbock, and S Voß. 2023. "Electronic Health Data in the Context of Patient Length-of-Stay Prediction: Using Generative Adversarial Nets for Synthetic Data Creation." In *Proceedings—2023 Congress in Computer Science, Computer Engineering, and Applied Computing, CSCE 2023, 1597–1604. Lottumstr.* 18a, Berlin, 10119, Germany: Institute of Electrical and Electronics Engineers Inc. https://doi.org/10.1109/CSCE60160.2023.00262.

Chadha, N, E Popil, J Gregory, L Armstrong-Davies, and G Justin. 2024. "How Do We Teach Generative Artificial Intelligence to Medical Educators? Pilot of a Faculty Development Workshop Using ChatGPT." *Medical Teacher* 47 (1): 160–162. https://doi.org/10.1080/0142159X.2024.2341806.

Chatterjee, A, M W Gerdes, A Prinz, M A Riegler, and S G Martinez. 2024. "Semantic Representation and Comparative Analysis of Physical Activity Sensor Observations Using MOX2-5 Sensor in Real and Synthetic Datasets: A Proof-of-Concept-Study." *Scientific Reports* 14 (4634). https://doi.org/10.1038/s41598-024-55183-6.

Chen, J, C Yi, H Du, D Niyato, J Kang, J Cai, and X Shen. 2024. “A Revolution of Personalized Healthcare: Enabling Human Digital Twin with Mobile AIGC.” *IEEE Network*, 38 (6): 234–242. https://doi.org/10.1109/MNET.2024.3366560.

Coucke, P. 2024. “Generative Artificial Intelligence and Large Language Models in Healthcare.” *Revue medicale de Liege* 79 (1): 54–59. https://www.scopus.com/inward/record.uri?eid=2-s2.0-85182544171&partnerID=40&md5=28950bdd88c1e677feb9da3b53b5694c.

Davis, Fred D. 1989. “Perceived Usefulness, Perceived Ease of Use, and User Acceptance of Information Technology.” *MIS Quarterly: Management Information Systems* 13 (3): 319–339. https://doi.org/10.2307/249008.

Denecke, K, R May, and O Rivera-Romero. 2024. “Transformer Models in Healthcare: A Survey and Thematic Analysis of Potentials, Shortcomings and Risks.” *Journal of Medical Systems* 48 (23). https://doi.org/10.1007/s10916-024-02043-5.

Golda, A, K Mekonen, A Pandey, A Singh, V Hassija, V Chamola, and B Sikdar. 2024. “Privacy and Security Concerns in Generative AI: A Comprehensive Survey.” *IEEE Access* 12: 48126–48144. https://doi.org/10.1109/ACCESS.2024.3381611.

Grinbaum, A, and L Adomaitis. 2024. “Dual Use Concerns of Generative AI and Large Language Models.” *Journal of Responsible Innovation* 11 (1): 1–18. https://doi.org/10.1080/23299460.2024.2304381.

Grupac, M, A Zauskova, and E Nica. 2023. “Generative Artificial Intelligence-Based Treatment Planning in Clinical Decision-Making, in Precision Medicine, and in Personalized Healthcare.” *Contemporary Readings in Law and Social Justice* 15 (1): 45–62. https://doi.org/10.22381/CRLSJ15120233.

Harrer, S. 2023. “Attention Is Not All You Need: The Complicated Case of Ethically Using Large Language Models in Healthcare and Medicine.” *EBioMedicine* 90. https://doi.org/10.1016/j.ebiom.2023.104512.

Hayward, R. 2023. “Generative Artificial Intelligence-Driven Healthcare Systems in Medical Imaging Analysis, in Clinical Decision Support, and in Patient Engagement and Monitoring.” *Contemporary Readings in Law and Social Justice* 15 (1): 63–80. https://doi.org/10.22381/CRLSJ15120234.

Hirosawa, T, and T Shimizu. 2024. “Enhancing Clinical Reasoning with Chat Generative Pre-Trained Transformer: A Practical Guide.” *Diagnosis* 11 (1): 102–105. https://doi.org/10.1515/dx-2023-0116.

Hobensack, M, H von Gerich, P Vyas, J Withall, L.-M. Peltonen, L J Block, S Davies, et al. 2024. “A Rapid Review on Current and Potential Uses of Large Language Models in Nursing.” *International Journal of Nursing Studies* 154. https://doi.org/10.1016/j.ijnurstu.2024.104753.

Horak, J, A Novak, and L C Voumik. 2023. “Healthcare Generative Artificial Intelligence Tools in Medical Diagnosis, Treatment, and Prognosis.” *Contemporary Readings in Law and Social Justice* 15 (1): 81–98. https://doi.org/10.22381/CRLSJ15120235.

Jayakumar, P, K D Oude Nijhuis, J H F Oosterhoff, and K J Bozic. 2023. “Value-Based Healthcare: Can Generative Artificial Intelligence and Large Language Models Be a Catalyst for Value-Based Healthcare?” *Clinical Orthopaedics and Related Research* 481 (10): 1890–1894. https://doi.org/10.1097/CORR.0000000000002854.

Jindal, J A, M P Lungren, and N H Shah. 2024. “Ensuring Useful Adoption of Generative Artificial Intelligence in Healthcare.” *Journal of the American Medical Informatics Association* 31 (6): 1441–1444. https://doi.org/10.1093/jamia/ocae043.

Kovacova, M, F Kevicky, and G H Popescu. 2023. “Generative Artificial Intelligence-Driven Healthcare Systems in Patient Record Analysis, in Disease Diagnosis and Monitoring, and in Customized Treatment Plans.” *Contemporary Readings in Law and Social Justice* 15 (1): 152–170. https://doi.org/10.22381/CRLSJ15120239.

Ktena, I, O Wiles, I Albuquerque, S.-A. Rebuffi, R Tanno, A G Roy, S Azizi, et al. 2024. "Generative Models Improve Fairness of Medical Classifiers under Distribution Shifts." *Nature Medicine* 30 (4): 1166–1173. https://doi.org/10.1038/s41591-024-02838-6.

Kumar, D, R Dhalwal, and A Chaudhary. 2024. "Exploring the Ethical Implications of Generative AI in Healthcare." In *The Ethical Frontier of AI and Data Analysis*, 180–195. Lovely Professional University, India: IGI Global. https://doi.org/10.4018/979-8-3693-2964-1.ch011.

Kuzlu, M, Z Xiao, S Sarp, F O Catak, N Gurler, and O Guler. 2023. "The Rise of Generative Artificial Intelligence in Healthcare." In *12th Mediterranean Conference on Embedded Computing, MECO 2023*. Old Dominion University, Electrical Engineering Technology, Norfolk, VA, United States: Institute of Electrical and Electronics Engineers Inc. https://doi.org/10.1109/MECO58584.2023.10155107.

Lang, O, D Yaya-Stupp, I Traynis, H Cole-Lewis, C R Bennett, C R Lyles, C Lau, et al. 2024. "Using Generative AI to Investigate Medical Imagery Models and Datasets." *EBioMedicine* 102. https://doi.org/10.1016/j.ebiom.2024.105075.

Mishra, N, and K K Mishra. 2024. *A Review Study on the Challenges and Opportunities in Implementing the Metaverse in Healthcare: An Asian Perspective. IGI Global.* IGI Global. https://doi.org/10.4018/979-8-3693-2019-8.CH018.

Nedbal, C, N Naik, D Castellani, V Gauhar, R Geraghty, and B K Somani. 2024. "ChatGPT in Urology Practice: Revolutionizing Efficiency and Patient Care with Generative Artificial Intelligence." *Current Opinion in Urology* 34 (2): 98–104. https://doi.org/10.1097/MOU.0000000000001151.

Novozhilova, E, K Mays, S Paik, and J E Katz. 2024. "More Capable, Less Benevolent: Trust Perceptions of AI Systems across Societal Contexts." *Machine Learning and Knowledge Extraction* 6 (1): 342–366. https://doi.org/10.3390/make6010017.

Oniani, D, J Hilsman, Y Peng, R K Poropatich, J C Pamplin, G L Legault, and Y Wang. 2023. "Adopting and Expanding Ethical Principles for Generative Artificial Intelligence from Military to Healthcare." *Npj Digital Medicine* 6 (1). https://doi.org/10.1038/s41746-023-00965-x.

Padoan, A, and M Plebani. 2024. "Dynamic Mirroring: Unveiling the Role of Digital Twins, Artificial Intelligence and Synthetic Data for Personalized Medicine in Laboratory Medicine." *Clinical Chemistry and Laboratory Medicine (CCLM)* 62 (11): 2156–2161. https://doi.org/10.1515/cclm-2024-0517.

Puriwat, W, and S Tripopsakul. 2021. "Explaining Social Media Adoption for a Business Purpose: An Application of the Utaut Model." *Sustainability (Switzerland)* 13 (4): 1–13. https://doi.org/10.3390/su13042082.

Razmi, R M. 2023. *AI Doctor: The Rise of Artificial Intelligence in Healthcare: A Guide for Users, Buyers, Builders, and Investors. Ai Doctor: The Rise of Artificial Intelligence in Healthcare: A Guide for Users, Buyers, Builders, and Investors.* Zoi Capital, United States: Wiley. https://doi.org/10.1002/9781394240197.

Reddy, S. 2024. "Generative AI in Healthcare: An Implementation Science Informed Translational Path on Application, Integration and Governance." *Implementation Science* 19 (27). https://doi.org/10.1186/s13012-024-01357-9.

Saban, M, and I Dubovi. 2024. "A Comparative Vignette Study: Evaluating the Potential Role of a Generative AI Model in Enhancing Clinical Decision-Making in Nursing." *Journal of Advanced Nursing*. https://doi.org/10.1111/jan.16101.

Salinas-Navarro, D E, E Vilalta-Perdomo, R Michel-Villarreal, and L Montesinos. 2024. "Designing Experiential Learning Activities with Generative Artificial Intelligence Tools for Authentic Assessment." *Interactive Technology and Smart Education* 21 (4): 708–734. https://doi.org/10.1108/ITSE-12-2023-0236.

Sarkar, U. 2024. "The More Things Change, the More They Stay the Same: Understanding the Safety of Outpatient Care." *Annals of Internal Medicine* 177 (6): 824–825. https://doi.org/10.7326/M24-0876.

Sullivan, D, V P Hall, and J Morrison. 2024. "Navigating the Future: Artificial Intelligence's Impact on Transformational Nurse Leadership." *Teaching and Learning in Nursing* 19 (3): 298–300. https://doi.org/10.1016/j.teln.2024.04.017.

Umer, F, and N Adnan. 2024. "Generative Artificial Intelligence: Synthetic Datasets in Dentistry." *BDJ Open* 10 (13). https://doi.org/10.1038/s41405-024-00198-4.

Wang, F. 2024. "The Application of Intelligent Information Systems Driven by 6G Big Data in Product Sales Traceability." *Wireless Personal Communications*. https://doi.org/10.1007/s11277-024-11210-3.

Xu, Y, Z Jiang, D S W Ting, A W C Kow, F Bello, J Car, Y.-C. Tham, and T Y Wong. 2024. "Medical Education and Physician Training in the Era of Artificial Intelligence." *Singapore Medical Journal* 65 (3): 159–166. https://doi.org/10.4103/singaporemedj.SMJ-2023-203.

Yu, I.-C., and J.-M. Guo. 2024. "The Generative Artificial Intelligence Revolution in Nursing: A New Chapter in Enhancing Care Quality and Education." *Journal of Nursing* 71 (2): 12–19. https://doi.org/10.6224/JN.202404_71(2).03.

Yu, P, H Xu, X Hu, and C Deng. 2023. "Leveraging Generative AI and Large Language Models: A Comprehensive Roadmap for Healthcare Integration." *Healthcare (Switzerland)* 11 (20): 1–19. https://doi.org/10.3390/healthcare11202776.

Zhang, S, Z Q G Liau, K L M Tan, and W L Chua. 2024. "Evaluating the Accuracy and Relevance of ChatGPT Responses to Frequently Asked Questions Regarding Total Knee Replacement." *Knee Surgery and Related Research* 36 (15). https://doi.org/10.1186/s43019-024-00218-5.

8 Advancing Healthcare through Artificial Intelligence

Pioneering Solutions and Impactful Applications

Jatin Kumar, Gurmeet Singh, Vishakha Saini, Amit Chaudhary, Aruna Sharma, and Deepak Sood

INTRODUCTION

In a recent National Academy of Medicine study on current and potential benefits of artificial intelligence (AI) in healthcare, the authors noted "unprecedented opportunities" to augment the care provided by professionals, and the assistance AI provides in exploring how to overcome or go beyond human limitations, to the dangers of machine mistake. Importantly, the article has shown that there is a lot of promise attached to these technologies even with a lot of caution that would be indulged in using these technologies (Matheny et al., 2019). AI in health is fast growing and advancing as a result of the fast digitization of data related to health and the fast adoption of new technologies (Hashimoto et al., 2018; Mayo & Leung, 2018; Topol, 2019). However, big integration-related hurdles that may possibly stand in the way of deploying AI in healthcare are protection, federated learning that involves making important advances in various areas, for example, distributed optimization, large-scale machine learning (ML), and confidentiality, and performance of models and bias (Hinton et al., 2019). The centrality of technology has increased substantially in the era, as well as the industrial revolution also in terms of the growth and output (Aerts & Bogdan-Martin, 2021; Ali et al., 2023). This trend is expected to continue. Kaplan and Haenlein study in 2020 about the technical evolution in machines and how these have replaced manual and cumbersome work; this way it is promoting the improved growth of the human being. AI is one of the most important technical innovations that allowed humans, with better levels of psychological and cognitive acumen, to substitute physical effort in many fields (Bansal et al., 2020; Chien et al., 2020; Kaplan & Haenlein, 2020; Kumar et al., 2023). The target of AI is to make smart software as well as computers capable of executing this stuff, which most human beings feel must require human thought. Because of this and for other

 DOI: 10.1201/9781003531272-8

reasons, the most interesting features of AI continue to be their ability to do many tasks that humans can and to learn from past experiences, hence adapting to new inputs and environments (Chee et al., 2021; Kaplan & Haenlein, 2020). Above all, self-regulation has already specifically benefited the control of the expansion of the medical industry brought about by AI. Recent technologies of AI implemented at the moment include robots, massive data, and learning application algorithms. This sector uses these technologies for the tracing, identification, assessment of the risks of systems, and benefits in it. Throughout various AI may provide recommendations for assessment, treatment or therapeutic perspectives, and strategies at different stages of illness and the diagnostic process in addition to prescribing and using drugs for symptom reduction and encouragement of early actions that deter further deterioration of patient state (Dharani, 2021; Hossen & Karmoker, 2020). Those actions can enhance the outcomes of patients. At present, modern hospitals are looking into deploying AI technologies for enhancing clinical correctness and to reduce the cost of operating procedures. AI has developed significantly in recent years and is being used in a wide range of disciplines, including the healthcare sector, to provide various benefits. AI has replaced manual health systems with digital ones that are automated in a variety of sectors; indeed, in some instances, the human role has been reduced to more routine tasks of patients and resource, with AI elements taking over or having to be supported by complex processing (Sqalli & Al-Thani, 2019; Zhou et al., 2020).

AI-based healthcare systems are very much-rapidly evolving in present years, with the vigorous evolution focusing highly on the areas of diagnosis and early identification (Dhieb et al., 2020; Merhi, 2023; Yu & Zhou, 2021). These are actually what make it possible for AI to manipulate activities that sometimes human beings cannot manage at the cheapest, with pace and clarity, dependability, as well as comprehensiveness. Information systems (IS) developers can overcome more barriers to the technological progression associated with health digitization when they are in a position of developing effective AI systems capable of executing some tasks (Tobore et al., 2019). Creative AI thus has to be created in expanding its effectiveness and efficiency in its healthcare sector without hiking its costs since a higher number of people would need quick delivery of healthcare services. AI remains to lead in this area by providing faster and creative solutions (Comito et al., 2020; Maduri et al., 2020). Modern AI solutions in health related to surveillance, identification, and measurement of risks and benefits include robots, big data, and machine-learning software (Ali et al., 2023; Dharani, 2021). AI has digitally substituted manual health systems with automated ones in a number of industries; in some cases, individuals are now just required to do more routine patient and resource management duties (Bernardini et al., 2021; Comito et al., 2020; Yu & Zhou, 2021).

APPLICATIONS OF AI IN MEDICAL FIELD

It is also fully recognized that the tools of AI will only support and extend human labor but not substitute it wholly, subsequently replacing the physicians and other health professionals. AI will contribute to helping medical practitioners in various fields, including patient outreach and clinical assessment, administrative processing, and special assistance in image examination and monitoring patients with the help of automation of medical devices and much more. There are different opinions on how AI will be applied within the healthcare sector, though. According to Forbes' estimates, the key industries for 2018 will be in image analysis, robotic surgery, clinical decision support, administrative processes, and virtual assistants (Marr, 2018). Other topics around the ones on the above were dosages error reduction, networked equipment, and Cybersecurity; this was done by a paper published in 2018 by Accenture (Kalis et al., 2018). The following sectors were identified in a 2019 McKinsey study as relevant: electroceuticals, robotics-assisted surgery, targeted and personalized medicine, and cognitive gadgets (Carlton, 2020). The general prominent application of AI in the healthcare industry is discussed below and can be seen in Figure 8.1.

Virtual Nursing Assistance

The goal of computer science, with a specialization in artificial intelligence or AI, is to build robots that can undertake all of the above activities commonly carried out by the human brain: recognizing speech, translating languages, visual recognition, and decision-making. How AI is used in medicine is a growing trend. Moreover, global investment is inclined to be more than US $36 billion by 2025 based on continued growth, so that AI is able to incorporate the practice of medicine at the mainstream level. Some examples that are either being tested or already implemented in the health industry, and in particular the nursing sector, are predictive analytics based on ML, robotic equipment, and virtual healthcare assistant applications (Sakarovitch et al., 2014). ML is a subset of AI where normal algorithms are used to make sense of data without direct programming. The machine learns from the data and tunes its output based on the kind of data input into the machine-learning program. As such, in this regard, predictive analytics uses ML by deriving trends out of the data and predicting future health outcomes and the risk at which a patient has developing pressure ulcers. Predictive analytics have been embedded in advanced health service software to predict changes in patient diagnoses within both hospital and community contexts (Cramer et al., 2019; Sakarovitch et al., 2014). This provides nurses with an early opportunity to act and begin the appropriate treatment. In a Canadian home health service, virtual health assistant software, or chatbots, are utilized by nurses to assist individuals with mental health diagnoses (Chawla, 2020). In addition to that, Japan's nurses in their hospitals and long-term care (LTC) centers use AI-based robots to take care of patients' daily duties and to foster social contact (Maalouf et al., 2018).

Drug Delivery

AI and ML algorithms are playing an increasingly large role in biomedical research, presenting new opportunities for the optimization of drug delivery. AI could be utilized to model the mechanisms of drug delivery in an effective manner such that the best possible therapeutic effects are ascertained. AI could also be implemented

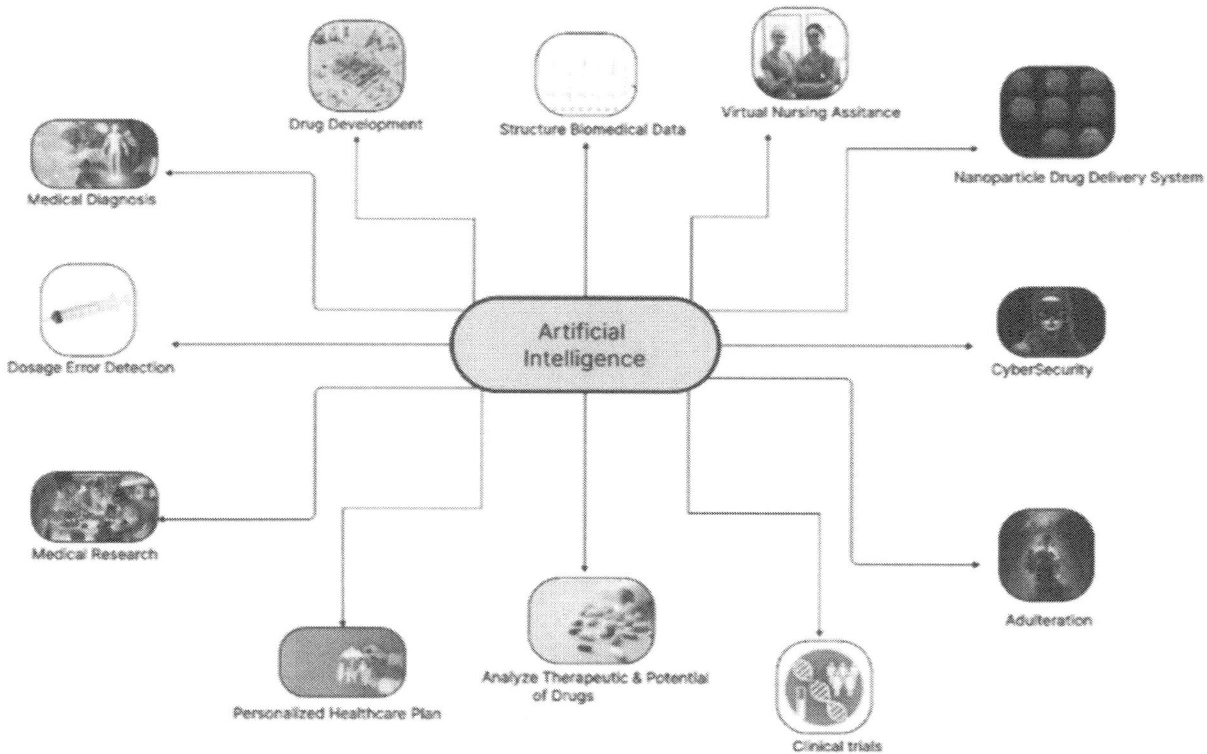

FIGURE 8.1 AI application in healthcare sector

Source: Authors' conceptualization.

for the identification of structure-function relationships between formulation factors and release kinetics (Hassanzadeh et al., 2019; Mirvakili & Langer, 2021). For example, a computer model cascade was fabricated for the prediction of the diffusivity of drugs obtained from different mucoadhesive compounds in one study (Lee et al., 2015). AI has miles to go in practical application, although it has the potential to radically change the way medicines could be presented. There is a lot more yet to do in offering improvements, providing suggestions on how to actually go about picking a ML model, and taking the bar even higher by collecting that level of data which will make the connotation of this capability of AI in the delivery of healthcare understood. Excitingly new is the direction of combining soft electronics with, say, chips, sensors, micro- or nano-robots, an external or internal power source, and drug delivery. An example is the innteliCap [AAPS] that contains temperature and pH sensors plus a microprocessor that controls both the pump and a motor that drives the release of medication (Becker et al., 2014). Another instance would be a chipped pill using a liquid auto-injector that demonstrated it can maximize the bioavailability of biologic medication, such as peptides or proteins when taken through the oral route, to up to 80% (Abramson, et al., 2022). The long-acting drug-formulation platforms to follow could be uniquely benefitted by being able to have continuously accessible data allowed with chip-to-cloud technology, based on safe, low-power microchips. This would allow the patient and the physician to monitor the release profile and implement changes as needed (Mirvakili & Langer, 2021). For example, a computer-based programmer communicating via a wireless link was used to test a drug delivery microchip designed to deliver microgram quantities of an antiosteoporosis drug once frequently for as many as three weeks to determine whether it was working as expected (Farra et al., 2012).

Cyber Security

One of the main causes by which the establishment of AI in the care system can pose a potential risk to patient safety, compromise the data pertaining to the patient, and intervene in vital health procedures is the increase in cyberattacks (Al-Mistarehi et al., 2023; Alotaibi et al., 2020). Predictive algorithms can be used to recognize and stay clear of some forms of cyberthreats. Cyber risk environment and cybersecurity related to healthcare systems will require a cautious review to protect the patients' privacy and sustain the integrity of the system itself (Alotaibi et al., 2020; Radanliev & De Roure, 2021). After all, due to the rising numbers and patterns of cyber threats, health-based organizations are forced to scale up cyber defense mechanisms. An important improvement in the field of cybersecurity could result from the use of AI in detecting and responding to threats by health organizations. Among the greatest challenges to healthcare cybersecurity is the fact that attack surfaces are on the rise, while threats multiply with a speed that has no precedent. Healthcare networks are complex ecosystems, which are multi-accessed and geographically dispersed in a number of locations. They handle untold numbers of outside suppliers and service providers. For that reason, most devices pose challenges for a security team to visualize the whole network and spot any potential vulnerabilities in their course (Telo, 2017; Zeadally et al., 2020).

Clinical Trials

Establishing safety and effectiveness of a pharmaceutical product in humans for a specific disease condition requires six to seven years' worth of clinical trials, coupled with a big investment. However, only 10% of the compounds that pass these trials get market authorization, leading to a massive loss for the industry (Hay et al., 2014). Such failures may result from poorly developed infrastructure, lack of technological standards, or inadequate patient selection. AI can, however, give back a solution in reducing such inaccuracies due to the enormous volumes of digital medical data at our disposal. As a result of increased complexity of the data and the use of contract research organizations, however, sponsor monitoring of clinical trials is becoming difficult and expensive (Harrer et al., 2019). Because risk-based monitoring (RBM) is not fully effective, with an uneven use and postponed data assessment, the advantages of this technique in terms of clarity over conventional techniques are clearer. In addition, retrospective assessments being carried out for present data quality monitoring do not effectively permit proactive risk reduction. A possible way of improving the monitoring of trials but yet reducing costs advanced is through the use of technologies that are AI/ML-assisted. These technologies, by providing real-time quality control over trial data and performance of the sites, will have the capacity to enhance present RBM procedures. Such technologies learn continuously from accumulated trial results in order to enhance risk prediction and signal identification by integrating innovative machine-learning methodologies with predictive analytics. The AI/ML systems can apply advanced analytics, quick and accurate key endpoint identification, to ensure right and complete clinical data in its entirety when evaluating data quality. In a related strain, the same technologies could be used in effective detection of problematic sites for site performance monitoring by means of adaptive learning and preset risk indicators (Paul et al., 2021; Sertkaya et al., 2016).

Analyse Therapeutic Potential of Drug

Two areas where AI-based modeling may be useful are in reducing side effects and optimizing dosing schedules. For instance, AI algorithms can help embed patient-specific information, clinical considerations, and drug release patterns into computer models so that the resulting program simulates the pharmacokinetics and pharmacodynamics of the medication (Keutzer et al., 2022). They model the predicted safety and efficacy of a drug across different dosing regimens, depending on input parameters—for example, drug concentrations in the body, dosing schedules, and patient characteristics. AI algorithms empower such research in optimizing dosing regimens to derive maximal therapeutic benefit and minimal adverse effect. Furthermore, AI can help in the identification of possible side effects or drug interactions by using vast data and identifying patterns that are not obvious through the usual methods. For better safety of the patient, the clinicians can use this data in helping them to finally decide in choosing confidently combinations or even on changing the dosage (Salas et al., 2022). Dissolution rate is a process of measuring the rate at which a dissolved medicine is likely to become accessible to its biological fluid, and therefore the magnitude to which it might be absorbed and produce a therapeutic effect. AI has made giant strides in the dissolution rates of theoretically predicted technology, which not only aid in making drugs but also in the process of fine-tuning their dosages. AI models help in reaching important physicochemical parameters and molecular features that can affect the dissolving procedure since they sort through large volumes of experimental statistics. The ML approach in the algorithms leads to the development of accurate projections as it helps in interpreting intricate correlations and patterns in the properties of the medications and the dissolution rates. While AI has many insights on the behavior of different drug formulations once they enter the process of dissolution, it is thus easy to identify formulation strategies that are effective in improving drug delivery and, at the same time, leading in the development of better systems of drug delivery (An et al., 2023). The application of AI transforms the pharmaceutical industry in numerous ways and plays a critical part in justifying the demonstrated therapeutic potentials by pharmaceuticals. One such critical area is in the research and development of novel drugs, where most algorithms within AI go through extensive data to pick the possible candidates for drugs at a searching pace faster than the conventional approach (An et al., 2023). The use of AI can accelerate the identification of new drug candidates through prediction of the interactions between particular chemicals and biological targets by analyzing biological information. Moreover, virtual screening carried out based on AI-powered algorithms can simulate molecular interactions to identify high-potential, active drug candidates. Further applications of AI include the repurposing of existing drugs by analyzing their molecular structure and biological effect for novel therapeutic uses (Naseem et al., 2020). During clinical trials, for example, AI allows for smoother patient recruiting by combing through vast datasets to quickly identify a pool of suitable candidates and to predict the response of these candidates to treatment, thus optimizing the design of the trials and thereby cutting the costs of these processes (Camarinha et al., 2014). AI contributes to pharmacovigilance through the monitoring of real-world data to detect adverse reactions and ensure drug safety for marketed pharmaceutical products. Besides, precision medicine using AI enables personalized treatment approaches to be achieved according to the data of an individual patient, taking into account such characteristics as genetically and environmentally predetermined and lifestyle-modified features. In the search for new treatments, bringing AI into use in the clinic and the making of drugs typically leads to improved patient outcomes by raising productivity and boosting innovation (Johnson et al., 2021).

Personalized Healthcare

Individualized medicine is sometimes referred to as precision healthcare or tailor-made precision health surgery. Personalized medicine in healthcare involves tailoring a patient's care and treatment options to the individual characteristics of a patient. Its customized strategy aims at resultant improved patient outcomes with more focused, economical, and secure therapies (Quazi, 2022; Subramanian et al., 2020). AI has significant importance in the field of personalized therapy since it can analyse large and complex datasets, predict outcomes, and improve therapeutic techniques. The latter issue, of precision medicine, is a medical approach where a healthcare provider (HCP) can uncover and share data that issues support for a change of a medical decision based on individual patient circumstances rather than simply the proof for a typical patient (Hartmaier et al., 2017; van der Schee et al., 2018). This allows medical practitioners to provide customized care to individual patients. It provided a gateway for opportunities that would not have existed otherwise. Two practical benefits of precision medicine early diagnosis of diseases and highly individualized treatment plan have already been taking place in the medical center (Hartmaier et al., 2017; van der Schee et al., 2018). The latest of the emerging areas is personalized treatment, which brings out the huge potential of precision medicine (Johnson et al., 2021). In another study, a ML model based on patient gene expression data was studied and it predicted treatment outcomes with high accuracy. AI has been largely devoted to diagnosis and treatment associated with detecting diseases, as far back as at least the 1970s when Stanford developed MYCIN to detect blood-borne bacterial illnesses. Such pioneering rule-based systems, among others, were applied in clinical practice even though they showed promise for accurate detection and treatment of illnesses. They did not outperform human diagnosticians and had poor integration with clinical procedures and medical record systems (Sheu et al., 2023).

Dosage Error Detection

Drug safety is the most important of the patient safety indices. Patients who incur hazardous side effects because the wrong drug is administered may be a subject to a medical malpractice suit (Rodziewicz et al. 2018) Issues related to inappropriate doses of high-alert drugs out of the totality of all pharmaceuticals are a grave cause of serious concern for the Joint Commission on Accreditation of Healthcare Organizations (JCAHO). Before it became available in the United States, physicians were using dosing nomograms based on AI and tested by researchers already published in the literature (Hu and colleagues, 2012). But nomograms are based only on the age of the patient and the international nationalized ratio (INR). For example, in drugs like warfarin, which belongs to the class of narrow therapeutic scope and in which loading levels (LLs) are very pharmacologically dense, the reference available to adjust the dose is very much unsatisfactory. Recently, most researchers have built warfarin dose prediction models upon medical and genetic data, extracted through quantitative or, more exactly, ML methods. Models for predicting dosage with warfarin were created using ML techniques based on ensemble techniques (Asiimwe et al., 2021; Zhang et al., 2022). A few ensemble techniques are applied properly to enhance the forecast accuracy with an ultimate view of developing a highly reliable prediction model (Levinson & Wu, 2021). In such instances where drugs are overdosed or underdosed in that order, drugs in excessive or minimal doses are accumulated and this results in a plethora of deleterious effects on the efficacy of some organs in the body (Bauman et al., 2007). AI has been practiced in a lot of clinical trials toward the estimation of drug dosage of digoxin, warfarin, and insulin among others (Hu et al., 2018; Simon et al., 2013).

Medical Diagnostic

Since at least the 1970s when Stanford developed MYCIN to detect blood-borne bacterial illnesses, AI has mostly concentrated on sickness diagnosis and treatment. These and other groundbreaking systems developed under the paradigms of the rules though reported to be not used in real-world clinical practice, they exhibited potential for providing precise diagnosis and treatment of the diseases. They did not outperform human diagnosticians and had poor integration with clinical procedures and medical record systems. In this regard, the emphasis that IBM's Watson has given to precision medicine in the identification and management of cancer has attracted a lot of media coverage in recent times (Bush, 2018). The most common approaches in image analysis related to cancer linked to or involving cancer are deep learning and radiomics. These computerized image analysis technologies, often referred to as CAD, appear to give better accuracy in analysis when coupled as compared to the former generation (Vial et al., 2018). Utilizing AI or big data to inform a more accurate diagnosis and treatment regime then could be provided by a human being. Most of these inferences are based on radiological image analysis (N. H. S. R. C. S. D. M. Programme & Group, 2012), although some—such as retinal scanning or genetic-based precision medicine—make use of entirely different forms of pictures (Schmidt-Erfurth et al., 2018). As such, the development of new kinds of medicine based on such statistically-conclusive ML models ought finally to usher in an entirely new era: an era usually viewed in a positive light but which necessarily poses some concomitant challenges with respect to patient-clinician interaction/medical ethics (Aronson & Rehm, 2015; Davenport & Kalakota, 2019).

Medication Discovery

Medicinal chemistry has, therefore, received quite a bit of attention with reference to AI in the sense that it is a possible game-changer for the health industry: in dealing with much testing, an arduous, and lengthy process to search for and develop new drugs in history using techniques that require much labor (Paul et al., 2021). Lately, authors have described that efficacy prediction of pharmaceutical drugs by using deep learning has been found accurate (Zhuang & Ibrahim, 2021). AI-based techniques may also predict potential toxicity of a drug candidate (Pu et al., 2019). Such and many other studies have shown that AI can potentially increase the ability, along with the accuracy, of the drug development process. However, there are limitations and constraints of AI applications for the development of new bioactive molecules. Conclusion: In the end, what AI has to offer and the difficulties it exerts can only be better understood when the field is further studied along with the ethical issues that are being addressed in the field of AI (Sakarovitch et al., 2014). Whether or not these challenges can be surpassed, the thought that the input from AI will be a telling one when it comes to the future development of new drugs and treatments cannot be denied.

Structural Biomedical Data

AI particularly plays a critical role in the biomedical health field, where it goes a long way in the transformation of patient care, diagnosis, and therapy. It is capable of sifting through large amounts of biomedical data at speeds and levels of accuracy previously unheard of through the use of complex algorithms and ML approaches, thus to provide quick diagnostic and individual treatment plans in interventions

(Alowais et al., 2023). AI-empowered imaging systems enhance the level of interpretation in medical images by enabling the clinician to identify subtle abnormalities that may be missed otherwise, thus contributing to diagnostic accuracy (Eskandar, 2023; Krishnan et al., 2023). Further, when genomics, proteomics, and clinical data resources are integrated at scale, AI algorithms are capable of uncovering novel biomarkers and therapeutic targets. AI-enabled decision support systems help clinicians select the best possible line of therapy based on the specifics of any patient's medical condition, among other relevant factors. Further, AI in patient monitoring and prediction allows for timely, proactive intervention to avoid the development of a particular disease and other adverse outcomes. All in all, AI has enormous potential to enhance biological healthcare by providing every working physician with effective tools for substantially improving patient outcomes and speeding up care delivery (Bates et al., 2021).

ADVANTAGES OF ADOPTING AI IN HEALTHCARE

Indeed, people can greatly benefit from AI in numerous ways, including easier decision-making, early diagnosis, health surveillance, and process simplification (Comito et al., 2020; Deng et al., 2019; Jahan & Tripathi, 2021; Khan et al., 2020; Ladgham et al., 2013; Minz & Mahobiya, 2017; Rahman et al., 2020; Sakkos et al., 2021; Sasubilli et al., 2020; Seeböck et al., 2018; Sqalli & Al-Thani, 2019; Strachna & Asan, 2020; Wong et al., 2019). AI has already been proven to be an effective tool in analyzing massive amounts of data and coming up with new suggestions that would be meaningful and worthwhile for the medical personnel. Eventually, these valuable suggestions would make a difference in the way the patients are managed, along with their appraisal and treatment choices. AI could be very helpful in examining such massive bulk information. Generally, a lot can be taken off in terms of time and effort while making a diagnosis and deciding as to what line of treatment to follow. Now that AI has the ability to derive decisions on their own with little to no intervention by humans, it must offer a viable solution for this problem. Indeed, it's for this effect hence presents the best tool to conquer this limitation. In this regard, as pointed out by Kaur et al. (2021), AI has even been observed to exhibit superiority over humans in some medical applications such as radiology, cardiology, and tumor diagnosis. We could assist the members of the population better cope with their chronic illnesses and reduce many of the hospital visits. This system incorporates biometric data collection devices, AI models to present health-related insights, and exclusively developed visual analytics applications to present the fetched data both textually and graphically. (Murray et al., 2019). Murray et al. observe AI has been used to tackle a wide range of issues in many studies. Another area where AI may find future use in the healthcare segment is in detecting false claims. The fraud entailed by health insurance does become a severe menace to the insurance business. The growing amount of data also grows harder and harder while trying to find fraudulent activity. Fake claims in the health insurance market identification also is a research concern to many authors (Anbarasi & Dhivya, 2017; Bagde & Chaudhari, 2016; Dhieb et al., 2020). Many benefits go to further the use of AI technology in the health field. It helps in cutting down the amount of resources and time and the cost of therapy (Rahman et al., 2021). Secondly, it minimizes the time it would take to detect an illness hence also cutting down on the time taken to make decisions. This really affects the treatment procedures and, in its most extreme outcomes, it could save a life. In the healthcare sector, there is a necessity of data sharing by different medics for the well-being of the people (Paranjape et al., 2019).

CHALLENGES OF ADOPTING AI IN HEALTHCARE

AI integration in the healthcare becomes a haystack with a myriad of obstacles and drawbacks that must be taken care of to make sure its effective and ethical utilization; for instance, the prime significant concern is the accessibility and quality of the data. In spite of its potentially strong capacity to analyse big data for prediction modeling and even decision-making, accessing databases in the healthcare setting is limited because of issues of patient records confidentiality (Lee et al., 2018; Schmidt-Erfurth et al., 2018). It is typical that institutions place a restriction on free access to health information that could potentially accelerate the development and improvement of AI algorithms. Furthermore, the latest statistics on the development of AI systems may not be readily available, which would be an obstruction to the ongoing effectiveness of the AI. Information security and confidentiality issues need also to be taken into account, combined with the sensitive nature of heath records and data gathered and accumulated surreptitiously without the consent of patients (Lee et al., 2018). Cases such as the outcry that surrounded Google's acquisition of DeepMind, and their subsequent fallouts due to privacy violations, have thus commanded the importance of stringent laws and ethical considerations in healthcare ventures using AI: Recently researchers found that even though the problems related to biases are on a large scale occurring due to the data collection process, and then feeding them into the algorithms in making decisions, the issues are both ethical and operational (Ji et al., 2020). In contrast, the biases in datasets, for instance, underrepresenting minorities, can cause these distorted results and sub-double predictive value, meaning poor-quality patient care all the more (Food & Administration, 2018; Khan et al., 2023). Furthermore, AI has a risk of overfitting, learning only specific relations of spurious data, and making incorrect predictions, which debilitates its generalization and robustness (Fernandes et al., 2020; Neill, 2013). Even more critically, most AI algorithms run as a "black box," which means that understanding and transparency of the decision process are minimal, hence a possible source of mistrust from their users toward the system they support in their operations (Wolff et al., 2020). Ethical issues further ensue on accountability and responsibility levels within an AI-driven healthcare system—for instance, uncertainty regarding liability during failures or errors in the system. In addition to these, there is no standardized guideline followed in the utilization of ethical aspects of AI in healthcare, which further increases the need for continuous efforts in frame-setting universal ethical standards and regulatory frameworks (Alami et al., 2021). Moreover, social concerns like fears of job replacement and suspicion of AI technologies also impede their general acceptation and integration into practice. The further limitation toward the realization of AI-based therapy application and full implementation inside a healthcare setting is the lack of real data for confirming their effectiveness during the conduction of a clinical study (Díaz et al., 2019). There are many issues on which work should be done in order to have AI seamlessly integrated, for example problems with user-friendliness and stakeholder engagement and how to fit it properly into existing clinical workflows (Alami et al., 2021). Furthermore, biased and discriminatory algorithms contribute to more inequality and exclusion, reiterating the importance of diversity in development teams in order to partly neutralize such bias, besides the data sources so that decisions are balanced and fair (Hagendorff, 2020).

ADOPTION OF AI IN HEALTHCARE: LEGAL AND ETHICAL CONSIDERATIONS

Through AI in healthcare, patients have significantly been taken good care of, development of therapy, and diagnosis of sickness. Minor adjustments within the sector have come along with it, though, such as the difficulties encountered when it comes to the morality and legality of its quick expansion. Major ethical issues arise through the application of algorithms based on deep learning (Moon et al., 2023). There are laws which are required for the healthcare industry to take care of such as ethical and right use of the AI technology. Investment of the private as well as the public sector for developing AI and other digital health advancement is increasing around the globe (Bozorgi, 2023). Nevertheless, issues related to the ethical concerns raised in both the development and the application of AI in medicine have not received many attentions. Liability legislation should answer the question of who is responsible for poor judgments when it comes to the use of AI in healthcare services. Ethical standards and legal and regulatory frameworks need to be developed and further enhanced to deal with the potential ethical and legal implications of the application of AI to healthcare issues. Public health issues surrounding the application of AI are mostly classified under the ethical concerns of openness, privacy, security, and responsibility.

THE FUTURE OF AI IN HEALTHCARE

AI in healthcare has the potential to vastly revolutionize patient, diagnostic, and treatment management in the future. With the increased acceptance of precision medicine, large data volumes generated from patients will be analyzed by AI systems in order to enable tailored treatment programs designed based on individual unique biological, lifestyle, and environmental features, in a way that will help reduce any adverse effects and enhance the outcomes for patients. AI-powered analysis of images will enhance diagnostic capabilities through easier detection of illnesses at early stages and the more accurate interpretation of medical representations. AI-driven methods for the development and discovery of new drugs will also hasten the process of finding new treatments, optimizing drug compositions for optimal and safe performance. Telemedicine and remote monitoring technologies are rapidly being developed to reach the point of providing personalized health advice and continuous monitoring of vital signs of both primary and underserved populations, even in remote areas. Robotic technologies would enable surgeons to perform difficult procedures more precisely and much more efficiently, whereas clinical decision support systems would further guide healthcare clinicians in making well-informed choice of treatment. Partnerships in research and innovation are set to push these frontiers even higher into the future, as solutions are sought for ethical and regulatory issues which provide privacy for the patients, information security, and algorithm transparency. Lastly, AI has the potential to change the very paradigms of healthcare service delivery into a more patient-centric, effective, and efficient framework.

REFERENCES

Abramson, A., Frederiksen, M. R., Vegge, A., Jensen, B., Poulsen, M., Mouridsen, B., Jespersen, M. O., Kirk, R. K., Windum, J., & Hubálek, F. (2022). Oral delivery of systemic monoclonal antibodies, peptides and small molecules using gastric auto-injectors. Nature Biotechnology, 40(1), 103–109.

Aerts, A., & Bogdan-Martin, D. (2021). Leveraging data and AI to deliver on the promise of digital health. International Journal of Medical Informatics, 150, 104456.

Al-Mistarehi, A.-H., Mijwil, M. M., Filali, Y., Bounabi, M., Ali, G., & Abotaleb, M. (2023). Artificial intelligence solutions for health 4.0: Overcoming challenges and surveying applications. Mesopotamian Journal of Artificial Intelligence in Healthcare, 2023, 15–20.

Alami, H., Lehoux, P., Denis, J.-L., Motulsky, A., Petitgand, C., Savoldelli, M., Rouquet, R., Gagnon, M.-P., Roy, D., & Fortin, J.-P. (2021). Organizational readiness for artificial intelligence in health care: Insights for decision-making and practice. Journal of Health Organization and Management, 35(1), 106–114.

Ali, O., Abdelbaki, W., Shrestha, A., Elbasi, E., Alryalat, M. A. A., & Dwivedi, Y. K. (2023). A systematic literature review of artificial intelligence in the healthcare sector: Benefits, challenges, methodologies, and functionalities. Journal of Innovation & Knowledge, 8(1), 100333.

Alotaibi, S., Mehmood, R., Katib, I., Rana, O., & Albeshri, A. (2020). Sehaa: A big data analytics tool for healthcare symptoms and diseases detection using Twitter, Apache Spark, and Machine Learning. Applied Sciences, 10(4), 1398.

Alowais, S. A., Alghamdi, S. S., Alsuhebany, N., Alqahtani, T., Alshaya, A. I., Almohareb, S. N., Aldairem, A., Alrashed, M., Bin Saleh, K., & Badreldin, H. A. (2023). Revolutionizing healthcare: The role of artificial intelligence in clinical practice. BMC medical education, 23(1), 689.

An, Q., Rahman, S., Zhou, J., & Kang, J. J. (2023). A comprehensive review on machine learning in healthcare industry: Classification, restrictions, opportunities and challenges. Sensors, 23(9), 4178.

Anbarasi, M., & Dhivya, S. (2017). Fraud detection using outlier predictor in health insurance data. 2017 International Conference on Information Communication and Embedded Systems (ICICES), Chennai.

Aronson, S. J., & Rehm, H. L. (2015). Building the foundation for genomics in precision medicine. Nature, 526(7573), 336–342.

Asiimwe, I. G., Zhang, E. J., Osanlou, R., Jorgensen, A. L., & Pirmohamed, M. (2021). Warfarin dosing algorithms: A systematic review. British Journal of Clinical Pharmacology, 87(4), 1717–1729.

Bagde, P. R., & Chaudhari, M. S. (2016). Analysis of fraud detection mechanism in health insurance using statistical data mining techniques. IJCSIT, 7(2), 925–927.

Bansal, A., Padappayil, R. P., Garg, C., Singal, A., Gupta, M., & Klein, A. (2020). Utility of artificial intelligence amidst the COVID 19 pandemic: A review. Journal of Medical Systems, 44, 1–6.

Bates, D. W., Levine, D., Syrowatka, A., Kuznetsova, M., Craig, K. J. T., Rui, A., Jackson, G. P., & Rhee, K. (2021). The potential of artificial intelligence to improve patient safety: A scoping review. NPJ Digital Medicine, 4(1), 54.

Bauman, J. L., DiDomenico, R. J., & Galanter, W. L. (2007). Mechanisms, manifestations, and management of digoxin toxicity in the modern era. American Journal of Cardiovascular Drugs, 6, 77–86.

Becker, D., Zhang, J., Heimbach, T., Penland, R. C., Wanke, C., Shimizu, J., & Kulmatycki, K. (2014). Novel orally swallowable IntelliCap® device to quantify regional drug absorption in human GI tract using diltiazem as model drug. AAPS PharmSciTech, 15, 1490–1497.

Bernardini, M., Romeo, L., Frontoni, E., & Amini, M.-R. (2021). A semi-supervised multitask learning approach for predicting short-term kidney disease evolution. IEEE Journal of Biomedical and Health Informatics, 25(10), 3983–3994.

Bozorgi, M. (2023). The impact of procedural law on artificial intelligence by improving the healthcare systems. In Integrating Digital Health Strategies for Effective Administration (pp. 172–192). IGI Global.

Bush, J. (2018). How AI is taking the scut work out of health care. Harvard Business Review, 5.

Camarinha-Matos, L. M., & Afsarmanesh, H. (Eds.). (2014). Collaborative Systems for Smart Networked Environments: 15th IFIP WG 5.5 Working Conference on Virtual Enterprises, PRO-VE 2014, Amsterdam, The Netherlands, October 6–8, 2014, Proceedings (Vol. 434). Springer.

Carlton, S. (2020). The era of exponential improvement in healthcare? Telehealth and Medicine Today, 5(1). Retrieved from https://telehealthandmedicinetoday.com/index.php/journal/article/view/166

Chawla, N. (2020). AI, IOT and wearable technology for smart healthcare—A review. International Journal of Recent Research Aspects, 7(1), 9–13.

Chee, M. L., Ong, M. E. H., Siddiqui, F. J., Zhang, Z., Lim, S. L., Ho, A. F. W., & Liu, N. (2021). Artificial intelligence applications for COVID-19 in intensive care and emergency settings: A systematic review. International Journal of Environmental Research and Public Health, 18(9), 4749.C

Chien, C.-F., Dauzère-Pérès, S., Huh, W. T., Jang, Y. J., & Morrison, J. R. (2020). Artificial intelligence in manufacturing and logistics systems: Algorithms, applications, and case studies. International Journal of Production Research 58(9), 2730–2731.

Comito, C., Falcone, D., & Forestiero, A. (2020). Current trends and practices in smart health monitoring and clinical decision support. 2020 IEEE International Conference on Bioinformatics and Biomedicine (BIBM), Seoul, South Korea.

Cramer, E. M., Seneviratne, M. G., Sharifi, H., Ozturk, A., & Hernandez-Boussard, T. (2019). Predicting the incidence of pressure ulcers in the intensive care unit using machine learning. eGEMs, 7(1), Article no. 49, 1–11.

Davenport, T., & Kalakota, R. (2019). The potential for artificial intelligence in healthcare. Future Healthcare Journal, 6(2), 94.

Deng, Y., Sun, Y., Zhu, Y., Xu, Y., Yang, Q., Zhang, S., Wang, Z., Sun, J., Zhao, W., & Zhou, X. (2019). A new framework to reduce doctor's workload for medical image annotation. IEEE Access, 7, 107097–107104.

Dharani, N. (2021). ANN based COVID-19 prediction and symptoms relevance survey and analysis. 2021 5th international conference on computing methodologies and communication (ICCMC), Tamil Nadu, India.

Dhieb, N., Ghazzai, H., Besbes, H., & Massoud, Y. (2020). A secure AI-driven architecture for automated insurance systems: Fraud detection and risk measurement. IEEE access, 8, 58546–58558.

Díaz, Ó., Dalton, J. A., & Giraldo, J. (2019). Artificial intelligence: A novel approach for drug discovery. Trends in Pharmacological Sciences, 40(8), 550–551.

Eskandar, K. (2023). Artificial intelligence in healthcare: Explore the applications of AI in various medical domains, such as medical imaging, diagnosis, drug discovery, and patient care. Series of Medical Science, 4(1), 37–53.

Farra, R., Sheppard Jr, N. F., McCabe, L., Neer, R. M., Anderson, J. M., Santini Jr, J. T., Cima, M. J., & Langer, R. (2012). First-in-human testing of a wirelessly controlled drug delivery microchip. Science Translational Medicine, 4(122), 122ra121–122ra121.

Fernandes, M., Vieira, S. M., Leite, F., Palos, C., Finkelstein, S., & Sousa, J. M. (2020). Clinical decision support systems for triage in the emergency department using intelligent systems: A review. Artificial Intelligence in Medicine, 102, 101762.

Food, U., & Administration, D. (2018). FDA permits marketing of artificial intelligence-based device to detect certain diabetes-related eye problems. News Release, April.

Hagendorff, T. (2020). The ethics of AI ethics: An evaluation of guidelines. Minds and Machines, 30(1), 99–120.

Harrer, S., Shah, P., Antony, B., & Hu, J. (2019). Artificial intelligence for clinical trial design. Trends in Pharmacological Sciences, 40(8), 577–591.

Hartmaier, R. J., Albacker, L. A., Chmielecki, J., Bailey, M., He, J., Goldberg, M. E., Ramkissoon, S., Suh, J., Elvin, J. A., & Chiacchia, S. (2017). High-throughput genomic profiling of adult solid tumors reveals novel insights into cancer pathogenesis. Cancer Research, 77(9), 2464–2475.

Hashimoto, D. A., Rosman, G., Rus, D., & Meireles, O. R. (2018). Artificial intelligence in surgery: Promises and perils. Annals of Surgery, 268(1), 70.

Hassanzadeh, P., Atyabi, F., & Dinarvand, R. (2019). The significance of artificial intelligence in drug delivery system design. Advanced Drug Delivery Reviews, 151, 169–190.

Hay, M., Thomas, D. W., Craighead, J. L., Economides, C., & Rosenthal, J. (2014). Clinical development success rates for investigational drugs. Nature Biotechnology, 32(1), 40–51.

Hinton, G., Obermeyer, Z., Emanuel, E., LeCun, Y., Bengio, Y., Hinton, G., Hasin, Y., Seldin, M., Lusis, A., & Sun, S. (2019). AI in health: State of the art, challenges, and future directions. Yearbook of Medical Informatics, 28(01), 016–026.

Hossen, M. S., & Karmoker, D. (2020). Predicting the probability of Covid-19 recovered in south Asian countries based on healthy diet pattern using a machine learning approach. 2020 2nd International Conference on Sustainable Technologies for Industry 4.0 (STI), Bangladesh.

Hu, Y. H., Tai, C. T., Tsai, C. F., & Huang, M. W. (2018). Improvement of adequate digoxin dosage: an application of machine learning approach. Journal of Healthcare Engineering, 2018(1), 3948245.

Hu, Y. H., Wu, F., Lo, C. L., & Tai, C. T. (2012). Predicting warfarin dosage from clinical data: A supervised learning approach. Artificial Intelligence in Medicine, 56(1), 27–34.

Jahan, R., & Tripathi, M. M. (2021). Brain tumor detection using machine learning in MR images. 2021 10th IEEE International Conference on Communication Systems and Network Technologies (CSNT), Bhopal, India.

Ji, S., Gu, Q., Weng, H., Liu, Q., Zhou, P., Chen, J., Li, Z., Beyah, R., & Wang, T. (2020). De-Health: All your online health information are belong to us. 2020 IEEE 36th International Conference on Data Engineering (ICDE), Texas, USA.

Johnson, K. B., Wei, W. Q., Weeraratne, D., Frisse, M. E., Misulis, K., Rhee, K., Zhao, J., & Snowdon, J. L. (2021). Precision medicine, AI, and the future of personalized health care. Clinical and Translational Science, 14(1), 86–93.

Kalis, B., Collier, M., & Fu, R. (2018). 10 promising AI applications in health care. Harvard Business Review, 2–5.

Kaplan, A., & Haenlein, M. (2020). Rulers of the world, unite! The challenges and opportunities of artificial intelligence. Business Horizons, 63(1), 37–50.

Kaur, A., Garg, R., & Gupta, P. (2021). Challenges facing AI and Big data for Resource-poor Healthcare System. 2021 Second International Conference on Electronics and Sustainable Communication Systems (ICESC), Tamil Nadu, India.

Keutzer, L., You, H., Farnoud, A., Nyberg, J., Wicha, S. G., Maher-Edwards, G., Vlasakakis, G., Moghaddam, G. K., Svensson, E. M., & Menden, M. P. (2022). Machine learning and pharmacometrics for prediction of pharmacokinetic data: Differences, similarities and challenges illustrated with rifampicin. Pharmaceutics, 14(8), 1530.

Khan, B., Fatima, H., Qureshi, A., Kumar, S., Hanan, A., Hussain, J., & Abdullah, S. (2023). Drawbacks of artificial intelligence and their potential solutions in the healthcare sector. Biomedical Materials & Devices, 1(2), 731–738.

Khan, M., Yaseen, Q., Mumtaz, A., Saleem, A., Ishaq, S., & Udeen, H. (2020). Severe analysis of cardiac disease detection using the wearable device by artificial intelligence. 2020 IEEE International Conference for Innovation in Technology (INOCON), Bangalore, India.

Krishnan, G., Singh, S., Pathania, M., Gosavi, S., Abhishek, S., Parchani, A., & Dhar, M. (2023). Artificial intelligence in clinical medicine: Catalyzing a sustainable global healthcare paradigm. Frontiers in Artificial Intelligence, 6.

Kumar, P., Sharma, S. K., & Dutot, V. (2023). Artificial intelligence (AI)-enabled CRM capability in healthcare: The impact on service innovation. International Journal of Information Management, 69, 102598.

Ladgham, A., Torkhani, G., Sakly, A., & Mtibaa, A. (2013). Modified support vector machines for MR brain images recognition. 2013 International Conference on Control, Decision and Information Technologies (CoDIT), Tunisia.

Lee, S.-I., Celik, S., Logsdon, B. A., Lundberg, S. M., Martins, T. J., Oehler, V. G., Estey, E. H., Miller, C. P., Chien, S., & Dai, J. (2018). A machine learning approach to integrate big data for precision medicine in acute myeloid leukemia. Nature Communications, 9(1), 42.

Lee, Y., Khemka, A., Acharya, G., Giri, N., & Lee, C. H. (2015). A cascade computer model for mocrobicide diffusivity from mucoadhesive formulations. BMC Bioinformatics, 16, 1–12.

Maalouf, N., Sidaoui, A., Elhajj, I. H., & Asmar, D. (2018). Robotics in nursing: A scoping review. Journal of Nursing Scholarship, 50(6), 590–600.

Maduri, P. K., Dewangan, Y., Yadav, D., Chauhan, S., & Singh, K. (2020). IoT based patient health monitoring portable Kit. 2020 2nd International Conference on Advances in Computing, Communication Control and Networking (ICACCCN), Greater Noida, India.

Marr, B. (2018). How is AI used in healthcare-5 powerful real-world examples that show the latest advances. Forbes, July, 27.

Matheny, M., Israni, S. T., Ahmed, M., & Whicher, D. (2019). Artificial Intelligence in Health Care: The Hope, the Hype, the Promise, the Peril. Washington, DC: National Academy of Medicine, 10.

Mayo, R. C., & Leung, J. (2018). Artificial intelligence and deep learning–Radiology's next frontier? Clinical Imaging, 49, 87–88.

Merhi, M. I. (2023). An evaluation of the critical success factors impacting artificial intelligence implementation. International Journal of Information Management, 69, 102545.

Minz, A., & Mahobiya, C. (2017). MR image classification using adaboost for brain tumor type. 2017 IEEE 7th International Advance Computing Conference (IACC), Hyderabad, India.

Mirvakili, S. M., & Langer, R. (2021). Wireless on-demand drug delivery. Nature Electronics, 4(7), 464–477.

Moon, G., Yang, J. H., Son, Y., Choi, E. K., & Lee, I. (2023). Ethical Principles and Considerations concerning the Use of Artificial Intelligence in Healthcare. Korean Journal of Medical Ethics, 26(2), 103–131.

Murray, M., Macedo, M., & Glynn, C. (2019). Delivering health intelligence for healthcare services. 2019 First International Conference on Digital Data Processing (DDP), United Kingdom.

Naseem, M., Akhund, R., Arshad, H., & Ibrahim, M. T. (2020). Exploring the potential of artificial intelligence and machine learning to combat COVID-19 and existing opportunities for LMIC: A scoping review. Journal of Primary Care & Community Health, 11, 2150132720963634.

Neill, D. B. (2013). Using artificial intelligence to improve hospital inpatient care. IEEE Intelligent Systems, 28(2), 92–95.

National Health Service Right Care Shared Decision Making Programme and Capita Group. (2012). Measuring shared decision making: A review of research evidence. In: NHS London.

Paranjape, K., Schinkel, M., Panday, R. N., Car, J., & Nanayakkara, P. (2019). Introducing artificial intelligence training in medical education. JMIR Medical Education, 5(2), e16048.

Paul, D., Sanap, G., Shenoy, S., Kalyane, D., Kalia, K., & Tekade, R. K. (2021). Artificial intelligence in drug discovery and development. Drug Discovery Today, 26(1), 80.

Pu, L., Naderi, M., Liu, T., Wu, H. C., Mukhopadhyay, S., & Brylinski, M. (2019). e toxpred: A machine learning-based approach to estimate the toxicity of drug candidates. BMC Pharmacology and Toxicology, 20, 1–15.

Quazi, S. (2022). Artificial intelligence and machine learning in precision and genomic medicine. Medical Oncology, 39(8), 120.

Radanliev, P., & De Roure, D. (2021). Epistemological and bibliometric analysis of ethics and shared responsibility—Health policy and IoT systems. Sustainability, 13(15), 8355.

Rahman, M. A., Abualsaud, K., Barnes, S., Rashid, M., & Abdullah, S. M. (2020). A natural user interface and blockchain-based in-home smart health monitoring system. 2020 IEEE International Conference on Informatics, IoT, and Enabling Technologies (ICIoT), Doha, Qatar.

Rahman, M. M., Khatun, F., Uzzaman, A., Sami, S. I., Bhuiyan, M. A.-A., & Kiong, T. S. (2021). A comprehensive study of artificial intelligence and machine learning approaches in confronting the coronavirus (COVID-19) pandemic. International Journal of Health Services, 51(4), 446–461.

Rodziewicz, T. L., Houseman, B., Vaqar, S., & Hipskind, J. E. (2018). Medical error reduction and prevention. n: StatPearls [Internet]. Treasure Island (FL): StatPearls Publishing; 2025 Jan-. Available from: https://www.ncbi.nlm.nih.gov/books/NBK499956/

Sakkos, D., Mccay, K. D., Marcroft, C., Embleton, N. D., Chattopadhyay, S., & Ho, E. S. (2021). Identification of abnormal movements in infants: A deep neural network for body part-based prediction of cerebral palsy. IEEE access, 9, 94281–94292.

Salas, M., Petracek, J., Yalamanchili, P., Aimer, O., Kasthuril, D., Dhingra, S., Junaid, T., & Bostic, T. (2022). The use of artificial Intelligence in pharmacovigilance: A systematic review of the literature. Pharmaceutical Medicine, 36(5), 295–306.

Sasubilli, S. M., Kumar, A., & Dutt, V. (2020). Machine learning implementation on medical domain to identify disease insights using TMS. 2020 International Conference on Advances in Computing and Communication Engineering (ICACCE), United States.

Schmidt-Erfurth, U., Bogunovic, H., Sadeghipour, A., Schlegl, T., Langs, G., Gerendas, B. S., Osborne, A., & Waldstein, S. M. (2018). Machine learning to analyze the prognostic value of current imaging biomarkers in neovascular age-related macular degeneration. Ophthalmology Retina, 2(1), 24–30.

Seeböck, P., Waldstein, S. M., Klimscha, S., Bogunovic, H., Schlegl, T., Gerendas, B. S., Donner, R., Schmidt-Erfurth, U., & Langs, G. (2018). Unsupervised identification of disease marker candidates in retinal OCT imaging data. IEEE Transactions on Medical Imaging, 38(4), 1037–1047.

Sertkaya, A., Wong, H.-H., Jessup, A., & Beleche, T. (2016). Key cost drivers of pharmaceutical clinical trials in the United States. Clinical Trials, 13(2), 117–126.

Sheu, Y.-h., Magdamo, C., Miller, M., Das, S., Blacker, D., & Smoller, J. W. (2023). AI-assisted prediction of differential response to antidepressant classes using electronic health records. NPJ Digital Medicine, 6(1), 73.

Simon, A. C., Holleman, F., Gude, W. T., Hoekstra, J. B., Peute, L. W., Jaspers, M. W., & Peek, N. (2013). Safety and usability evaluation of a web-based insulin self-titration system for patients with type 2 diabetes mellitus. Artificial Intelligence in Medicine, 59(1), 23–31.

Sqalli, M. T., & Al-Thani, D. (2019). AI-supported health coaching model for patients with chronic diseases. 2019 16th International Symposium on Wireless Communication Systems (ISWCS), Finland.

Strachna, O., & Asan, O. (2020). Reengineering clinical decision support systems for artificial intelligence. 2020 IEEE International Conference on Healthcare Informatics (ICHI), Germany.

Subramanian, M., Wojtusciszyn, A., Favre, L., Boughorbel, S., Shan, J., Letaief, K. B., ... & Chouchane, L. (2020). Precision medicine in the era of artificial intelligence: implications in chronic disease management. Journal of Translational Medicine, 18, 1–12.

Telo, J. (2017). AI for enhanced healthcare security: An investigation of anomaly detection, predictive analytics, access control, threat intelligence, and incident response. Journal of Advanced Analytics in Healthcare Management, 1(1), 21–37.

Tobore, I., Li, J., Yuhang, L., Al-Handarish, Y., Kandwal, A., Nie, Z., & Wang, L. (2019). Deep learning intervention for health care challenges: Some biomedical domain considerations. JMIR mHealth and uHealth, 7(8), e11966.

Topol, E. J. (2019). High-performance medicine: The convergence of human and artificial intelligence. Nature medicine, 25(1), 44–56.

van der Schee, M., Pinheiro, H., & Gaude, E. (2018). Breath biopsy for early detection and precision medicine in cancer. ecancermedicalscience, 12.

Vial, A., Stirling, D., Field, M., Ros, M., Ritz, C., Carolan, M., Holloway, L., & Miller, A. A. (2018). The role of deep learning and radiomic feature extraction in cancer-specific predictive modelling: A review. Translational Cancer Research, 7(3), 803–816.

Wolff, J., Pauling, J., Keck, A., & Baumbach, J. (2020). The economic impact of artificial intelligence in health care: Systematic review. Journal of Medical Internet Research, 22(2), e16866.

Wong, D. L. T., Yu, J., Li, Y., Deepu, C. J., Ngo, D. H., Zhou, C., Singh, S. R., Koh, A., Hong, R., & Veeravalli, B. (2019). An integrated wearable wireless vital signs biosensor for continuous inpatient monitoring. IEEE Sensors Journal, 20(1), 448–462.

Wu, H., & Levinson, D. (2021). The ensemble approach to forecasting: A review and synthesis. Transportation Research Part C: Emerging Technologies, 132, 103357.

Yu, H., & Zhou, Z. (2021). Optimization of IoT-based artificial intelligence assisted telemedicine health analysis system. IEEE Access, 9, 85034–85048.

Zeadally, S., Adi, E., Baig, Z., & Khan, I. A. (2020). Harnessing artificial intelligence capabilities to improve cybersecurity. IEEE Access, 8, 23817–23837.

Zhang, F., Liu, Y., Ma, W., Zhao, S., Chen, J., & Gu, Z. (2022). Nonlinear machine learning in warfarin dose prediction: Insights from contemporary modelling studies. Journal of Personalized Medicine, 12(5), 717.

Zhou, L., Li, Z., Zhou, J., Li, H., Chen, Y., Huang, Y., Xie, D., Zhao, L., Fan, M., & Hashmi, S. (2020). A rapid, accurate and machine-agnostic segmentation and quantification method for CT-based COVID-19 diagnosis. IEEE Transactions on Medical Imaging, 39(8), 2638–2652.

Zhuang, D., & Ibrahim, A. K. (2021). Deep learning for drug discovery: a study of identifying high efficacy drug compounds using a cascade transfer learning approach. Applied Sciences, 11(17), 7772.

9 The XAI Factor in the Age of AI

Does It Enhance AI Augmented Decision-Making Quality in HealthCare HR

Saladi Jaswanth Seshasai and K D Balaji

INTRODUCTION: EVOLUTION OF AI IN HEALTHCARE HR DECISION-MAKING

Early Stages: Foundational Automation

At the beginning of the artificial intelligence (AI) usage in healthcare human resources (HR), the approaches were more primitive, aimed at the automation of the most basic processes, including payroll and scheduling (Singla and Kumar 2024). It was evident that usage of AI systems was effective in automation of these processes to optimally free up the time of the HR professionals for more strategic work. This early phase became the foundational phase by demonstrating the usefulness of AI in the repetitive tasks of sorting data with precision. However, the focus on operations' productivity established the conditions and expectations of future evolutions, demonstrating how AI can revolutionize HR undertakings for healthcare environments. Hence, the initial phase of automation laid the ground for taking advantage of the possibilities that AI offers to increase the efficiency of resource utilization and consequently, the organizational efficiency in the HR departments (Singla 2024).

Mid-Stages: Predictive Insights and Strategic Planning

With the progression of AI technologies especially with the incorporation of explainable AI (XAI), healthcare HR decision-making moved from a descriptive analysis to one that was predictive and more in line with strategic planning. This stage received a boost from XAI in that deeper explanation of what AI was suggesting was provided and made easier to understand large numbers of data flows to recognizing glimpses of meaningful patterns about the employees' performance and turnover rate with various other aspects of the workforce. Finally, such a shift ensured that HR leaders could understand the rationale for AI-made proposals and consequently make informed decisions. Regarding operations and deliveries, predictive analytics

DOI: 10.1201/9781003531272-9

allowed for more effective quantitative predictions of staffing requirements and possible employee turnovers, as well as a multitude of detailed plans that could be strategically developed to meet organizational objectives. Thus, XAI-driven thinking can elevate the quality of the decision-making process besides encouraging proactive approach to organize HR in healthcare organizations.

IMPORTANCE OF TRANSPARENCY AND INTERPRETABILITY (XAI)

In the context of the healthcare HR field, using a relatively unexplored research orientation based on a phenomenological process facilitates getting to know how XAI impacts the quality of decisions. In this particular context, phenomenology examines different actors and their expectations, considerations, and perspectives of employing XAI within the HR field, the clinics' staff, and administration. Transparency and easier interpretability are the two main concepts that are closely associated with the role XAI has on the decision-making process. Another valuable contribution of phenomenology is that precise descriptions of AI algorithms help to increase trust and accountability among the stakeholders since it does not leave them in the dark regarding the logic behind the decisions made. This transparency also contributes to reinforcement of trust in the AI decisions besides ensuring compliance with the ethical and legal requirements (Liao, Yang, & Wan 2020).

Equally, phenomenology reveals how XAI reduces biases in traditional practices to select and promote people in the organization. Basically, through making the decision-making process transparent, XAI enables the revelation and modification of parameters that perhaps could lead to biased decision-making as a result of gender, ethnicity, or any other sensitive aspect (Holzinger et al. 2018). This approach ensures that there is balance and equality when it comes to the decisions that are made in the Human Resource Management (HRM) department for the workers, thus creating a favorable environment. Furthermore, as a result of interpretability, the organization can promptly address the areas that need enhancements in terms of HR practices. Phenomenological studies emphasize that getting an insight into the mechanisms for generating the recommendations facilitates the enhancement of the strategies and enables the HR professionals to align the decision-making process with organizational objectives. Such a process of continuous refinement is particularly relevant to deal with the shifting nature of healthcare settings and productivity of human labor (Topol 2019).

Moreover, the roles and interactions between the HR, clinical staff, and managers within the collaborative setting enabled by XAI are examined from phenomenological viewpoints. In particular, the present study highlights how through operating informational work and fostering common ground on AI ideas, effective communication enhances the complex processes of decision-making about the workforce planning, skill development, and succession planning which are critically important for patient care quality and organizational success. Therefore, by proposing the application of phenomenology when examining XAI in the context of healthcare's HR—one can see the magic of this approach. On the same note, XAI does not only make it possible to optimize the operational efficiencies since it increases transparency, reduces biases, encourages continual improvement, and promotes collaboration, but it also enhances ethical integrity in healthcare provision to deliver its services.

STATEMENT OF PROBLEM

The gap in the present understanding revolves around evaluating the consequences of XAI on the decision-making front in healthcare HR in the long run. While this paper outlined a trajectory of XAI and its early applications to tasks involving recruitment and performance evaluation, further research is still needed to understand how XAI's impacts might persistently manifest in other vital and fascinating HR strategies. Some of the areas that lack studies include: Whether it has a positive impact on the employee retention, career development, and in general on the formulation of healthcare HR policies. This lack of understanding prevents healthcare organizations from maximizing on XAI's application for enhancing the quality of the decisions made over time. Due to the lack of multifaceted guidelines and research findings, XAI may not be integrated into healthcare HRM professionals' strategic agendas in a way that would ensure its positive impact on organizational environment and workforce development while avoiding unethical approaches in the long term.

RESEARCH GAP

However, current investigation is mostly centered on examining XAI's effects on the short-term factors that affect tasks like recruitment and performance appraisal, aspects that have not been explored regarding strategic management, workforce development, and culture, especially in the context of healthcare organizations. In particular, there is insufficient research regarding how XAI may help supplemented long-term strategies for employee retention, advancement programs, and general HR practices redesign. Filling this void is important to establish inclusive frameworks that can enable the implementation of XAI in the healthcare HR practices to enhance its effectiveness of the useful information contents in facilitating ethically sound and operationally efficient decision-making processes in the appropriate future-related contexts.

REVIEW OF LITERATURE

The purpose of this paper is to highlight the importance of XAI in the applications that are crucial such as healthcare, law, and defense. From it, current XAI methods are discussed, with criticisms regarding to limitations in post-hoc methods and the absence of contrastive and counterfactual explanation. To fill these gaps, the study presents an ante-hoc methodology that uses argumentative reasoning, thus making the model's rationale more comprehensible to humans. Alzheimer's disease diagnostics highlighted here reveals its ability to solve decision performance and explainability from the case studies (Zeng et al. 2022).

This article provides a brief of the current state of research and development of XAI in healthcare, focusing on the capability of XAI to explain the hidden, thus reducing the doubt in the models. Carried out with reference to the PRISMA method on three databases including PubMed, Science Direct, and the Web of Science, the study assesses LIME, SHAP, and PDP XAI techniques on a diabetes dataset. It is also identified that there is still a lack of interpretability for more complex models and clearer explanations so as to help medical professionals and patients, therefore, stimulating more investigation in the biomedical usage of XAI (Gupta et al. 2024).

The paper focuses on what XAI is as well as its capabilities of improving the levels of transparency, trust, and understanding of the decisions made by artificial intelligence systems. Dividing XAI into methods such as feature importance analysis, model interpretability, and natural language explanation, the paper demonstrates these techniques' potential in areas like healthcare, finance, and self-driving cars. The work also discusses the shortcomings and constraints of XAI and also to state that there is a requirement for enhanced studies in order to comprehend the impact of utilizing various XAI solutions and to deal with the implementation obstacles in certain fields. (Tiwari 2023).

From Figure 9.1, this research proposes an implementation-oriented framework to assess XAI models for clinical decision-making applications. It highlights mixed outcomes: Whereas explanation makes medical service safer and more trustworthy toward healthcare providers (HCPs), such problems as confirmation bias or overdependence on these models appear. Nevertheless, these reasons reduce automation bias, help in the case of the ambiguous decision, and provide information to fewer experienced HCPs on how to treat patients and change their role in clinical facilities. (Wysocki et al. 2023).

This study focuses on XAI in the healthcare sector since it is important to have transparency in AI systems in important fields. It discusses XAI techniques including feature-based and human-centric techniques, and it brings out the importance of explaining AI systems. Thus, discussing healthcare issues, the work highlights the importance of XAI in safety-critical settings, intending to contribute to the development of a better understanding of its uses and experimental findings in this critical area (Sadeghi et al. 2024).

RESEARCH MODEL

Research Model

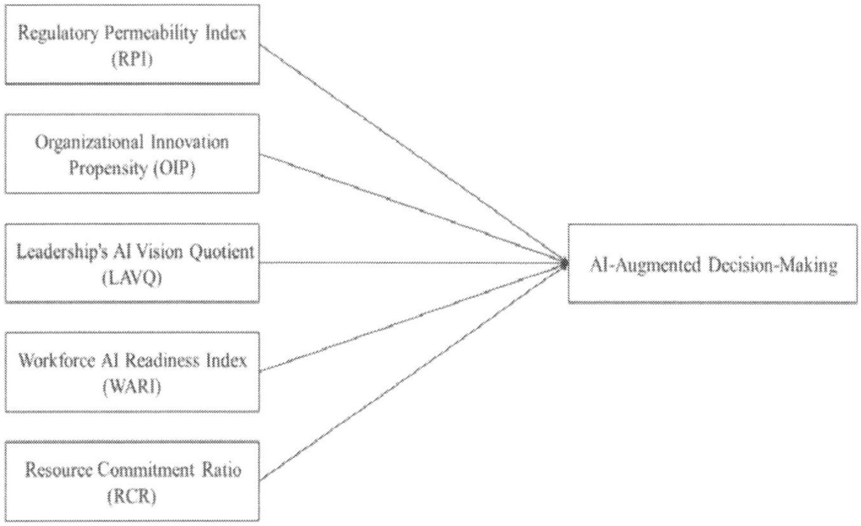

FIGURE 9.1 Research model on AI augmented decision-making.

Source: Authors' own research.

RESEARCH METHODOLOGY

From Table 9.1, the study sample comprised 268 participants with varied roles in the HR department, mainly general/specialist HR (28.7%) and recruiters (20.9%). The majority of the participants had 5–15 years of experience (60%), worked in medium-sized organizations (40.3%), and were employed in hospitals (44.8%). Half of the respondents had only a limited or moderate experience with AI in HR, which shows that while it is a developing field, it is not yet fully established. The gender distribution was slightly biased toward the male participants (53.4%). This diverse sample enables one to understand the views of different HR professionals on the application of AI in healthcare.

From Table 9.2, The organization is moderately ready for AI integration based on the average scores in all the dimensions. The regulatory environment index (RPI) is high and resource commitment index (RCR) also shows a favorable position; however, a small relative weakness is identified in workforce readiness index (WARI), which can be improved through training and skill development programs. Leadership vision (LAVQ) and AI-augmented decision-making (ADM) are moderate and can be

TABLE 9.1
Demographic Profile

Demographic Variable	Categories	Number of Participants (N)	Percentage (%)
Role	HR Manager/Director	42	15.70%
	HR Generalist/Specialist	77	28.70%
	Recruiter	56	20.90%
	Talent Management Professional	35	13.10%
	Other (Please Specify)	58	21.60%
Years of Experience in HR	Less than 5 years	62	23.10%
	5–10 years	88	32.80%
	11–15 years	73	27.20%
	16+ years	45	16.80%
Organization Size	Small (Less than 100 employees)	55	20.50%
	Medium (100–500 employees)	108	40.30%
	Large (501+ employees)	105	39.20%
Type of Healthcare Organization	Hospital	120	44.80%
	Clinic	75	28.00%
	Long-term care facility	43	16.00%
	Other (please specify)	30	11.20%
Familiarity with AI in HR	No prior experience	72	26.90%
	Limited experience	95	35.40%
	Moderate experience	66	24.60%
	Extensive experience	35	13.10%
Gender	Male	143	53.40%
	Female	125	46.60%

TABLE 9.2
Reliability Table

Regulatory Permeability Index (RPI)	0.742
Organizational Innovation Propensity (OIP)	0.719
Leadership's AI Vision Quotient (LAVQ)	0.712
Workforce AI Readiness Index (WARI)	0.699
Resource Commitment Ratio (RCR)	0.734
AI Augmented Decision-Making (ADM)	0.703

improved to maximize the use of AI. In general, the organization is ready for the introduction of AI with some emphasis on certain areas.

From Table 9.3, The results show a good variability of scores on all six indices and a fixed number of participants equal to 268. Average rating is usually between 6 and 25 to demonstrate that opinions are quite diverse. Nonetheless, although slightly negatively skewed, which means that the majority of the values are shifted toward higher values, the standard deviation is still consistently equal to 3.5, which shows that the data is reasonably spread out. The kurtosis values are approximately 3, which indicates that the distribution of scores for each measure is slightly more than the normal distribution and has heavier tails. In conclusion, these descriptive statistics give a positive impression of the dataset, the variability of which indicates that it could be useful for further analysis.

From Table 9.4, The correlation table shows that all the pairs of variables are positively correlated with one another. It is noteworthy that all coefficients of correlation are significant at $p < .001$ level. The highest value of the coefficient of determination is observed between LAVQ and ADM with the coefficient of determination of .768. Other pairs also show a high level of correlation; these

TABLE 9.3
Descriptive Statistics

Descriptive Statistics

	N	Minimum	Maximum	Std. Deviation	Skewness		Kurtosis	
	Statistic	Statistic	Statistic	Statistic	Statistic	Std. Error	Statistic	Std. Error
RPI	268	6.00	25.00	3.60332	−1.706	.149	2.984	.297
OIP	268	8.00	25.00	3.42552	−1.492	.149	2.160	.297
LAVQ	268	6.00	25.00	3.50353	−1.753	.149	2.974	.297
WARI	268	6.00	24.00	3.35203	−1.701	.149	2.928	.297
RCR	268	6.00	25.00	3.54207	−1.603	.149	2.719	.297
ADM	268	7.00	24.00	3.41183	−1.685	.149	2.670	.297
Valid N (listwise)	268							

TABLE 9.4
Correlation Table

		RPI	OIP	LAVQ	WARI	RCR	ADM
RPI	Pearson Correlation	1	.716**	.753**	.725**	.742**	.740**
	Sig. (2-tailed)		.000	.000	.000	.000	.000
	N	268	268	268	268	268	268
OIP	Pearson Correlation	.716**	1	.723**	.749**	.714**	.749**
	Sig. (2-tailed)	.000		.000	.000	.000	.000
	N	268	268	268	268	268	268
LAVQ	Pearson Correlation	.753**	.723**	1	.741**	.737**	.768**
	Sig. (2-tailed)	.000	.000		.000	.000	.000
	N	268	268	268	268	268	268
WARI	Pearson Correlation	.725**	.749**	.741**	1	.752**	.757**
	Sig. (2-tailed)	.000	.000	.000		.000	.000
	N	268	268	268	268	268	268
RCR	Pearson Correlation	.742**	.714**	.737**	.752**	1	.730**
	Sig. (2-tailed)	.000	.000	.000	.000		.000
	N	268	268	268	268	268	268
ADM	Pearson Correlation	.740**	.749**	.768**	.757**	.730**	1
	Sig. (2-tailed)	.000	.000	.000	.000	.000	
	N	268	268	268	268	268	268

include WARI and ADM (r = .757), RPI and LAVQ (r = .753), and WARI and RCR (r = .752). The rest of the correlations, although still generally considered strong, are slightly lower in value, ranging from .714 (OIP and RCR) to .749 (OIP and ADM, OIP and WARI). All in all, these findings indicate that the variables in this dataset are strongly correlated.

From Table 9.5, The regression model explains 71.4% of the variance in the dependent variable (R Square). The adjusted R square of .709 suggests this model's explanatory power is robust and not inflated by the number of predictors. The standard error of the estimate (1.84106) indicates the average distance the observed values

TABLE 9.5
Regression Table

Model Summary

					Change Statistics				
Model	R	R Square	Adjusted R Square	Std. Error of the Estimate	R Square Change	F Change	df1	df2	Sig. F Change
1	.845[a]	.714	.709	1.84106	.714	130.992	5	262	.000

[a] Predictors: (Constant), RCR, OIP, LAVQ, RPI, WARI

fall from the regression line. The change statistics reveal that including the predictors (RCR, OIP, LAVQ, RPI, WARI) significantly improved the model's ability to predict the dependent variable, as evidenced by the large F change value (130.992) with a p-value of .000.

ANOVA[a]

Model		Sum of Squares	df	Mean Square	F	Sig.
1	Regression	2219.982	5	443.996	130.992	.000[b]
	Residual	888.048	262	3.389		
	Total	3108.030	267			

[a] Dependent Variable: ADM

[b] Predictors: (Constant), RCR, OIP, LAVQ, RPI, WARI

The ANOVA table shows that the regression model is highly significant with F-Statistic of 130.992 and the p-value of .000. This means that the predictors (RCR, OIP, LAVQ, RPI, WARI) taken as a whole account for a significant proportion of the variation in the dependent variable, ADM. In particular, the model explains 2219.982 of the overall 3108. 030 sum of squares which indicates that the predictors used are useful in predicting ADM.

Coefficients[a]

Model		Unstandardized Coefficients		Standardized Coefficients		
		B	Std. Error	Beta	t	Sig.
1	(Constant)	1.175	.702		1.673	.096
	RPI	.150	.055	.158	2.726	.007
	OIP	.212	.056	.213	3.779	.000
	LAVQ	.251	.057	.258	4.399	.000
	WARI	.206	.061	.202	3.402	.001
	RCR	.114	.056	.119	2.033	.043

[a] Dependent variable: ADM.

The regression analysis shows that all the predictor variables (RPI, OIP, LAVQ, WARI, RCR) have a positive and significant relationship with the dependent variable, ADM at $p < .05$ level of significance except the constant term. Among them, OIP and LAVQ have the greatest impact on the results, while WARI, RPI, and RCR have a slightly smaller effect. In particular, the increase in OIP or LAVQ by 1 unit results in the decrease of the dependent variable by 0.212 or. An increase of 251 units in ADM and a 251 units increase in ADM, respectively. The model accounts for a good amount of variance in ADM, meaning these factors are relevant predictors.

FINDINGS

Demographics

- Diverse Roles: In line with the above, most of the HR professionals in the study served in different roles; generalists/specialists (n = 28.7%) and recruiters (n = 20.9%).
- Experienced Professionals: Majority of participants have 5 to 15 years of experience, although a few have up to 30 years' experience in HR, most of which are middle aged and educate profession, this makes the sample reasonable mature.
- Medium-Sized Organizations: Interestingly, the most numerous groups were the participants employed in medium-sized healthcare organizations, occupied from 100 to 500 people (40.3%).
- Hospital Setting: Hospitals were the most common locations with 44.8% of the participants.
- Growing AI Familiarity: Regarding the experience with AI in HR: 60% of the participants indicated they have limited or moderate experience, which may imply that this is a developing area.
- Gender Imbalance: With regards to the gender of the participants, more of the students were male (53.4%).

Organization's AI Preparedness

- Overall Preparedness: The level of preparedness for integrating AI in the company's operations was found to be moderately high in all the identified dimensions by the organization (Reliability from Figures 9.2 and 9.3).
- Strengths: This showed an exceptional position in regulatory receptiveness (RPI) as well as the resources control (RCR).
- Potential Growth Areas: Workforce readiness (WARI) provided the area for latent enhancement.
- Moderate Scores: The results reveal that LAVQ was moderately developed, as was ADM; both need future improvements.

Descriptive Statistics

- Wide Score Distribution: Regarding the responses from survey about six measures it ranged from 6 to 25 which is indicating the variability.
- Slight Negative Skew: Based on the analysis of the data we have found that the data was somewhat biased toward complex values which indicate that the perception of AI as seen by the participants is rather positive.
- Reasonable Spread: Standard deviation around 3.5 is considered as significant and described a good spread of data.
- Peaked Distribution: A value of kurtosis equal to 3 is considered to oblique somewhat additional a peaked distribution than normal.

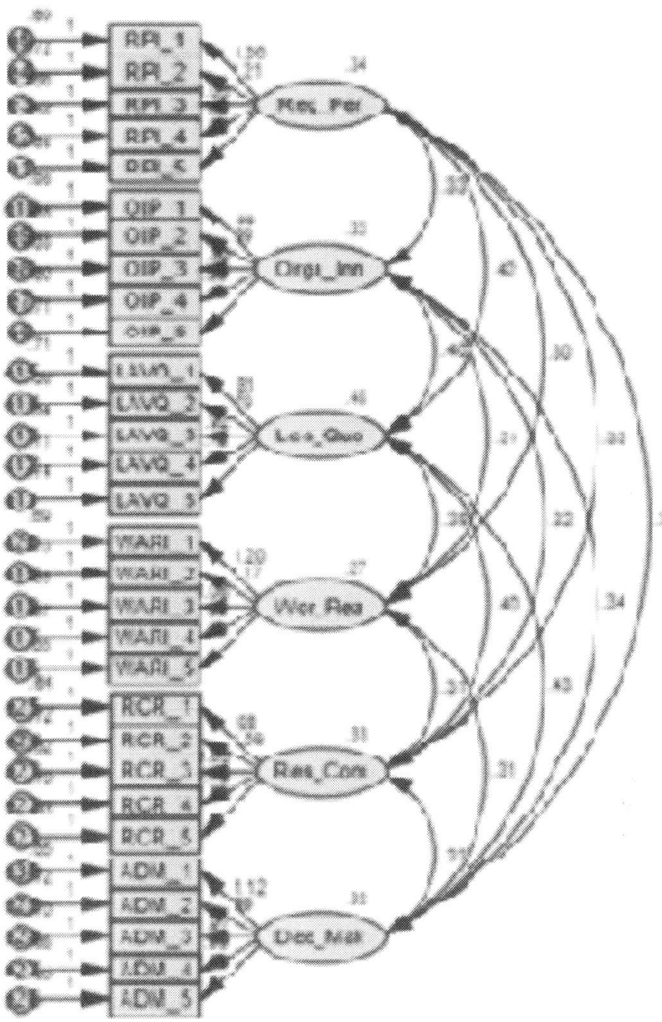

FIGURE 9.2 Confirmatory factor analysis.

Source: Authors' own research.

Correlations

- Strong Positive Relationships: The results revealed that all the pairs of the variables had a positive correlation, which implies that they move in the same direction.
- Strongest Correlations: The highest level of association was found between leadership's AI vision (LAVQ) and AI-augmented decision making (ADM). Other significant relationships were also noted between WARI and ADM, RPI and LAVQ, and WARI and RCR.

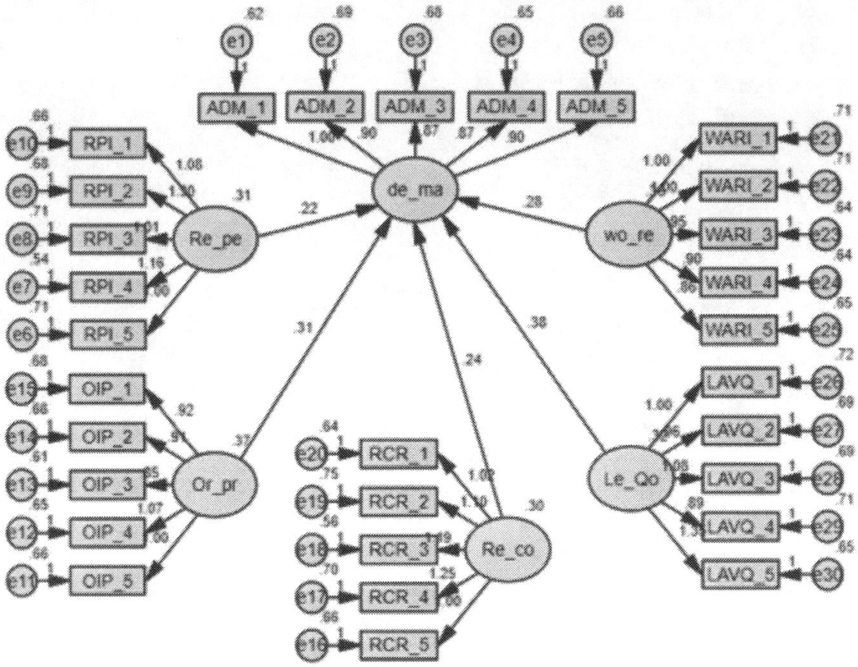

FIGURE 9.3 SEM model.

Source: Authors' own research.

Regression

- Significant Predictors: The results of the study indicated that all the independent variables (RPI, OIP, LAVQ, WARI, RCR) had a significant impact on the dependent variable, ADM which is the AI-augmented decision-making.
- Strongest Predictors: The results also depicted that the factors having the highest impact on ADM include organizational innovation propensity (OIP) and leadership's AI vision (LAVQ).
- Explanatory Power: The model explained 71% of the total score of the variables used in the study. These factors contribute to explaining AI use in decision-making, and they explain 4% of the variance in ADM.

FUTURE DIRECTIONS

Further research in the context could look at adopting new approaches like neurosymbolic AI to enhance the decision-making process in the healthcare HR. Evaluating the ethical issues and bias of XAI systems in the complicated medical environment will be important, as well as designing new AI structures that integrate deep learning with symbolic computation to enhance the interpretability of the model without compromising the model's performance. In addition, the ways of applying reinforcement learning in enhancing HR distribution depending on XAI results can upgrade the process of managing a workforce in healthcare. Exploring the possibilities of using quantum computing to improve XAI's computational speed and security for healthcare data may also be another interesting area of research. Last but not the least, it will be crucial to examine the possibilities of interdisciplinary cooperation between AI researchers, ethicists, and healthcare practitioners to address the multifaceted socio-technical nature of XAI in healthcare HR decision-making.

CONCLUSION

Consequently, this extensive study highlights the prospect of XAI as the key to revolutionize decision-making in healthcare HR for enhancing the transparency and credibility of AI. Hence, our study complexly theorizes how compliance, an innovative culture and vision in AI leadership, diversions in resource provisioning and organizational workforce preparedness define the successful application and impact of XAI. These contribute not only to the XAI inclusion but are also vitally important as the key moderators to the improvement of the quality and credibility of the decisions made with the help of AI in the sphere of healthcare HR. The results support highlighting the need for healthcare organizations to make XAI implementation a high-priority business goal. Therefore, through demanding and promoting the appropriate regulation for XAI and by continuing the culture of innovation in AI application, it is possible to benefit from effective AI use while dealing with the problem associated with explanations of algorithms. In this regard, developing leadership with AI literacy and guaranteeing adequate resources are cited as the most important factors that can enhance the utilization of XAI advantages by a skilled workforce. HR specialists will also benefit from the study because it underscores the need to gain experience in explaining and applying AI-driven decision-making, which would allow them to be efficient in multifaceted AI-mediated HR tasks. Thus, the frameworks intended for responsible use of AI are supposed to be studied thoroughly, allowing to avoid possible negative impacts on clinical environments. Finally, but importantly, the research contributes significantly to theoretical development while providing stakeholders with valuable recommendations to safely implement XAI in the process of improving the organizational decision-making process and innovation in healthcare HR fields.

REFERENCES

Holzinger, A., G. Langs, H. Denk, and K. Zatloukal. "Machine learning and artificial intelligence in bioinformatics." Journal of Computational Biology 25.4 (2018): 357–396.

Liao, P., T. Yang, and P. Wan. "Understanding the black box: A model-agnostic approach for interpretable machine learning." BMC Bioinformatics 21.suppl. 13 (2020): 382.

Sadeghi, Zahra, Roohallah Alizadehsani, Mehmet Akif CIFCI, Samina Kausar, Rizwan Rehman, Priyakshi Mahanta, Pranjal Kumar Bora et al. "A review of explainable artificial intelligence in healthcare." Computers and Electrical Engineering 118 (2024): 109370. https://doi.org/10.4018/ijabim.325229

Singla, B., and Shalender Kumar, eds. AI Healthcare Applications and Security, Ethical, and Legal Considerations. Hershey, PA: IGI Global, 2024. https://doi.org/10.4018/979-8-3693-7452-8

Singla, B., Shalender Kumar, and Stamer Katja, eds. Revolutionizing the Healthcare Sector with AI. Hershey, PA: IGI Global, 2024. https://doi.org/10.4018/979-8-3693-3731-8

Tiwari, Rudra. "Explainable AI (XAI) and its applications in building trust and understanding in AI decision making." International Journal of Scientific. Research in Engineering and Management 7 (2023): 1–13.

Topol, E. J. "High-performance medicine: The convergence of human and artificial intelligence." Nature Medicine 25.1 (2019): 44–56.

Wysocki, Oskar, Jessica Katharine Davies, Markel Vigo, Anne Caroline Armstrong, Dónal Landers, Rebecca Lee, and André Freitas. "Assessing the communication gap between AI models and healthcare professionals: Explainability, utility and trust in AI-driven clinical decision-making." Artificial Intelligence 316 (2023): 103839.

Zeng, A. G. X., S. Bansal, L. Jin, A. Mitchell, W. C. Chen, H. A. Abbas, M. Chan-Seng-Yue, V. Voisin, P. van Galen, A. Tierens, M. Cheok, C. Preudhomme, H. Dombret, N. Daver, P. A. Futreal, M. D. Minden, J. A. Kennedy, J. C. Y. Wang, and J. E. Dick. "A cellular hierarchy framework for understanding heterogeneity and predicting drug response in acute myeloid leukemia." Nature Medicine 28.6: 1212–1223. https://doi.org/10.1038/s41591-022-01819-x

10 AI Adoption Challenges in Healthcare

Sailee Chowdhury, Shayeri Chatterjee Ganguly, Ramesh Kumari Dasgupta, Priyanka Chakraborty, Banani Mondal, and Ananya Bhowmick

INTRODUCTION

The union of artificial intelligence (AI) and healthcare is poised to transform the well-being of patients, diagnostics, and treatment outcomes (Alowais et al. 2023). From drug discovery to personalized medicine, AI's potential to enhance healthcare delivery is immense. However, despite significant advancements, widespread adoption of AI in clinical settings remains hindered by a complex interplay of challenges. This chapter explores the key roadblocks that limit the incorporation of AI into the healthcare mainstream (Bajwa et al. 2021). It also examines the diversified role of AI in the field of healthcare, focusing on its contributions to the diagnosis, treatment, and multifaceted obstacles hindering the widespread in healthcare. One of the most significant hurdles in the adoption of AI is the scarcity of high-quality medical data. AI for healthcare needs massive amounts of clean, structured data to train and test its algorithms. Unfortunately, healthcare data is far from ideal. Medical records are scattered across different hospitals and clinics, often formatted inconsistently (Agrawal and Prabakaran 2020; Wang, Pershing, and Lee 2020). Even sharing this data is complicated due to privacy regulations. This lack of high-quality data creates a double threat. First, AI algorithms might inherit biases present in the data, worsening existing healthcare inequalities. Second, these algorithms might simply not work well in real-world situations because they haven't been trained on real-world data (David Rodriguez 2024; Schwendicke, Samek, and Krois 2020). Another challenge is the amalgamation of AI into prevailing clinical settings. Many healthcare facilities still grapple with outdated IT infrastructure, making it difficult to seamlessly integrate AI tools (Harnett 2018). Clinicians, already burdened by time constraints, may be resistant to adopting new technologies that require additional training or disrupt their established routines (Lunceford 2009; Safi, Thiessen, and Schmailzl 2018). Furthermore, a lack of clear guidelines and protocols for utilizing AI in decision-making can lead to confusion and hinder trust among healthcare professionals (Reddy et al. 2020). The issue of trust and transparency is paramount. AI algorithms are often complex "black boxes," rendering it troublesome for clinicians to comprehend how they attain their commendations (Bernal and Mazo 2022; Kiseleva, Kotzinos, and De Hert 2022; Mennella et al. 2024). This lack of transparency can breed skepticism and reluctance to rely on AI-generated insights (Wanner et al. 2022). Additionally, concerns regarding potential bias in algorithms,

DOI: 10.1201/9781003531272-10

particularly if trained on imbalanced datasets, can raise ethical and legal questions about fairness and patient safety. Regulatory hurdles are a major roadblock for the progression of AI in medical and pharmaceutical grounds (McKee and Wouters 2022; Mennella et al. 2024). Regulatory hurdles also pose a significant barrier. The rapidly evolving nature of AI technology often outpaces the ability of regulatory bodies to establish clear and comprehensive frameworks (Yu, Beam, and Kohane 2018). This creates uncertainty for developers and healthcare providers regarding compliance and liability issues. The lack of standardized regulations can also hinder the scalability and widespread adoption of AI solutions (Ahmed et al. 2023; Khan et al. 2023). The economic viability of AI in healthcare presents a complex issue (Khanna et al. 2022). While AI offers promising solutions for streamlining processes and reducing overall costs, upfront expenses for development, implementation, and maintenance can be significant. This can create a hurdle for healthcare institutions, which require a clear return on investment to justify such expenditures. The challenge lies in demonstrating this value proposition. AI's potential to improve efficiency and generate cost savings may not be immediately apparent, making it difficult to secure initial buy-in (Ricardo Costa Climent, Haftor, and Staniewski 2024). While AI offers tremendous potential in healthcare, the human touch remains irreplaceable. AI isn't meant to steal doctors' jobs, but rather become a powerful partner, augmenting their expertise for improved patient care. Addressing healthcare workers' concerns about AI replacing them is crucial (Castagno and Khalifa 2020). Let's focus on fostering a collaborative environment where AI empowers clinicians, eventually procuring improved patient outcomes (Chibugo et al. 2024). Collaboration among researchers, healthcare providers, policymakers, and technologists is essential to certify the accountable and ethical development and adoption of AI in healthcare (Ali et al. 2023).

APPLICATION OF AI IN HEALTHCARE SECTOR

Medical Imaging and Diagnostic Services

AI is such an image-processing technology that radiologists are utilizing to examine diseases at an early stage and decrease diagnostic errors in disease prevention. Likewise, it is a useful tool for assessing echocardiogram charts and ECG, implemented by cardiologists, for decision-making. Medical imaging, such as MRIs, X-rays, and CT scans, are well assessed by the algorithms of AI with more accuracy. This helps radiologists spot anomalies and diseases at an early stage. The Ultromics technology, reported in an Oxford hospital, uses artificial intelligence (AI) to analyze echocardiogram scans to diagnose ischemic heart disease (Dash et al. 2019). AI is an extensive and expanded field of algorithms, data, analytics, deep learning, neural networks, and acumens that is constantly developing and acclimatizing to meet the necessities of the healthcare system and the patients. Several sections of AI are there to demonstrate the working techniques of machine learning (ML) techniques in the diagnosis of diseases, like diabetes, cancer, Alzheimer's, chronic diseases, heart disease, cerebrovascular disease, stroke, and skin and liver diseases (Zhang et al. 2019). Algorithms of AI have the competence to methodically inspect medical images, aiding the radiologists in rapid detection of abnormalities or diseases initially (Alrefaei et al. 2022).

Disease Prediction by Patient Data

AI representations may scrutinize patient information like symptoms, medical history, and test results, to aid the doctors in producing precise diagnoses and in estimating the progress of diseases (Aria and Cuccurullo 2017). Biological procedures, principally the processing methodologies of input, in human brains, serve as inspiration for AI. AI can process data, learn, recognize patterns, make judgments, and predict (Howard et al. 2020). There are two main types of AI techniques: supervised and unsupervised learning. The former necessitates training on datasets to obtain necessary outputs. Training develops a model for future prediction. The latter clusters comparable data points (Guo 2020). The former is further divided into two types: classification, forecasting the final class labels, with both positive and negative results, and regression, constructing a predictive model from past data and detecting unlabeled data.

Extensive Dataset Analysis

AI algorithms are able to evaluate huge datasets to find probable medication candidates, forecast their efficacy, and improve the process of drug development, decreasing the cost and time needed to market new drugs (Baig et al. 2017).

Personalized Medicine

The arrival of high-tech strategies for conducting biomedical studies like sequencing of DNA using wireless devices and imaging protocols necessitates integration, analysis, and interpretation of the huge amount of produced data. A plethora of statistical methods can deal with the huge generated data; however, involvement of AI techniques indicates that they may be predominantly suitable (Briganti and Moine 2020). Furthermore, the use of data-specific biomedical technologies in research has discovered significant variation among persons at the biochemical, genetic, behavioral levels, and physiological exposure, mainly in terms of treatment of disease. This shows that it is frequently necessary to fine-tune, or "personalize," medicines to the refined and unique features of the individuals (Sanchez-Lengeling and Aspuru-Guzik 2018).

Optimization of Hospital Administration

AI can improve the healthcare system by optimizing hospital processes, restructuring administrative works, and refining resource distribution, leading to improved patient care at a lower cost. It can reduce administrative burdens by automating the generation of organized data sections from therapy, retrieving data from past medical records, and collecting documented patient encounters (Wani et al. 2022). For example, the regular nurse in the United States dedicates a quarter of the working duration to regulatory and managerial tasks. Voice text saves time for doctors and nurses. Although electronic health record (EHR) systems are used in collaboration with the existing system, they lack the accuracy of others (Ranchon et al. 2023).

Personalized Health Advice

Applications powered by AI and chatbots can provide individualized health advice, support behavior modification programs, and actively engage patients in controlling their own healthcare. Healthcare chatbots are intelligent assistants used by medical facilities and experts to help patients seek aid faster. They can assist with frequently asked questions, appointment scheduling, reminders, and other recurring questions or requests that sometimes overburden medical offices (Pietro Biancone et al. 2019).

Predictive Medicine

Disease prediction and diagnosis, as well as treatment results and prognoses, by AI and its capacity in detecting important relationships in raw data aids in diagnosing, treating, and forecasting outcomes in medical workflow. It allows healthcare professionals to address illness outbreaks. Furthermore, it is possible to develop forecasts for identifying risks and determinants for each patient, for more targeted therapeutic interventions. AI approaches can help in designing and developing new drugs, as well as patient monitoring and treatment plan customization for specific patients. Physicians benefit themselves by improving their decision-making associated with patients. The distribution of AI-enabled ML can alter the medicinal field by developing predictive replicas for drugs and diagnostic tests for monitoring patients throughout (Rahimian et al. 2018).

Virtual Patient Care

The growth of wearables, as well as ML and AI in healthcare, has already been studied. Thus, patient monitoring and management through simulated care using sensitive and active and wearables have become a genuineness and are under the standard of care. Furthermore, AI is used to control chronic disorders such as hypertension, diabetes mellitus, chronic bronchial asthma, and sleep apnea, using non-invasive sensored wearables (Smith et al. 2020).

Drug Discovery and Other Medical Researches

AI is adapted to analyzing the massive and complicated datasets utilized in the medical and pharmaceutical fields. Furthermore, it may be used to find scientific studies, combine different types of data, and promote the discovery of drug compounds (O'Mara-Eves et al. 2015). Pharmaceutical companies are focusing on AI to reorganize drug development. Predictive analytics can be used to identify suitable candidates for clinical trials and create precise models of biological processes. ML contributes to the pre-clinical phase by selecting the cohort, arranging volunteers, and gathering and analyzing data. It can improve the patient-oriented perspective, generalizability, efficacy, and success of clinical trials. However, therapeutic trials should place a greater emphasis on ML's functional and conceptual challenges. In addition to ML, the potential across boosting participant management in clinical trials has been revealed by natural language processing (NLP) (Shaik et al. 2023). Interlacing bio and nano-remediation can result in a suitable technology known as "nano bioremediation," which is predicted to eliminate the limitations of bioremediation. Furthermore, AI, a cutting-edge and sophisticated technique that uses digital software, has the potential to significantly transform the bioremediation process, resulting in a faster, more efficient, and robust method for reorienting systems contaminated by oil (Bala et al. 2022; Moussa et al. 2021).

Healthcare Robotics

Apart from medical personnel, few health robots can help patients. Just like exoskeleton robots help paralyzed people walk and become independent. A smart prosthesis or these bionic limbs contain sensors making them more responsive and accurate compared to natural parts of the body, and they can be covered and associated with the user's muscles. Surgery and rehabilitation are also aided by robots (Cruciger et al. 2014).

METHODS OF USING AI

Medical Imaging and Diagnostics

Medical imaging has been cutting-edge to be an indispensable part of modern medicine, assisting in diagnosis and therapy. Computed tomography (CT) scans, nuclear medicine, mammography, X-rays, and ultrasound are some examples (Zhou et al. 2021). In different medical contexts and at all levels of primary healthcare, medical imaging is essential. To confirm, record, and evaluate, the development of several diseases as well as how they respond to diagnostic imaging services and treatment are crucial (Lambin et al. 2017). In order to create technological solutions for better imaging services for diagnosis in remote areas, the WHO works with manufacturers and partners. Additionally, training courses on the administration and use of medical imaging are offered by the WHO and its partners, with a focus on patient safety.

Predictive Analytics

This has reshaped the healthcare industry by exploiting predictive models and data-enabled perceptions, due to which healthcare administrations can perceive possible problems even before they ascend and apprehend the requirements of their patients promptly. Predictive analytics empower healthcare professionals to predict patient outcomes and distribute resources, which renders enhanced care for patients and cuts down expenses (Wills 2014). Other applications using this type of analytics in healthcare include personalizing treatments, refining operational competence, and dropping hospital readmissions by primary interventions (Johnson et al. 2020). The possibilities are endless when it comes to leveraging predictive analytics for the assistance of both medical professionals as well as patients. With this technology now available, healthcare providers have a valuable tool to help improve the quality of care they can offer and ensure patient safety.

Personalized Medicine

The amalgamation of AI in healthcare has made the advent of personalized medicine, which promises more efficient and customized patient care. Conventional medical treatments often follow a one-size-fits-all kind of strategy; however, AI-enabled personalized medicine is revolutionizing the field by leveraging data, advanced analytics, and ML to produce customized treatment recommendations. Precision medicine, sometimes referred to as "personalized medicine," is a branch of medicine that tailors medical procedures, treatments, and supplies to the precise requirements of individual patients. The objective is to offer more efficacious treatments that minimize adverse effects and maximize results by considering the distinct genetic composition, medical background, and lifestyle of every patient.

Drug Discovery and Development

Many pharmacological compounds are developed from over 1060 molecules. The drug development process is limited by outdated technologies, making it a costly and laborious chore that can be resolved with AI. It can recognize compounds that are hits and leads, quickly validate therapeutic targets, and optimize drug structure design (Yu and MacKerell 2016). AI has many benefits, but it also has limitations when it comes to data, including data volume, growth, diversity, and uncertainty. Pharmaceutical businesses have access to datasets containing millions of molecules for medication development, which may be too large for conventional ML methods to handle. Simple physicochemical factors such as log D or P, or a huge number of compounds, can be quickly forecast using a computational model that is based on the quantitative structure-activity relationship (Batool, Ahmad, and Choi 2019).

Virtual Health Assistants

Virtual healthcare assistants are applications or software that assist individuals in using digital skills to deal with their well-being. It offers several features, including symptom tracking, regular healthcare prompts, and access to medical records. It may be accessed via a computer, tablet, or smartphone. Digital healthcare assistants work in the healthcare industry and do repetitive, everyday duties such as making appointments, responding to inquiries, organizing emails and lists of things to do, and sending out reminders. They can also be used by clinics to check patients' status remotely and to remind individuals to take their prescribed medications (Kao and Liebovitz 2017). In summary, AI, NLP, ML, and other technologies are utilized by digital healthcare assistants to offer easily available health management tools and aid people in maintaining their health. The use of digital health advisors in medical services is covered in more detail in the next section (Car et al. 2017).

Robotic Surgery

Through the use of small wounds for cameras and instruments, robotic surgery makes it possible to operate in deep anatomical regions (such as the synovial joints, the gastrointestinal tract, pelvic cavities, and others). Improved identification of anatomical features and devices is possible with real-time AI picture improvement. Intraoperative picture quality can vary significantly due to the dynamic nature of intraoperative visual surroundings during dissection or repair procedures. In response to these modifications, Ali et al. have created an online pre-processing system that improves intraoperative imaging in knee arthroscopy by denoising, blurring of images, as well as color-correcting real-time camera imagery. Their approach performed better than current picture enhancement and required a lot less time to compute before displaying the image (Knudsen et al. 2024). Electrocautery devices are frequently used by robotic surgeons for dissection and ligation operations. However, this procedure produces smoke that gets stuck in the anatomical region of interest and can momentarily obstruct vision until it is removed by suction. In order to produce an improved, smoke-free surgical image, Wang et al. have proposed using a convolutional neural network in conjunction with a Swim transformer. This is especially important in situations where a surgeon must move swiftly and see well, like in the case of a severe intraoperative hemorrhage (Zaffino et al. 2020).

EHR Management

The foundation of contemporary medicine is now EHRs, which have completely changed how medical professionals obtain and use patient data. AI has strengthened EHRs' capabilities by allowing for better decision support, individualized treatment, and increased productivity. An in-depth discussion of the importance of EHRs and how AI is changing healthcare delivery will be covered in this chapter (Wang, Sun, and Li 2023). EHRs are the foundation of contemporary medicine. The days of leafing through piles of paper in search of vital medical information are long gone. Healthcare professionals can now view a patient's entire medical history in a single setting thanks to EHRs. This contains information about demographics, illnesses, therapies, prescription drugs, outcomes of lab tests, and more. EHRs offer a thorough understanding of population health, treatment trends, and illness patterns. EHRs are the unsung heroes of the healthcare industry because of the priceless data they provide to public health specialists, enabling them to create efficient policies, programs, and interventions (Casey et al. 2016).

Clinical Decision Support Systems (CDSS)

CDSSs are AI-enabled systems that use analysis of data, foresight, and optimization among other AI techniques to help complex decision-making processes. By giving medical practitioners more precise and tailored information for diagnosis, risk assessment, monitoring, therapy optimization, and early caution of cardiovascular disease (CVD), AI-based CDSSs significantly improve patient care. These are only a few instances of how AI is being used for CVD systems that support decisions, which is a fast-developing field (Siontis et al. 2021). However, in order for such systems to be completely dependable and efficient, they must be thoroughly assessed by medical experts and taught using accurate data (Shiferaw and Zolfo 2012).

Telemedicine

The WHO defines telemedicine as "The use of information and communication technology to deliver medical treatment where a patient's distance is a significant consideration." To improve community health, the definition comprises numerous activities, including preventing, diagnosing, and treating illnesses, directing research, and contributing to continuing education for healthcare professionals (Jones, DeRuyter, and Morris 2020). For a healthcare approach rather than a technique, telemedicine can be implemented via a diversity of modalities, including real-time video consultations or store-and-forward messaging systems. Terms like "digital health" and "mobile health" provide a broader view of people's medical treatment in the digital age, while others, like "telemedicine" and "telehealth," have separate technical as well as regulatory definitions despite being used interchangeably.

Healthcare Operations and Management

The process of supervising, assisting, and enhancing all nonclinical processes within a healthcare company is known as healthcare operations management. This includes running the business, supervising the workforce, managing the spending, coordinating with payers and insurers, deploying technology, upholding compliance, and facilitating internal communication. Numerous jobs in healthcare operations can be made better or more efficient by carefully integrating AI. The market for AI-associated healthcare was estimated to be worth about $15.4 billion USD in 2022, and during the approaching years, it is expected to upsurge rapidly. Healthcare operation management is one of the specialties in healthcare that stands to gain the greatest benefits from AI in the coming years (Karpathakis, Morley, and Floridi 2024).

Mental Health Support

AI for mental health has been a revolutionary device for dealing with issues linked to mental health. The necessity for innovative and operative solutions is mounting as communities initiate to recognize the worth of mental health (Santosh and Gaur 2021). In this regard, incorporating AI presents a viable path for revolutionizing mental health services. For those looking for comprehensive and individualized services, AI provides a ray of hope for its efficacy in improving diagnosis, support, and treatment. Customized interventions, problem anticipation, and pattern identification are enhanced by sophisticated algorithms and data analysis. Though there is much potential in the application of AI to mental health, there are also important practical and ethical issues raised by this development. Thus, it's critical to maintain the proper balance between human engagement and technical advancement (Ahmad et al. 2021).

Genomics and Precision Medicine

Since the Human Genome Project was completed, the field of genomic medicine—an interdisciplinary medical specialty that uses genomic information—has grown quickly. Genetic markers, germline, intron, microarray, somatic, DNA, RNA, exon, exome, codon, genome, and biomarker are all defined in the fundamental idea of genomic medicine. It is estimated that there are 20,000–25,000 genes in humans, the minuscule units of heredity. One copy of the gene from each parent makes up the human genome. The genes that code for proteins and non-proteins make up the human genome. The number of DNA nucleotides in a gene might range from 100 to 2 million. Consequently, the complexity of gene networks and the quantity of genes are reflected in the genome (Quazi 2022). Precision medicine is also growing speedily. It was initially referred to by the National Research Council as "a New Taxonomy of human disease based on molecular biology." This movement in healthcare can be best understood as a revolution brought about by the discoveries made during the sequencing of the human genome. From then onward, the discipline has developed to understand the precision of health states, illness states, and treatment options for afflicted persons characterized by the junction of multi-omics data with medical records, environmental knowledge, and behavioral variables.

LIMITATIONS OF USING AI IN HEALTHCARE

AI-related responsibilities, creativity, and accuracy continue to provide significant ethical and legal difficulties. It is necessary to do more thorough evaluations of AI content and how it impacts human labor. Additionally, over-reliance on AI may lead to a deterioration in human involvement and critical thinking. It is common for current research to come up with a lack of fully examining the wider ramifications, leading to the need for taking a more inclusive tactic to understand the full extent and effects of incorporating AI into the health sector. Though uplifting, the usage of AI technologies in healthcare and medicine cannot be without its limitations. The possibility of errors in medical information supplied by AI systems, like ChatGPT or Meta, which are unable to completely understand complicated medical situations, is one major cause for concern. Inaccurate diagnoses or misinterpretations of patient history may result in serious medical errors. In addition, biases may be introduced by using training data to power AI systems, which might harm the accuracy and neutrality of the information formed. Alarms about the privacy of patient data, permission, and responsibility for material formed by AI, lead to ethical questions. The unavailability of dynamic learning and real-time updates in these systems disseminates obsolete medical information. The encouragement for integrating AI tools in medicine and healthcare systems progresses patient care, clinical decision-making processes, and medical research. AI tool users can obtain medical information more easily and with greater empowerment provided by NLP, as these skills are incorporated into the interface. Healthcare workers benefit from its capacity to examine vast volumes of medical material as it keeps them informed about the most recent findings and available treatments. For healthcare practitioners, AI may help provide clear and precise medical paperwork, which will simplify their administrative duties.

Furthermore, it enhances medical education, facilitates distant consultations, and optimizes clinical operations. However, there are still some significant drawbacks to data-based patient interaction as opposed to human practical decision-making when ethically managing patient safety (Younis et al. 2024).

Limitation on Clinical Implementation of Artificial Intelligence

The prime hindrance of AI-enabled drugs is the unavailability of practical indications approving their effectiveness in prearranged clinical trials. The majority of research on AI implementation has been in the corporate area; therefore, the idea on its impact on patient's outcome is limited. AI-based research concerning health has been steered in non-clinical settings, indicating that generalizing study outcomes might be problematic. The most widely used method in medicinal and pharmaceutical research, randomized controlled clinical trials, is not successful in showing how AI progresses in healthcare. Due to the scarcity of beneficial data and unpredictable studies, there lies the drawback of AI in healthcare (Alami, Lehoux, et.al. 2021). AI has been incorporated into medical procedures for better application for gaining extensive acceptance. Load reduction effectively is affected by the ease of accessibility of information systems. AI-enabled therapies shouldn't hinder physicians' capability to review or examine EHRs. The cost of the technology utilizes capital with money needed for training the medical practitioners to utilize it properly. There are some examples of assimilating AI into clinical medicine; the majority of these situations are in the preliminary level. On several occasions of the implementation of innovations, the primary barriers to successful integration have been the involvement of stakeholders throughout the development phase. Developing a resolution that can be merged into a clinical platform requires input from a diverse variety of people. During the Ebola as well as the SARS pandemics, a lot of AI research was done for modifying outcomes by earlier diagnosis or precise epidemiological estimation. Though these advancements possess certain limitations, their significance is affected by their integration into current practices without confusing AI-untrained physicians. Furthermore, clinical trials or research has come across algorithm-dependent issues (Damschroder et al. 2009).

Biased and Discriminatory Algorithms

The problem of "bias" exists in the technology sphere as well as the social and cultural ones. Technology artifacts and biased software can be the consequence of inadequate design or erroneous or imbalanced data entered into algorithms. Thus, AI just serves to reinforce the age, gender, and racial discrimination that already permeates our society, thereby expanding the wealth divide. As reported, Amazon researched a few years ago with a less conventional approach to hiring. The applicant search tool used AI to rate candidates on a one- to five-star rating system, similar to how Amazon shoppers rate products. Amazon's computer model favored male applicants over female ones (Hagendorf 2020). The skewed data utilized for product design and the deficiency of variety across development teams were the major issues. Their cultural prejudices and misinterpretations get deep-seated in the very fabric of technical progress as a result of a lack of diversity. Therefore, companies that do not embrace diversity face the risk of producing goods or services that are inaccessible to significant percentages of the public. Four years ago, research found that over 33% of black women and fewer than 1% of white males were incorrectly identified by several facial recognition algorithms. Despite all the firmness from the host, about the excellence of the program, the majority of participants—more than 77% male and 83% white—were used to measure the program's efficacy.

Limitations on Data Collection by AI Tools

First, the inaccessibility of pertinent data created the problem. For ML and DL models to predict a lot of tasks, enormous datasets are required. Industries with access to such datasets have advanced immensely in ML, producing specific and neat algorithms. Hence, accessing data is a complex drawback in the healthcare sector (Ji et al. 2020). Organizations generally do not share health-related data willingly, as confidentiality needs to be maintained. Data accessibility, after being used for once, becomes challenging. ML would improve with the addition of more data to the training set, which is again another source of challenge. Thus, a paradigm transformation from the treatment of patients to the modification of healthcare is obligatory for the active deployment of AI and IT in the healthcare sector. In contrast to diversified learning, few modern algorithms can work on an unimodal or lesser scale, and the inverse issue of storage of always-growing datasets can be alleviated with increasing utilization of cloud computing servers. AI-based systems also raised the issue of privacy and data security. Hackers repeatedly target health records during data cracks due to the sensitivity and vitality of information. Thus, it is vital to preserve the confidentiality of medical records (Baowaly et al. 2018). As AI advances, customers can confuse AI systems for real people and settle for more concealed data collection, which poses major privacy problems. Patient permission is a crucial aspect of data privacy concerns, as medical professionals may allow extensive usage of patient data for AI research without unambiguous agreement from patients. Regulations that limit the utilization, accumulation, and distribution of personal data, like the General Computational Regulations of Europe and the Health Research Regulations, have been effective in 2018 and are a sample of regulation. However, for training AI systems, discretion rules created as a solution may limit the availability worldwide since diverse laws from diverse nations make questions of collaboration and cooperative research more complex. If we intend to avoid these limitations impeding industrial innovation, we need stricter data security rules and regulations. Increasing client-based encryption of data is one approach, while using merged knowledge for training sample models, without dispersing data is another approach.

Moreover, analyzing the data quality for creating algorithms is also difficult. Considering that patient-related data has approximately ½ of four months, certain prediction algorithms might not project future outcomes effectively, due to replication of the past. Additionally, due to the inaccuracy of medical records and inconsistent storage, they are seldom cleanly structured. In spite of all the efforts, AI-based dataset systems still have unpredicted gaps. The extensive usage of electronic medical records aids in addressing this issue, but monitoring concerns and connectivity among institutions limits the data quantity needed to create effective algorithms.

Algorithms Developmental Drawbacks

Prejudices in data-gathering trials for guiding model building may lead to biased outcomes such as poor prediction performance arising from the under-representation of minorities due to racial prejudices in making the dataset. AI models, like the stereotypical neural network handle the prejudice on their own. After collecting data, the emergence of AI poses a problem. Overfitting is caused if the algorithm determines inappropriate associations between the characteristics of the patients and their results. When several factors affect the outcome, the algorithm makes incorrect predictions. Consequently, even if the algorithm achieves well in the training dataset, it may produce imperfect outcomes. Data leak is another area of alarm. When the algorithm obtains terrific accuracy, its predictability out of the training dataset is condensed. To solve this, another new dataset is required (Neill 2013). The so-called "black-box" issue is one common critique directed against AI systems. In most cases, deep learning algorithms are not able to produce compelling reasoning for their predictions. The system has no legal defense if the suggestions are incorrect. Scientists find it more difficult to comprehend how the data is associated with the predictions. Moreover, the "black box" can reduce confidence in the medical field. Though this is still an ongoing discussion, it is important to note that most doctors only have a cursory understanding of imaging tools for diagnosis like CT scans and MRI, and that the mechanism of action of many commonly prescribed drugs is poorly understood. Google has recently released a device to aid in the ongoing research into creating AI systems that are understandable by humans (Wolff et al. 2020).

Social Acceptance

People are concerned about the replacement of their employment by AI in the healthcare industry. Some people are against AI-based approaches for fear of getting replaced. Medical procedures are fundamentally random and human-centric; thus, they cannot always be as specific or organized like an algorithm. Although reasonable to a certain extent, skepticism about AI averts the technology from wide acceptance. Ignorance might lead to magnified prospects about the impact and efficacy of AI. To change false perceptions among people, public conversation concerning the importance of AI in the healthcare field is required (Cruciger et al. 2014).

Ethical Issues

AI is occasionally supposed as a "black box" that considers that the interpretation of the algorithm might be problematic. The interrogation of liability is significant when considering the scope of AI aiming to progress medical consequences. Due to this, the detection of defaulters is unclear, in case of system breakdown. It might be incorrect to consider the doctor accountable as they were not involved in the progress or monitoring of the algorithm. On the other hand, the developer cannot be considered at fault. As the ethical implementation of AI in the healthcare sector is not defined, there are still some ambiguities left. In this context, the Food and Drug Administration (FDA) has contributed to upholding the ideals for evaluating the safekeeping and efficiency of AI-based systems. In Hong Kong and China, AI is forbidden to make moral decisions in the healthcare industry (Khan et al. 2023). The problem has worsened since there are benchmarks for the ethical implementation of AI-ML in healthcare. The efficacy of AI-enabled solutions to avert complications has been demonstrated by the NHS. Public discussion regarding these problems is equally crucial in emerging a global custom that is advantageous to the people (Schmidt-Erfurth et al. 2018).

CHALLENGES FACED DUE TO AI ADOPTION IN HEALTHCARE

AI in healthcare brings forth certain exceptional challenges that can be encountered. As assimilating AI into healthcare suggests that an extensive arena of individuals will engage with AI, we should anticipate some bias from AI users because of the insight of "dangerous AI" that has permeated popular culture. Additionally, without formal IT expertise, and inadequate AI knowledge, people often decide on the integration of technologies. Raising public knowledge and dispelling widespread misconceptions about AI will be the first steps in solving this issue. Second, governments will need to be persuaded of the value of integrating technology by persuasively expressing ideas (Miller and Brown 2018).

Legal Perspective

The query of "whether a new category with its special features and implications needs to be developed, or whether AI fits within existing legal categories" is always debated. Healthcare could be greatly enhanced by using AI in clinical settings, but there are also moral concerns that must be addressed. Data privacy, biases, algorithmic fairness, transparency, safety, informed consent to the usage of data, and algorithmic biases are all crucial considerations are such examples (Gerke, Minssen, and Cohen 2020) that must be resolved for AI in the healthcare sector. The aim is to aid legislators in assuring that the ethically challenging situations due to AI in healthcare backgrounds are addressed initially (Morley et al. 2020). These discussions around AI have emphasized the drawbacks of algorithmic transparency. AI in risky situations needs fair, transparent, and responsible design and supremacy. The two utmost vital components of transparency are the information's accessibility and comprehensibility.

Ethical Considerations

The viability, ethics, and design of lethal autonomous weapon systems (LAWS) have all increased in recent years. These devices would be capable of killing and harming people in addition to having the enormous discretion of AI autonomy. Although there may be many benefits to these developments, there have been concerns expressed about the morality of creating and utilizing LAWS (Taylor 2020). Selection prejudice in datasets that are used to build AI systems is an ordinary issue. According to

Buolamwini and Gebru, the datasets and the robotic recognition of the face that goes along with it are biased, which makes it harder to identify people with darker skin, especially women. A vast amount of data is needed for ML, and the most frequently utilized clinical trial research databases are sourced from specific populations. The association for the development of AI states that AIs should be assessed and authenticated. Before being put into use, it is imperative to test, establish, and evaluate the presentation, reliability, well-being, and compliance of AI systems. As stated earlier, clinical rules of professional conduct do not permit unaccountable behavior. However, it has been assumed that lack of transparency is not restricted to AIS and it can be in doctors. Supervisors of AIS users must elucidate that doctors cannot dodge accountability by blaming the AIS (Smith 2020).

STRATEGIES TO OVERCOME THE ISSUES CAUSED DUE TO AI ADOPTION

AI is revolutionizing healthcare with rapidly diagnosing conditions and developing futuristic visualization tools. However, even though health AI investment is still surging, adoption in healthcare settings may be too sluggish to keep up with the expectations of the industry. It's difficult to introduce cutting-edge technology into an industry as complicated and tightly regulated as healthcare.

Regulation

Needless to mention, we strictly adhere to medical device regulations. However, these rules are typically drafted with physical devices in mind. We must do more than just abide by the regulations. It is necessary that we collaborate with regulatory agencies to develop new frameworks specifically designed for AI. Post-market surveillance constructive feedback streams will aid in the development and improvement of AI technologies (Wang et al. 2021).

Privacy

Healthcare professionals are privy to the most personal information about their patients, and we assume a great deal of responsibility in doing that. There is always more that we, as digital health companies, can do to safeguard the information of our users. When privacy rules aren't strict enough already, we must work with organizations and authorities in the legal system to strengthen them (Vatansever et al. 2020).

REPRESENTATION

AI in health needs to be accessible to everyone. However, a population's health demands are as varied as its members. If we don't use diverse datasets when developing AI solutions, we can't expect them to function for everyone. Although there isn't any neutral data, we may try to ensure that the data we collect and use reflects the variety of the communities we want to serve, like remote patient monitoring using AI (Shaik et al. 2023).

Sustainability

Users want the technologies to be both safe and efficient. But in AI, there is a special problem. The goal is to assist numerous people. To balance the interests of the health system and the person, we must, nevertheless, take certain measures. AI systems that check otherwise healthy individuals for certain illnesses, for example, may result in an uncontrollably large number of patients visiting clinics. We must continue conducting research and publishing thorough clinical evaluation studies in order to meet this problem head-on. To make sure that health systems and doctors have the resources and tools necessary to handle any growth in demand, we must collaborate with them (Păvăloaia and Necula 2023).

Clarity

The reasoning behind the AI that doctors employ must be understood by them. Therefore, wherever possible, we must give concise explanations. Its openness is essential to fostering confidence in AI. Decisions may get harder to explain when algorithms—like neural networks, for example—become more complex. We must be clear when this occurs so that individuals can choose the instruments they use with knowledge. We can reduce the degree to which transparency is impacted by complexity by retaining human oversight throughout development.

Sociocultural

Knowledge in medicine doubles every few months. That's a lot to remain vigilant about. Sadly, this implies that unless they have a special interest, the majority of doctors don't have the time to keep up with AI advancements (Veinot, Ancker, and Bakken 2019). Furthermore, medical schools typically do not provide a thorough education on developing technology. Certain medical professionals are reluctant to adopt new technologies because of this unfamiliarity. We must endeavor to ensure that rising technologies, innovation, and digitization are taught in higher education and first training. In this manner, we may establish familiarity and trust from the beginning of a physician's career. It's serious to be reminded that opposition to change in the healthcare industry isn't motivated by technophobia or fear. Patient and user protection is the top priority for stakeholders in the healthcare industry (Veinot, Ancker, and Bakken 2019).

CONCLUSION

AI has made massive progress in the field of healthcare system, catering to every stratum of people in society. In spite of its advancements, challenges do exist, which therefore requires judicious and rightful implementation of AI, in pharmacy, medicine, and healthcare. As stated in this comprehensive study, it is clearly indicated that there can be huge consequences if AI is not leveraged in the proper way. Hence, it needs to be exploited with adequate knowledge and insightfulness of the subject, in which AI is to be used. Moreover, the exploitation of AI with human resource is always a better strategy, which would potentially bring out better and safer outcomes, if compared with the complete replacement of manpower, with AI. Moreover, certain effective approaches have been found to be fruitful in order to counter the drawbacks caused due to AI adoption. Therefore, the proper way of leveraging AI and exploitation of mindful overcoming strategies would definitely prove to be advancing the stretch of the healthcare system.

REFERENCES

Agrawal, Raag, and Sudhakaran Prabakaran. 2020. "Big Data in Digital Healthcare: Lessons Learnt and Recommendations for General Practice." *Heredity* 124 (4): 525–534. doi:https://doi.org/10.1038/s41437-020-0303-2.

Ahmad, Zubair, Shabina Rahim, Maha Zubair, and Jamshid Abdul-Ghafar. 2021. "Artificial Intelligence (AI) in Medicine, Current Applications and Future Role with Special Emphasis on Its Potential and Promise in Pathology: Present and Future Impact, Obstacles Including Costs and Acceptance among Pathologists, Practical and Philosophical Considerations. A Comprehensive Review." *Diagnostic Pathology* 16 (24). doi:https://doi.org/10.1186/s13000-021-01085-4.

Ahmed, Molla Imaduddin, Brendan Spooner, John Isherwood, Mark A Lane, Emma Orrock, and Ashley Dennison. 2023. "A Systematic Review of the Barriers to the Implementation of Artificial Intelligence in Healthcare." *Cureus* 15 (10). Cureus, Inc. doi:https://doi.org/10.7759/cureus.46454.

Alami, Hassane, Pascale Lehoux, Jean-Louis Denis, et al. "Organizational Readiness for Artificial Intelligence in Health Care: Insights for Decision-Making and Practice." *Journal of Health Organization and Management*. 2020 (ahead-of-print):10.1108/JHOM-03-2020-0074. doi:10.1108/JHOM-03-2020-0074

Ali, Omar, Wiem Abdelbaki, Anup Shrestha, Ersin Elbasi, Mohammad Abdallah Ali Alryalat, and Yogesh K Dwivedi. 2023. "A Systematic Literature Review of Artificial Intelligence in the Healthcare Sector: Benefits, Challenges, Methodologies, and Functionalities." *Journal of Innovation & Knowledge* 8 (1): 100333. doi:https://doi.org/10.1016/j.jik.2023.100333.

Alowais, Shuroug A, Sahar S Alghamdi, Nada Alsuhebany, Tariq Alqahtani, Abdulrahman Alshaya, Sumaya N Almohareb, Atheer Aldairem, et al. 2023. "Revolutionizing Healthcare: The Role of Artificial Intelligence in Clinical Practice." *BMC Medical Education* 23 (1). BioMed Central. doi:https://doi.org/10.1186/s12909-023-04698-z.

Alrefaei, Abdulmajeed F., Yousef M. Hawsawi, Deyab Almaleki, Tarik Alafif, Faisal A. Alzahrani, and Muhammed A. Bakhrebah. 2022. "Genetic Data Sharing and Artificial Intelligence in the Era of Personalized Medicine Based on a Cross-Sectional Analysis of the Saudi Human Genome Program." *Scientific Reports* 12 (1): 1405. doi:https://doi.org/10.1038/s41598-022-05296-7.

Aria, Massimo, and Corrado Cuccurullo. 2017. "Bibliometrix: An R-Tool for Comprehensive Science Mapping Analysis." *Journal of Informetrics* 11 (4): 959–975. doi:https://doi.org/10.1016/j.joi.2017.08.007.

Baig, Mirza Mansoor, Hamid GholamHosseini, Aasia A. Moqeem, Farhaan Mirza, and Maria Lindén. 2017. "A Systematic Review of Wearable Patient Monitoring Systems – Current Challenges and Opportunities for Clinical Adoption." *Journal of Medical Systems* 41 (7). doi:https://doi.org/10.1007/s10916-017-0760-1.

Bajwa, Junaid, Usman Munir, Aditya Nori, and Bryan Williams. 2021. "Artificial Intelligence in Healthcare: Transforming the Practice of Medicine." *Future Healthcare Journal* 8 (2): e188–94. doi:https://doi.org/10.7861/fhj.2021-0095.

Bala, Saroj, Diksha Garg, Banjagere Veerabhadrappa Thirumalesh, Minaxi Sharma, Kandi Sridhar, Baskaran Stephen Inbaraj, and Manikant Tripathi. 2022. "Recent Strategies for Bioremediation of Emerging Pollutants: A Review for a Green and Sustainable Environment." *Toxics* 10 (8): 484. doi:https://doi.org/10.3390/toxics10080484.

Baowaly, Mrinal Kanti, Chia-Ching Lin, Chao-Lin Liu, and Kuan-Ta Chen. 2018. "Synthesizing Electronic Health Records Using Improved Generative Adversarial Networks." *Journal of the American Medical Informatics Association* 26 (3): 228–241. doi:https://doi.org/10.1093/jamia/ocy142.

Batool, Maria, Bilal Ahmad, and Sangdun Choi. 2019. "A Structure-Based Drug Discovery Paradigm." *International Journal of Molecular Sciences* 20 (11): 2783. doi:https://doi.org/10.3390/ijms20112783.

Bernal, Jose, and Claudia Mazo. 2022. "Transparency of Artificial Intelligence in Healthcare: Insights from Professionals in Computing and Healthcare Worldwide." *Applied Sciences* 12 (20): 10228. doi:https://doi.org/10.3390/app122010228.

Bi, Xin, Xiangguo Zhao, Hong Huang, Deyang Chen, and Yuliang Ma. 2019. "Functional Brain Network Classification for Alzheimer's Disease Detection with Deep Features and Extreme Learning Machine." *Cognitive Computation* 12 (3). Springer Science+Business Media: 513–527. doi:https://doi.org/10.1007/s12559-019-09688-2.

Briganti, Giovanni, and Olivier Le Moine. 2020. "Artificial Intelligence in Medicine: Today and Tomorrow." *Frontiers in Medicine* 7 (27). doi:https://doi.org/10.3389/fmed.2020.00027.

Car, Josip, Woan Shin Tan, Zhilian Huang, Peter Sloot, and Bryony Dean Franklin. 2017. "EHealth in the Future of Medications Management: Personalisation, Monitoring and Adherence." *BMC Medicine* 15 (1). doi:https://doi.org/10.1186/s12916-017-0838-0.

Casey, Joan A., Brian S. Schwartz, Walter F. Stewart, and Nancy E. Adler. 2016. "Using Electronic Health Records for Population Health Research: A Review of Methods and Applications." *Annual Review of Public Health* 37 (1): 61–81. doi:https://doi.org/10.1146/annurev-publhealth-032315-021353.

Castagno, Simone, and Mohamed Khalifa. 2020. "Perceptions of Artificial Intelligence among Healthcare Staff: A Qualitative Survey Study." *Frontiers in Artificial Intelligence* 3 (October). doi:https://doi.org/10.3389/frai.2020.578983.

Chibugo, Francisca, Roseline Ebulue, Charles Chukwudalu, and Sylvester Ekesiobi. 2024. "The Role of Artificial Intelligence In Healthcare: A Systematic Review of Applications and Challenges." *International Medical Science Research Journal* 4 (4). Fair East Publishers: 500–508. doi:https://doi.org/10.51594/imsrj.v4i4.1052.

Climent, Ricardo Costa, Darek M Haftor, and Marcin W Staniewski. 2024. "AI-Enabled Business Models for Competitive Advantage." *Journal of Innovation & Knowledge* 9 (3). Elsevier BV: 100532–100532. doi:https://doi.org/10.1016/j.jik.2024.100532.

Cruciger, Oliver, Thomas A. Schildhauer, Renate C. Meindl, Martin Tegenthoff, Peter Schwenkreis, Mustafa Citak, and Mirko Aach. 2014. "Impact of Locomotion Training with a Neurologic Controlled Hybrid Assistive Limb (HAL) Exoskeleton on Neuropathic Pain and Health Related Quality of Life (HRQoL) in Chronic SCI: A Case Study." *Disability and Rehabilitation: Assistive Technology*, November, 1–6. doi:https://doi.org/10.3109/17483107.2014.981875.

Damschroder, Laura J., David C. Aron, Rosalind E. Keith, Susan R. Kirsh, Jeffery A. Alexander, and Julie C. Lowery. 2009. "Fostering Implementation of Health Services Research Findings into Practice: A Consolidated Framework for Advancing Implementation Science." *Implementation Science* 4 (1).

Dash, Sabyasachi, Sushil Kumar Shakyawar, Mohit Sharma, and Sandeep Kaushik. 2019. "Big Data in Healthcare: Management, Analysis and Future Prospects." *Journal of Big Data* 6 (1): 1–25. doi:https://doi.org/10.1186/s40537-019-0217-0.

Gerke, Sara, Timo Minssen, and Glenn Cohen. 2020. "Ethical and Legal Challenges of Artificial Intelligence-Driven Healthcare." *Artificial Intelligence in Healthcare* 1 (1): 295–336. doi:https://doi.org/10.1016/B978-0-12-818438-7.00012-5.

Guo, Lingling. 2020. "Under the Background of Healthy China: Regulating the Analysis of Hybrid Machine Learning in Sports Activities to Control Chronic Diseases." *Measurement* 164 (November): 107847. doi:https://doi.org/10.1016/j.measurement.2020.107847.

Hagendorff, Thilo. 2020. "The Ethics of AI Ethics: An Evaluation of Guidelines." *Minds and Machines* 30 (1): 99–120. doi:https://doi.org/10.1007/s11023-020-09517-8.

Harnett, Patrick John. 2018. "Improvement Attributes in Healthcare: Implications for Integrated Care." *International Journal of Health Care Quality Assurance* 31 (3): 214–227. doi:https://doi.org/10.1108/ijhcqa-07-2016-0097.

Howard, Newton, Naima Chouikhi, Ahsan Adeel, Katelyn Dial, Adam Howard, and Amir Hussain. 2020. "BrainOS: A Novel Artificial Brain-Alike Automatic Machine Learning Framework." *Frontiers in Computational Neuroscience* 14 (March). doi:https://doi.org/10.3389/fncom.2020.00016.

Ji, Shouling, Qinchen Gu, Haiqin Weng, Qianjun Liu, Pan Zhou, Jing Chen, Zhao Li, Raheem Beyah, and Ting Wang. 2020. "De-Health: All Your Online Health Information Are Belong to Us." *IEEE Xplore*. April 1. doi:https://doi.org/10.1109/ICDE48307.2020.00143.

Johnson, Kevin B., Wei-Qi Wei, Dilhan Weeraratne, Mark E. Frisse, Karl Misulis, Kyu Rhee, Juan Zhao, and Jane L. Snowdon. 2020. "Precision Medicine, AI, and the Future of Personalized Health Care." *Clinical and Translational Science* 14 (1). https://www.ncbi.nlm.nih.gov/pmc/articles/PMC7877825/.

Jones, Mike, Frank DeRuyter, and John Morris. 2020. "The Digital Health Revolution and People with Disabilities: Perspective from the United States." *International Journal of Environmental Research and Public Health* 17 (2): 381. doi:https://doi.org/10.3390/ijerph17020381.

Kao, Cheng-Kai, and David M. Liebovitz. 2017. "Consumer Mobile Health Apps: Current State, Barriers, and Future Directions." *PM&R* 9 (5): S106–S115. doi:https://doi.org/10.1016/j.pmrj.2017.02.018.

Karpathakis, Kassandra, Jessica Morley, and Luciano Floridi. 2024. "A Justifiable Investment in AI for Healthcare: Aligning Ambition with Reality." *Social Science Research Network*, January. RELX Group (Netherlands). doi:https://doi.org/10.2139/ssrn.4795198.

Khan, Bangul, Hajira Fatima, Ayatullah Qureshi, Sanjay Kumar, Abdul Hanan, Jawad Hussain, and Saad Abdullah. 2023. "Drawbacks of Artificial Intelligence and Their Potential Solutions in the Healthcare Sector." *Biomedical Materials & Devices* 1 (36785697): 1–8. doi:https://doi.org/10.1007/s44174-023-00063-2.

Khanna, Narendra N., Mahesh A. Maindarkar, Vijay Viswanathan, Jose Fernandes E. Fernandes, Sudip Paul, Mrinalini Bhagawati, Puneet Ahluwalia, et al. 2022. "Economics of Artificial Intelligence in Healthcare: Diagnosis vs. Treatment." *Healthcare* 10 (12): 2493. doi:https://doi.org/10.3390/healthcare10122493.

Kiseleva, Anastasiya, Dimitris Kotzinos, and Paul De Hert. 2022. "Transparency of AI in Healthcare as a Multilayered System of Accountabilities: Between Legal Requirements and Technical Limitations." *Frontiers in Artificial Intelligence* 5 (May). doi:https://doi.org/10.3389/frai.2022.879603.

Knudsen, J. Everett, Umar Ghaffar, Runzhuo Ma, and Andrew J. Hung. 2024. "Clinical Applications of Artificial Intelligence in Robotic Surgery." *Journal of Robotic Surgery* 18 (1). Springer Science+Business Media. doi:https://doi.org/10.1007/s11701-024-01867-0.

Lambin, Philippe, Ralph T.H. Leijenaar, Timo M. Deist, Jurgen Peerlings, Evelyn E.C. de Jong, Janita van Timmeren, Sebastian Sanduleanu, et al. 2017. "Radiomics: The Bridge between Medical Imaging and Personalized Medicine." *Nature Reviews Clinical Oncology* 14 (12): 749–762. doi:https://doi.org/10.1038/nrclinonc.2017.141.

Lunceford, Brett. 2009. "Reconsidering Technology Adoption and Resistance Observations of a Semi-Luddite" 8 (1): 29–48. doi:https://doi.org/10.1386/eme.8.1.29_1.

McKee, Martin, and Olivier J. Wouters. 2022. "The Challenges of Regulating Artificial Intelligence in Healthcare Comment on 'Clinical Decision Support and New Regulatory Frameworks for Medical Devices: Are We Ready for It? – a Viewpoint Paper.'" *International Journal of Health Policy and Management*, September. doi:https://doi.org/10.34172/ijhpm.2022.7261.

Mennella, Ciro, Umberto Maniscalco, Giuseppe De Pietro, and Massimo Esposito. 2024. "Ethical and Regulatory Challenges of AI Technologies in Healthcare: A Narrative Review." *Heliyon* 10 (4). Elsevier BV: e26297–e26297. doi:https://doi.org/10.1016/j.heliyon.2024.e26297.

Miller, D. Douglas, and Eric W. Brown. 2018. "Artificial Intelligence in Medical Practice: The Question to the Answer?" *The American Journal of Medicine* 131 (2): 129–133. doi:https://doi.org/10.1016/j.amjmed.2017.10.035.

Morley, Jessica, Caio C.V. Machado, Christopher Burr, Josh Cowls, Indra Joshi, Mariarosaria Taddeo, and Luciano Floridi. 2020. "The Ethics of AI in Health Care: A Mapping Review." *Social Science & Medicine* 260 (113172): 113172.

Moussa, Zeiad, Bahaa Eldin, Salma Saleh Alrdahe, and A. Saber. 2021. "Innovative Artificial-Intelligence- Based Approach for the Biodegradation of Feather Keratin by Bacillus Paramycoides, and Cytotoxicity of the Resulting Amino Acids." *Frontiers in Microbiology* 12 (October). Frontiers Media. doi:https://doi.org/10.3389/fmicb.2021.731262.

Neill, Daniel B. 2013. "Using Artificial Intelligence to Improve Hospital Inpatient Care." *IEEE Intelligent Systems* 28 (2): 92–95. doi:https://doi.org/10.1109/mis.2013.51.

O'Mara-Eves, Alison, James Thomas, John McNaught, Makoto Miwa, and Sophia Ananiadou. 2015. "Using Text Mining for Study Identification in Systematic Reviews: A Systematic Review of Current Approaches." *Systematic Reviews* 4 (1). doi:https://doi.org/10.1186/2046-4053-4-5.

Păvăloaia, Vasile-Daniel, and Sabina-Cristiana Necula. 2023. "Artificial Intelligence as a Disruptive Technology—a Systematic Literature Review." *Electronics* 12 (5): 1102. doi:https://doi.org/10.3390/electronics12051102.

Pietro Biancone, Paolo, Silvana Secinaro, Valerio Brescia, and Davide Calandra. 2019. "Data Quality Methods and Applications in Health Care System: A Systematic Literature Review." *International Journal of Business and Management* 14 (4): 35. doi:https://doi.org/10.5539/ijbm.v14n4p35.

Quazi, Sameer. 2022. "Artificial Intelligence and Machine Learning in Precision and Genomic Medicine." *Medical Oncology* 39 (8). doi:https://doi.org/10.1007/s12032-022-01711-1.

Rahimian, Fatemeh, Gholamreza Salimi-Khorshidi, Amir H. Payberah, Jenny Tran, Roberto Ayala Solares, Francesca Raimondi, Milad Nazarzadeh, Dexter Canoy, and Kazem Rahimi. 2018. "Predicting the Risk of Emergency Admission with Machine Learning: Development and Validation Using Linked Electronic Health Records." Edited by Aziz Sheikh. *PLOS Medicine* 15 (11): e1002695. doi:https://doi.org/10.1371/journal.pmed.1002695.

Ranchon, Florence, Sébastien Chanoine, Sophie Lambert-Lacroix, Jean-Luc Bosson, Alexandre Moreau-Gaudry, and Pierrick Bedouch. 2023. "Development of Artificial Intelligence Powered Apps and Tools for Clinical Pharmacy Services: A Systematic Review." *International Journal of Medical Informatics* 172 (April): 104983. doi:https://doi.org/10.1016/j.ijmedinf.2022.104983.

Reddy, Sandeep, Sonia Allan, Simon Coghlan, and Paul Cooper. 2020. "A Governance Model for the Application of AI in Health Care." *Journal of the American Medical Informatics*

Association 27 (3): 491–497. https://academic.oup.com/jamia/advance-article-abstract/doi/10.1093/jamia/ocz192/5612169.

Rodriguez, David. 2024. "AI for Healthcare: Opportunities, Challenges, and Future Directions." *International Meridian Journal* 6 (6). https://meridianjournal.in/index.php/IMJ/article/view/51.

Safi, Sabur, Thomas Thiessen, and Kurt J.G. Schmailzl. 2018. "Acceptance and Resistance of New Digital Technologies in Medicine: Qualitative Study." *JMIR Research Protocols* 7 (12): e11072. doi:https://doi.org/10.2196/11072.

Sanchez-Lengeling, Benjamin, and Alán Aspuru-Guzik. 2018. "Inverse Molecular Design Using Machine Learning: Generative Models for Matter Engineering." *Science* 361 (6400): 360–365. doi:https://doi.org/10.1126/science.aat2663.

Santosh, K.C., and Loveleen Gaur. 2021. *Artificial Intelligence and Machine Learning in Public Healthcare. SpringerBriefs in Applied Sciences and Technology*. doi:https://doi.org/10.1007/978-981-16-6768-8.

Schmidt-Erfurth, Ursula, Hrvoje Bogunovic, Amir Sadeghipour, Thomas Schlegl, Georg Langs, Bianca S. Gerendas, Aaron Osborne, and Sebastian M. Waldstein. 2018. "Machine Learning to Analyze the Prognostic Value of Current Imaging Biomarkers in Neovascular Age-Related Macular Degeneration." *Ophthalmology Retina* 2 (1): 24–30. doi:https://doi.org/10.1016/j.oret.2017.03.015.

Schwendicke, F., W. Samek, and J. Krois. 2020. "Artificial Intelligence in Dentistry: Chances and Challenges." *Journal of Dental Research* 99 (7): 769–774. doi:https://doi.org/10.1177/0022034520915714.

Shaik, Thanveer, Xiaohui Tao, Niall Higgins, Lin Li, Raj Gururajan, Xujuan Zhou, and U. Rajendra Acharya. 2023. "Remote Patient Monitoring Using Artificial Intelligence: Current State, Applications, and Challenges." *WIREs Data Mining and Knowledge Discovery* 13 (2). doi:https://doi.org/10.1002/widm.1485.

Shiferaw, Fassil, and Maria Zolfo. 2012. "The Role of Information Communication Technology (ICT) towards Universal Health Coverage: The First Steps of a Telemedicine Project in Ethiopia." *Global Health Action* 5 (1): 15638. doi:https://doi.org/10.3402/gha.v5i0.15638.

Siontis, Konstantinos C., Peter A. Noseworthy, Zachi I. Attia, and Paul A. Friedman. 2021. "Artificial Intelligence-Enhanced Electrocardiography in Cardiovascular Disease Management." *Nature Reviews Cardiology* 18 (7): 465–478. doi:https://doi.org/10.1038/s41569-020-00503-2.

Smith, Anthony C., Emma Thomas, Centaine L. Snoswell, Helen Haydon, Ateev Mehrotra, Jane Clemensen, and Liam J. Caffery. 2020. "Telehealth for Global Emergencies: Implications for Coronavirus Disease 2019 (COVID-19)." *Journal of Telemedicine and Telecare* 26 (5): 1357633X2091656. doi:https://doi.org/10.1177/1357633x20916567.

Smith, Helen. 2020. "Clinical AI: Opacity, Accountability, Responsibility and Liability." *AI & Society* 36 (July). doi:https://doi.org/10.1007/s00146-020-01019-6.

Taylor, Isaac. 2020. "Who Is Responsible for Killer Robots? Autonomous Weapons, Group Agency, and the Military-Industrial Complex." *Journal of Applied Philosophy* 38 (2). doi:https://doi.org/10.1111/japp.12469.

Vatansever, Sezen, Avner Schlessinger, Daniel Wacker, H. Ümit Kaniskan, Jian Jin, Ming-Ming Zhou, and Bin Zhang. 2020. "Artificial Intelligence and Machine Learning-Aided Drug Discovery in Central Nervous System Diseases: State-Of-The-Arts and Future Directions." *Medicinal Research Reviews* 41 (3): 1427–1473. doi:https://doi.org/10.1002/med.21764.

Veinot, Tiffany C., Jessica S. Ancker, and Suzanne Bakken. 2019. "Health Informatics and Health Equity: Improving Our Reach and Impact." *Journal of the American Medical Informatics Association* 26 (8-9): 689–695. doi:https://doi.org/10.1093/jamia/ocz132.

Wang, Feng, Xinan Sun, and Jinhua Li. 2023. "Surgical Smoke Removal via Residual Swin Transformer Network." *International Journal of Computer Assisted Radiology and Surgery* 18 (8). Springer Science+Business Media: 1417–1427. doi:https://doi.org/10.1007/s11548-023-02835-z.

Wang, Qiang, Min Su, Min Zhang, and Rongrong Li. 2021. "Integrating Digital Technologies and Public Health to Fight Covid-19 Pandemic: Key Technologies, Applications, Challenges and Outlook of Digital Healthcare." *International Journal of Environmental Research and Public Health* 18 (11): 6053. doi:https://doi.org/10.3390/ijerph18116053.

Wang, Sophia Y., Suzann Pershing, and Aaron Y. Lee. 2020. "Big Data Requirements for Artificial Intelligence." *Current Opinion in Ophthalmology* 31 (5): 318–323. doi:https://doi.org/10.1097/icu.0000000000000676.

Wani, Shahid Ud Din, Nisar Ahmad Khan, Gaurav Thakur, Surya Prakash Gautam, Mohammad Ali, Prawez Alam, Sultan Alshehri, Mohammed M. Ghoneim, and Faiyaz Shakeel. 2022. "Utilization of Artificial Intelligence in Disease Prevention: Diagnosis, Treatment, and Implications for the Healthcare Workforce." *Healthcare* 10 (4): 608. doi:https://doi.org/10.3390/healthcare10040608.

Wanner, Jonas, Lukas-Valentin Herm, Kai Heinrich, and Christian Janiesch. 2022. "The Effect of Transparency and Trust on Intelligent System Acceptance: Evidence from a User-Based Study." *Electronic Markets* 32 (October): 2079–2102. doi:https://doi.org/10.1007/s12525-022-00593-5.

Wills, Mary J. 2014. "Decisions through Data: Analytics in Healthcare." *Journal of Healthcare Management* 59 (4): 254–262. doi:https://doi.org/10.1097/00115514-201407000-00005.

Wolff, Justus, Josch Pauling, Andreas Keck, and Jan Baumbach. 2020. "Systematic Review of Economic Impact Studies of Artificial Intelligence in Health Care." *Journal of Medical Internet Research* 22 (2): e16866. doi:https://doi.org/10.2196/16866.

Younis, Hussain A., Taiseer Abdalla Elfadil Eisa, Maged Nasser, Thaeer Mueen Sahib, Ameen A. Noor, Osamah Mohammed Alyasiri, Sani Salisu, Israa M. Hayder, and Hameed AbdulKareem Younis. 2024. "A Systematic Review and Meta-Analysis of Artificial Intelligence Tools in Medicine and Healthcare: Applications, Considerations, Limitations, Motivation and Challenges." *Diagnostics* 14 (1): 109. doi:https://doi.org/10.3390/diagnostics14010109.

Yu, Kun-Hsing, Andrew L. Beam, and Isaac S. Kohane. 2018. "Artificial Intelligence in Healthcare." *Nature Biomedical Engineering* 2 (10): 719–731. doi:https://doi.org/10.1038/s41551-018-0305-z.

Yu, Wenbo, and Alexander D. MacKerell. 2016. "Computer-Aided Drug Design Methods." *Methods in Molecular Biology* 1520 (November): 85–106. doi:https://doi.org/10.1007/978-1-4939-6634-9_5.

Zaffino, Paolo, Sara Moccia, Elena De Momi, and Maria Francesca Spadea. 2020. "A Review on Advances in Intra-Operative Imaging for Surgery and Therapy: Imagining the Operating Room of the Future." *Annals of Biomedical Engineering* 48 (8): 2171–2191. doi:https://doi.org/10.1007/s10439-020-02553-6.

Zhang, Caifeng, Rui Ma, Shiwei Sun, Yujie Li, Yichuan Wang, and Zhijun Yan. 2019. "Optimizing the Electronic Health Records through Big Data Analytics: A Knowledge-Based View." *IEEE Access* 7: 136223–136231. doi:https://doi.org/10.1109/access.2019.2939158.

Zhou, S. Kevin, Hayit Greenspan, Christos Davatzikos, James S. Duncan, Bram van Ginneken, Anant Madabhushi, Jerry L. Prince, Daniel Rueckert, and Ronald M. Summers. 2021. "A Review of Deep Learning in Medical Imaging: Imaging Traits, Technology Trends, Case Studies with Progress Highlights, and Future Promises." *Proceedings of the IEEE* 109 (5): 1–19. doi:https://doi.org/10.1109/jproc.2021.3054390.

11 Training Next-Generation Healthcare Professionals in the Era of AI

Nidhi Gupta, Jyoti Chauhan, Swati Chawla, and Shalaghya Sharma

INTRODUCTION

Artificial intelligence (AI) is developing at a very fast pace, and today, one of the cornerstones of healthcare is innovation in a very diverse array of medical disciplines. From radiology to genomics, AI technologies are used to extend professional capability in healthcare. High-accuracy diagnostic tools, effective treatment methods, and those which result in a great outcome of patient care are all part of what has been known to be integrated with AI in healthcare. Integration of AI in healthcare not only refers to technological advancement but also portray paradigmatic changes towards more precise, efficient, and personalized medicine. There is great scope for AI in healthcare. Machine learning algorithms scan extremely large datasets and identify patterns and correlations that otherwise lie outside human observation. For example, they have analysed tens of thousands of radiological images in the quest to detect anomalies at a pace much faster than traditional methods (Esteva et al., 2017). Contrarily, AI-driven models in oncology predict the response of patients to therapies; such customized treatment plans raise the survival scale of patients (Johnson et al., 2018). Also, AI improves predictive analytics through which it predicts outbreaks of diseases and even patient admission, therefore facilitating resource allocation and management. Natural Language Processing (NLP) is a subdivision of AI, which transforms the medials data management. NLP algorithms bring out all the information one would require from clinical unstructured notes. Therefore, they can manage the patients in the best possible way and make all the critical decisions (Rajkomar et al., 2019). Additionally, the usage of AI-controlled robotic systems will be very helpful during operations where they can provide precision with control so that the risk and time for recovery may get minimized. Taken all together, these developments demonstrate the revolutionizing role of AI in healthcare: a future where technology and expertise will conflate to yield superior care.

Importance of Training Next-Generation Healthcare Professionals

Integration of AI into healthcare systems calls for deep change in the education and training of health professionals. Conventional medical education has concentrated on biological sciences and clinical competencies; now, it will need to change towards the adoption of AI-related competencies. As AI continues to spread into

 DOI: 10.1201/9781003531272-11

every healthcare field, there is an emerging need for the next generation of healthcare professionals to become competent in harnessing these technologies effectively and ethically. The simplest requirements are that all those involved in healthcare have to understand how AI and machine learning work; this includes the development, validation, and application of algorithms clinically. Basic knowledge of data science is a critical factor in the practitioner being able to further appraise AI tools and output. For example, it will be very critical to understand the limitations and potential biases of an AI model so that there are no misdiagnosis or other injustices done to patients, as described by Obermeyer et al. (2019) Moreover, it is worth pointing out that it is relevant to develop ethical dimensions of AI in healthcare in training curricula. There are a number of critical ethical concerns related to AI use in the healthcare domain, for example, privacy concerns with health data, bias in algorithms, and probably that AI can further health disparities. Healthcare professionals must be trained to navigate such ethical challenges. Finally, ethical training should also cover the implications of AI in decision-making processes, focused on human supervision and accountability. Another important area of AI training for healthcare professionals is interdisciplinary collaboration. In most cases, applications of AI to healthcare require close collaboration between clinicians, data scientists, and engineers. In that respect, an interdisciplinary learning atmosphere will be fostered. For that reason, every healthcare professional should know how to collaborate with AI experts, speak their language, and integrate their insights into clinical practice. Only in this way the tools of AI will be developed and implemented so that they align with the clinical needs to improve the care of patients. Furthermore, there is the issue of continuous professional development in this fast-changing area of AI. Under these circumstances, healthcare professionals are forced to acquire lifelong learning skills so as to keep up with the improving technologies. These include workshops, online courses, and conferences on AI in healthcare. Continuous learning should be facilitated by the institution through the availability of resources to update knowledge and skills periodically. The role of training in AI for the next generation of healthcare professionals cannot be overemphasized. With AI taking over the future of health, professionals equipped with AI expertise are better poised to deliver quality care, innovate in their fields, and handle the emerging complex challenges brought about by the technologies. The primary objective of this chapter is to understand the role of training and AI for the next-generation healthcare professionals. The chapter explores the current state, benefits, and challenges of AI in healthcare. The chapter also sheds light on the required skills for next-generation healthcare professionals and how the training of next generation should be designed and assessed. Finally, the chapter concludes with the real-world applications, cases, and implications.

CHANGING LANDSCAPE OF HEALTHCARE: IMPACT OF AI

The Current State of AI Adoption in Healthcare

Diagnostic Imaging and Radiology

AI applications in diagnostic imaging and radiology have really made great strides. Evidence has shown that AI algorithms could actually equal and even surpass human radiologists in various tasks. Currently, AI tools have wide usage in detecting and diagnosing conditions from medical images like X-rays, CT scans, and MRIs. A study has demonstrated that AI systems detected breast cancer from mammograms with a sensitivity and specificity rivalling that of radiologists, making it possible to identify diseases at their earliest stages and thus assuring better patient outcomes.

Predictive Analytics and Patient Management

Predictive analytics is another area in which AI has made a big impact. AI algorithms analyse Electronic Health Records for predicting patient outcomes, hospital readmissions, or the progression of diseases. As per Esteva et al. (2022), AI could predict, with a high degree of accuracy, the onset of diabetic retinopathy from EHR data, and early interventions reduced the risk of blindness. AI-driven predictive models will also be applied to hospital workflows by optimizing their procedures, resource allocation, and betterment in patient management.

Personalized Medicine

AI applied to personalized medicine has already changed treatment planning to individualize therapies considering patients' genetic, environmental, and lifestyle factors. In this respect, AI algorithms analyse genomic data for the selection of the most effective treatments in cancer patients, avoiding a trial-and-error approach often associated with oncology. One important example is the use of AI in deciphering complex genetic information to determine personalized treatment plans that improves patient outcomes and reduces toxic side effects.

Natural Language Processing (NLP)

Increasingly, NLP technologies have found a place in processing and analysing healthcare's unstructured clinical data. NLP algorithms extract useful information from clinical notes, improving patient documentation and aiding clinical decision-making. NLP uses the identification of patterns in the symptoms and treatment responses of patients to get more accurate diagnoses and realize personalized care plans.

AI in Surgery

The development of AI-assisted robotic systems changes the role of AI in surgery. Such a system increases the accuracy and deliberation of surgeons while at work and results in improved surgical outcomes and shortens recovery time. According to Haidegger et al. (2022), the issue of AI integration in robotic surgery has developed significantly both minimally invasive procedures and surgical training. The AI-driven robots can thus perform complicated surgery with high precision; therefore, reducing human error as well as providing safety to the patients.

Challenges and Considerations

Despite all these improvements, there are still several challenges towards the diffusion of AI in healthcare. Other challenges to adoption also include data privacy and bias within the algorithms, as well as a requirement for rigorous validation and regulatory approval. Ethical and proper use of AI and transparency in decisions taken by AI are central to engaging the trust of both health experts and patients. lack of continuous education and training to health professionals is another very serious problem of healthcare sector in incorporating AI into clinical practice.

Benefits of AI in Healthcare

Improved Diagnostic Accuracy

AI algorithms demonstrate high accuracy in diagnosing diseases from medical images and clinical data. A study by Gulshan et al. (2021) indicated that AI systems can detect diabetic retinopathy with very high accuracy and often outperform human clinicians, which results in improved diagnosis accuracy and hence improved outcome for patients.

Personalized Medicine

AI allows the computation of more personalized treatment plans since it considers genetics information alongside clinical data to provide therapies for particular patients. A study indicates that AI-driven precision medicine improved treatment outcomes of cancer patients through the prediction of their response to certain drugs (Wang et al., 2016).

Operational Efficiency

AI helps in optimizing the workflow of hospitals by predicting admissions of patients and thus makes administrative work smoother. According to a recent review, applications of AI in hospital management have led to better resource allocation, reduced waiting times, and improved patient satisfaction (Haddad et al., 2022).

Predictive Analytics

AI-powered predictive analytics can predict outbreaks of diseases, readmission to hospitals, and deteriorations in patients' health, thereby enabling interventions earlier. As per Wilminket al. (Wilmink et al. (2020), AI models were much more accurate at predicting the onset of sepsis, which enabled timely treatments that could save lives. AI-assisted robotic systems enhance the accuracy of surgeries and reduce human errors, thereby promoting a faster recovery rate in patients. There have been tremendous improvements and advancements in robotic surgery, wherein integration of AI into surgery has been associated with improved surgical outcomes and low complication rate (Chatterjee et al., 2024).

Challenges of AI in Healthcare

Data Privacy and Security

Application of AI in healthcare means dealing with a great deal of critical information about patients; therefore, there are problems relating to the privacy and security of data. This makes ensuring conformance to regulations such as the General Data Protection Regulation (GDPR) and Health Insurance Portability and Accountability Act (HIPAA) very important.

Algorithmic Bias

Since AI systems rely on data-driven instructions, they generally represent biases carried within the training datasets. It might be projected into unequal treatment outcomes. A study explained that AI algorithms with racial and gender biases that are to be used for clinical decision-making can lead to substandard clinical results and healthcare disparities, and the development of fair and unbiased AI models is necessary (Obermeyer et al., 2019).

Regulatory and Ethical Concerns

Deployment of AI in healthcare requires rigorous validation and regulatory approval, which can be time-consuming and complex. Apart from these, concerns are raised over AI decision ethics and patient informed consent. Amann et al. (2023) recommended clear regulatory frameworks and ethical guidelines that have to be established for the use of AI in healthcare. Problems related to the integration of AI tools with existing systems, interoperability issues, and the reluctance by the healthcare providers to embrace change generate challenges.

Continuous Learning and Adaptation

The system has to undergo continuous learning and adaptation to ensure that it remains relevant for the fast-evolving medical knowledge and practices. Inherently, this would thus entail keeping the models of AI updated with continuous retraining of resource-intensive models. A 2024 study underscored that continuous learning frameworks are very instrumental in maintaining AI tools' accuracy and reliability within healthcare settings (Gomes et al., 2024).

Emerging Trends and Technologies

In many respects, AI will develop patient-centered care and advocacy:

- Tailored Medicine: AI will administer a treatment plan according to the needs, preferences, and values of individual patients.
- Predictive Analytics: AI recognizes which patients are at high risk and is able to intervene early so that problems do not arise.
- Chatbots and Virtual Assistants: AI-powered chatbots will assist patients emotionally through empathetic support, answer their questions, and guide them through issues with ease.
- NLP: AI enables NLP, promoting easier communication between patients and healthcare providers.
- Patient Engagement Platforms: AI-based patient engagement platforms allow patients to engage actively in their healthcare, thus enhancing patient-centredness.
- Care Coordination: The application of AI into care coordination allows for the ease of transitions without errors being committed.
- Patient Advocacy Support: AI identifies patients who require patient advocacy support, therefore ensuring early intervention.

- Mental Health Support: AI-based resources provide mental health support and crisis intervention.
- Improvement in Health Literacy: AI-based applications ensure patients understand complicated medical information more easily.
- Real-Time Feedback from Patients: AI enables real-time feedback so that healthcare providers can adapt and improve.
- Cultural Competence and Awareness: AI will enable healthcare providers to understand and cope with cultural differences and preferences.
- Accessibility and Inclusivity: AI-based tools make healthcare more accessible to those with disabilities, language barriers, or limited health literacy. By leveraging AI, healthcare providers can deliver more patient-centred, empathetic, and effective care, ultimately improving patient outcomes and experiences.

ESSENTIAL SKILLS FOR NEXT-GENERATION HEALTHCARE PROFESSIONALS

The essential skills for next-generation healthcare professionals in the digital environment are as follows:

Data Analysis and Interpretation

Data analysis and interpretation skills in the healthcare setup are imperative because they help health professionals analyse data of their patients in order to establish trends, patterns, and correlations that later help in informing treatment decisions or enhancing recovery. Whittaker et al. (2015) found that using data insights will drive evidence-based decision-making, cost reduction, and efficient resource allocation This scope of analytics looks at the effectiveness of treatment data and points out the best practices and areas for improvement. Predictive analytics in healthcare helps in forecasting of patient outcomes, hence allowing for the implementation of self-initiated solutions and customized care. It also helps in detecting any potential safety risks and puts in place data-driven interventions to reduce those risks. It analyses data for opportunities where resource allocation could be optimized, hence reducing waste and improving efficiency. The insights from data can be used in personalization for better patient engagement strategies, which will improve patient satisfaction and health outcomes. It will also contribute to medical research and development by examining data to find areas of innovation. Predictive analytics nvolves the study of trends in population health to create public health initiatives and policy decisions. From data-driven insights, identify areas for cost reduction that will make healthcare more affordable. The data analysis and interpretation skills are vital for healthcare professionals to enable them to drive improvement in patient care, operational efficiency, and economic sustainability—directly enhancing the overall quality of healthcare services.

Digital Literacy and Technology Adoption

The professionals in the healthcare sector can support in improving patient care. Healthcare professionals have easy access to appropriate and timely information, which aids in better diagnosis and treatment. It also allows for better patient engagement, education, and empowerment. This will help streamline clinical workflows, thereby improving efficiency and reducing errors. This technology also supports remote healthcare services. Telemedicine and remote monitoring facilitate healthcare services, especially in places considered remote or underserved populations. Digital data analytics support informed evidence-based decisions and improve healthcare outcomes. It is helpful to ensure good communication and collaboration between different professionals concerned with the care of a patient. Digital tools optimize medication administration to reduce medication errors and related adverse events and to facilitate medication administration in the best interest of every patient. Such digital resources keep health professionals updated about the latest medical knowledge and guidelines. Digitalization and automation can reduce administrative burdens, thus minimizing costs.

Critical Thinking and Problem-Solving

Critical thinking and problem-solving in a digital era are significant healthcare skills in the digital age. The reason is that critical thinking allows for the analysis of online resources, research, and data, which aids in decision-making. This also aids in the analysis of complex and large volumes of data from electronic health records, medical devices, and other digital sources. These skills allow for the characterization of possible biases in AI-driven diagnostic tools and considering multiple perspectives. Critical thinking can be applied towards the integration of digital information with clinical expertise to develop appropriate treatment plans. In the rapidly evolving landscape of digital healthcare, there is a need for constant updating of knowledge and skills. Healthcare professionals should do critical evaluation of digital systems and protocols that safeguard sensitive patient information. These skills will improve work efficiency with the help of digital health tools, including telemedicine platforms, and multidisciplinary teams that provide all-inclusive care. Huselid (2015) also concluded in their studies that by combining critical thinking and problem-solving skills with digital literacy, healthcare professionals can provide high-quality patient care, improve health outcomes, and thrive in the digital era.

Emotional Intelligence and Empathy

Emotional intelligence (EI) helps healthcare workers use digital means of communication to clearly and empathetically convey the right message across patients, families, and colleagues. This will help build trust between the patients and a professional since patients may even feel vulnerable while sharing their problems online. Sharma and Kumar (2023) revealed that empathy in digital health has to do with understanding the feeling and concerns of patients remotely. This will help the health expert to maintain their tone and language compassionate while communicating digitally. The ability of resolving conflict or misunderstanding, in case of rising from digital miscommunication, rests with EI and empathy. Sadiku et al. (2020a, b) opined that empathic professionals may provide patients with emotional support and resources during mental crises. EI and empathy enable professionals to acknowledge and value cultural backgrounds and their diversified cultural values in the digital realm. Logasakthi et al. (2023) explained that EI ensures effective teamwork amongst healthcare professionals and fosters sustainable HR practices for better management. Empathy ensures patient-centred care by addressing the needs and concerns of the person as an individual. EI empowers professionals to manage their own emotions in this digitally demanding environment and prevents burnout. With EI, health professionals can foster the much-needed empathy to drive compassion through the delivery of patient-centred care in the digital age, critical in driving better health outcomes and stronger relationship.

Adaptability and Continuous Learning

The field of research in AI is evolving, and professionals must continuously adapt to new tools and updates. AI-driven insight helps professionals respond to such emerging needs and preferences of the patients. Continuous learning helps the professional interpret and apply new data and analytics that come from the AI tools. The integration of AI with current workflow ensures seamless integration of AI tools into existing clinical processes. Lera et al. (2020) examined that continuous learning enables professionals to recognize the potential limitations and biases of AI decision-making and hence act against them. One has to adapt to changes in regulations and guidelines that are enacted on the use of AI in healthcare. It enables one to have an interdisciplinary level of effective teamwork with other teams using AI tools. In addition to that, continuous learning can also help professionals gain further skills in the interpretation of AI results and critical thinking. Therefore, adaptability and continuous learning will enable professionals to utilize AI for the benefit of patients and improve their outcomes. Continuous professional growth and development occur when professionals embrace AI and continuous learning. Considering the present and future use of AI, embracing adaptability and continuous learning enables healthcare professionals to harness AI tools in improving patient care and keeping pace with a rapidly changing digital healthcare landscape. The study by Hachoumi et al. (2023) analysed that for all health professions, lifelong and continuous learning is essential, as professionals are committed to delivering expert and poised care.

Cultural Competence and Diversity Awareness

For better healthcare outcome, understanding of diverse backgrounds and cultural aspects of patients helps healthcare professionals adopt tailor-made approach that provides better care to patients. Clear correspondence is guaranteed by keeping away from errors or distortion through social mindfulness. To build patient trust so that they can share their concerns and follow their treatment plan as per their health care instructors, it is important to have cultural competencies in healthcare professionals; it will help them to reduce cultural inequalities and differences. Cultural competence improves collaboration and employee satisfaction by encouraging inclusive teamwork. It assists an expert with grasping the social settings; it likewise helps an expert intending to social determinants of wellbeing. Socially delicate consideration prompts expanded patient fulfilment, reliability, and positive encounters. Social ability supports adherence to regulations, guidelines, and principles of license. Social ability enhances the individual and healthcare expert understanding towards each other.

Leadership and Management

The healthcare industry has realized that good leadership and management are critical in this age of digital disruption. One of the fundamental abilities is understanding digital technologies and how they are used in the healthcare industry, adopting and putting into practice cutting-edge solutions like data analytics, telemedicine, and AI tools that provide data-driven insights, which help in strategic action to improve results. It also ensures patient data security and privacy in a digital environment. In the light of the digital transition, leaders in healthcare industry oversee and direct organizational change, draw in, nurture, and hold onto professionals with digital expertise, cooperation, data distribution, and sharing throughout healthcare systems and stakeholders. To adapt digital technologies for patient empowerment, education, and involvement there is a need ofeffective leadership skills that foster collaboration and data sharing across healthcare systems and stakeholders. Transformational leaders look forward to leverage digital tools to enhance patient engagement, education, and empowerment. These leaders play an important role in ensuring ethical considerations and governance in the use of digital technologies and ensure that their team will upgrade with the latest digital trends, technologies, and best practices in healthcare.

Entrepreneurship and Innovation

Digital entrepreneurship and innovation are important skills, as through them one can stay ahead both as a person and as an organization. Entrepreneurial skills help turn new ideas into products and services that disrupt markets and result in new opportunities. Development of innovative solutions enhances care, experience, and outcomes for the patients. The entrepreneurial mindset will enable innovation in new ways for process streamlining, cost reduction, and productivity improvement through digital innovation. In a changing healthcare environment, professionals need an entrepreneurial mindset, attitude, and competencies that would foster experimentation, risk-taking, and lifelong learning within organizations. The development of creative solutions to a number of complex healthcare challenges needs to be worked out with regard to access, affordability, and quality. Embracing innovation opens up the power of digital technologies such as AI, blockchain, and the Internet of Things that drive healthcare betterment. Healthcare professionals or experts should learn how to collaborate with startups, academia, and industry partners in the pursuit of driving innovation and growth. It helps them come up with innovative business models that answer the arising market needs and trends. The healthcare professionals remain versatile and strong, thereby continuously adapt to changes in the market environment, technologies, and customer needs. Through the adoption of entrepneurship and innovation, there can be success for individuals and organizations in the digital era to change health outcomes for good. These skills are essential for healthcare professionals; they enable economic growth and development in several ways:

Improved Health Outcomes: Improved patient care and outcomes lead to greater productivity and economic growth.

Efficiency: Digital literacy and technology implementation make the whole process easier, cut costs, and improve resource allocation.

Innovation and Entrepreneurship: Healthcare innovation and entrepreneurship result in new products, services, and jobs that better provide patient care at reasonable costs.

Better Decision-making: It permits analysis and interpretation of data to support policy and resource allocation in healthcare.

Development of a Working Relationship: Improvement in communication and collaboration capabilities fosters partnerships that boost economic prosperity through collective actions.

Workforce Development: A skilled health workforce is key for investment attraction, stimulation of economic activity, and competitiveness enhancement.

Healthier Population: Improved social determinants of health are enhanced by cultural competence and awareness of diversity leading to a healthier workforce and reduced healthcare expenses.

Leadership and Management: It consists of all the factors that run healthcare organizations successfully and make a difference in local economies.

Patient-Centred Care: It enhances patient satisfaction with services provided as the core motive of business development and economic growth.

Flexibility and Continuing Education: Lifelong learning enshrines in professional healthcare workers the ability to be flexible and change with ever-changing horizons, driving innovation and economic growth.

By having these core competencies, next-generation healthcare professionals will greatly contribute to a much more efficient, effective, and innovative healthcare delivery system that is a significant contributor to economic growth and development.

CURRICULUM DESIGN AND DEVELOPMENT

It needs to be implemented with an interdisciplinary approach whereby several subjects such as computer science, biology, ethics, and clinical practice are convergent to appropriately train the subsequent generation of healthcare personnel. In this manner, students are assured of acquiring not only technical expertise in AI but also an appreciation of its impacts and applications in healthcare. Integrating knowledge from other disciplines, according to Jiang et al. (2017), fosters an integrated understanding and empowers healthcare professionals to apply AI technologies in ethical and efficient ways. Such an example is the confluence of medical studies with courses on data science and machine learning. The interdisciplinary amalgamation will equip medical students with the capabilities needed to scan giant datasets for trending and data-driven decision-making. Other legal and ethical studies similarly empower the students to operate in the complex regulatory space that surrounds AI in healthcare.

Interdisciplinary Approaches to AI Education

What is also known as "integrating AI into existing healthcare curricula" is the inclusion of AI concepts and tools into traditional medical education. This can be done step-by-step: first, introducing simple modules on AI, then gradually adding more complex topics as they expand their grasp. According to Topol (2019), even minor exposure to AI tools may help enhance the diagnostic and treatment-planning skills of medical students to a significant extent. For instance, AI-based technologies can be utilized to allow students to better visualize hard structures and understand spatial relationships in anatomy classes. AI can also be used in patient simulation during clinical education; in this way, students have a risk-free environment in which they can learn how to make decisions. These relationships strengthen education and prepare students for the future of AI-administered healthcare.

Crossing Over AI with Healthcare Curricula

New programmes that focus on AI in healthcare must be introduced to the curriculum to enhance education with practical skills training for the professional. Classes would cover several topics from foundational theories of AI to the state-of-the-art applications in genomics, personalized medicine, and medical imaging. According to Rajpurkar et al. (2018), "specialized AI courses for health care workers will significantly strengthen their ability to understand and use AI-generated insights at the point of care". Some of the ways by which educational institutions can provide healthcare AI include certificate programmes, master's degrees, and continuing education courses. The courses should offer opportunities for research and innovation, partnerships with industries, and hands-on practice with AI tools and platforms. They ensure medical professionals are both the users and developers of AI technology through this step.

Case Studies and Actual Applications

Case studies should be integrated in the curriculum to develop a better understanding and usage of AI in healthcare education. case studies amongst other relevant applications should be integrated in the curriculum. Through case studies, students can understand real-world applications of AI in healthcare, operations, and decision-making processes. They can use knowledge built through lab exercises and projects to develop their practical skills. Consider a case for diagnosing diabetic retinopathy by AI, for example, which offers benefits and challenges in its clinical application. Examples of practical activities include developing machine learning models that would predict illness outcomes or using AI technologies to analyse patient data. It is through these experiences that students are better equipped to use AI in the workplace, and healthcare innovation will be inspired.

PEDAGOGICAL APPROACHES FOR AI EDUCATION

AI is growing fast as a technology, which has heavy impacts on many industries, including education. The demand for integrating AI into the curricula of learning increased with more effective progress in developing the technology to instruct students about opportunities and dilemmas of the near future. Proper pedagogical approaches related to AI education would be required for students to get deep knowledge about AI concepts, applications, and their ethical implications. These approaches enable students to make potentially ethically good contributions to the field as they both endow them with the technical skills required to explore the AI ecosystem and further foster critical thinking and ethical awareness. Effective learning in AI context requires learners to develop an ability to learn interdisciplinarity and solve problems through practice in the real world (Holmes et al., 2019).

Flipped Classrooms and Interactive Learning

Flipped classrooms encourage the participation of students in learning; hence, they are a good pedagogical strategy for AI education. The use of pre-recorded lectures or online resources makes it possible for the students to get introduced to the AI principles outside the classroom. Immediately following this, in-class activities include group discussions, problem-solving exercises, and practical projects. Roehl et al. (2013) assert that a study on letting students use their knowledge in groups reveals that flipped classrooms increase learning outcomes and improve student engagement. This can be very helpful in AI education since it enables students to learn tricky subjects as well as gain real-world experience in an interactive, hands-on type of learning.

Gamification and Simulation-based Training

AI principles and their applications in health domain can best be learned through gamification and simulation-based training. Gamification refers to the inclusion of features (such as leaderboards, badges, and points) of game playing to promote and engage students in the learning process. Simulation-based learning, through the use of virtual settings and real-time situations, enables learners to personally experience AI tools and methods in use. According to a study, it has been discovered that a medical learning process is largely enhanced by gamification and simulation-based learning. Examples include AI-driven simulations, wherein the situation produced can closely mimic real-time clinical settings; hence these lend them a safe environment for mastering diagnostic and treatment planning skills. These methods make better recall of advanced AI-related concepts, but also make it even more fun to learn.

Virtual Reality and Immersion Learning

Virtual reality and immersion learning are new approaches to facilitate the learning of AI in healthcare education. Virtual reality is an interactive space for students to explore applications of AI, which may include virtual patient consultations, surgical simulations, and anatomy visualizations. Students will be able to learn in a much deeper and wider scope of AI technology and its potential applications in healthcare by going through an immersion learning experience. Based on the study conducted by Merchant et al. (2014), the use of immersive learning technologies, for instance, virtual reality, improves students' understanding and retention, particularly when more complex comprehension is involved. These technologies thus keep the learner in the AI learning domain, with hands-on experience with AI tools and approaches that enable an insight into their limitations and practical applications.

Project-based Learning and Hackathons

Hackathons as well as project-based learning are valuable methods of learning AI in healthcare. It emphasizes the spirit of creativity, teamwork, and problem-solving skills. In project-based learning, students work on real projects requiring the application of AI principles and methods. Through this practical work, students get trained to deal with complex problems and cultivate practical expertise. Hackathons-class intense group activities where participants create original answers to the given problems are effective in the teaching of AI. These activities encourage a collaborative and competitive learning environment for students as they have the opportunity to work with peers, mentors, and experts in the field. Mendez et al. (2020) state that hackathons stimulate learning through innovation, collaboration, and rapid development of AI solutions.

ASSESSMENT AND EVALUATION STRATEGIES

In the era of AI, the exercise of monitoring and assessing the education of the next generation of providers must be multifaceted, blending advanced instructional methods with scientific breakthroughs. The above training for these healthcare professionals can be evaluated in a few ways:

Competency-based Assessments and Evaluations

The competency-based assessment aims at determining to what extent healthcare professionals can apply their knowledge in real-world scenarios (Sallam et al., 2024). Some of the competency-based assessment methods include:

- Clinical Simulations: Develop realistic clinical environments where students can demonstrate their competencies through AI-enhanced simulations.
- Objective Structured Clinical Examinations (OSCEs): With AI, it becomes feasible to utilize dynamic, adaptive OSCEs for skills-assessment purposes.
- E-portfolios: Offer opportunities to the students to develop a digital portfolio with a variety of multimedia components that display their competencies.
- Rubrics: Design inclusive rubrics that assess achievement within competency areas in a balanced manner.

Mechanism of Feedback

Another way in which such training can be effective is through assessing timely feedback and evaluation. Techniques to be used include:

- AI-Driven Feedback Systems: Use AI to provide real-time, personalized feedback about students' achievements.

360-Degree Feedback: To present a complete view of the performance of a student, the method must include classmate and teacher feedback along with self-appraisals.
Regular Meetings: Plan out the frequency at which students and mentors should hold frequent one-on-one discussions about progress and areas to improve.
Peer Reviewing: For peer learning and self-improvement, encourage peer evaluations (Le et al., 2024).

Continuous Improvement for Goal Enhancement

Some of the most effective techniques for goal enhancement are:

Data Analytics: It follows the pattern of performances and tracks where improvements are needed through AI and data analytics.
Curricular Innovation: The curriculum is continuously upgraded with changing practices, technologies, and stakeholder feedback.
Teacher Professional Development: Teachers are continuously equipped with continuous learning to keep abreast of the newly emerging developments in AI and pedagogic practices.
Quality Improvement Cycles: Use Plan-Do-Study-Act (PDSA) cycles to iteratively try and refine education interventions (Khan et al., 2024).

Student Learning Objectives

To what extent the students have achieved the learning objectives of the programme can be known by student learning outcomes. These can be measured as follows:

Standardized Tests: AI-deepened standardized tests are used to measure knowledge and abilities objectively.
Performance Measures: Monitor patient outcomes and other clinical performance measures to gauge how well skills are being used in the real world.
Self-evaluation Tools Using the Support of AI: Self-evaluation tools help students assess themselves and be able to identify the need for improvement.
Long-term Tracking: Track graduates in long term for the assessment of professional performance changes over time that the training could have led to (Van der Vegt et al., 2024).

Determining the Effectiveness of Programme Results

Measuring the degree to which training prepares graduates to function well in real healthcare settings is highly important. Some of the key techniques for determining the effectiveness of the programme are:

Alumni Surveys: Ask the alumni how well the training has prepared them for their profession by conducting surveys with them and find out what the employers think about graduates' performance and preparedness.

Outcome-Based Metrics: Assess the success of a programme by looking at outcomes such as career advancement, employment placement, and certification passage rates.

Benchmarking: Compare achievements of a programme to national or international standards to discover areas of excellence and opportunities for improvement.

Techniques for Implementing AI in Assessment and Evaluation

AI Algorithm Grading: AI is used in grading to create more uniformity and ensure objectivity by using an AI algorithm for assignments and tests evaluation.

Predictive Analytics for Slow Learners: Predictive analytics can be used to identify students who may be weak at their studies and take proactive action to help them out.

NLP of Subjective Paper Analysis: NLP analysis will be applied to paper evaluations, essays, and feedback for better comprehension of students' understanding and flaws.

Healthcare education organizations will be able to ensure that the next generation of healthcare professionals is better equipped to meet the challenges of an AI-driven healthcare future by deploying these strategies to better train and assess the new professional (Kökver et al., 2024).

REAL-WORLD APPLICATION OF AI IN THE HEALTHCARE INDUSTRY

Artificial Intelligence Real-World Practices and Examples

AI is increasingly being integrated into clinical practice and healthcare operations, improving patient care and administrative efficiency. Below are some real-world applications:

AI-Powered Radiology: AI algorithms developed by Zebra Medical Vision and Aidoc analyse medical pictures to diagnose fractures, tumours, and brain haemorrhages with faster and more accurate results than human radiologists.

Personalised Medicine and Drug Development: IBM Watson for Genomics helps doctors personalize cancer treatment strategies by finding mutations and offering targeted medicines.

Patient Risk Stratification through Predictive Analytics Johns Hopkins University employs AI-based models to predict patient deterioration, readmissions, amongst other hazards with the goal of acting even in time and enabling person-centred treatment regimens.

Virtual Health Assistants: Buoy Health and Babylon Health work based on AI-powered chatbots for symptom checks, medical advice, and health monitoring. This helps relieve the healthcare workers of much burden while strengthening patient engagement.

Workflow Optimization for Efficient Administration: AI is used in Mayo Clinic for optimizing operating room schedules to allow reduced waiting times and optimum usage of available resources.

Remote Monitoring and Telehealth: Teladoc Health uses AI to analyse patient data from wearable devices and deliver real-time insights, allowing for remote monitoring and prompt interventions.

Clinical Decision Support Systems (CDSS): The Cleveland Clinic uses IBM Watson Health to help physicians diagnose and treat diseases with evidence-based recommendations and insights from medical literature.

AI in Pathology: PathAI analyses tissue samples and identifies anomalies to help pathologists make accurate diagnoses.

AI-Enhanced Surgical Robots: The da Vinci Surgical System uses AI to help surgeons execute minimally invasive treatments with greater precision and control.

AI for Public Health: Kaiser Permanente analyses massive datasets to find patterns and prevent outbreaks.

EHR Management: Epic systems uses AI to optimize operations, minimize administrative workloads, and improve patient record accuracy (Pauling et al., 2024).

Lessons Learned and Best Practices from Early Adopters

Integration Challenges: Integrating AI into existing healthcare systems might be challenging owing to compatibility difficulties and required process adjustments. There is a need to create effective integration strategies with rigorous testing, personnel training, and phased rollouts to reduce interruption.

Data Quality and Availability: AI systems rely on enormous amounts of high-quality data, yet incomplete, inconsistent, or siloed data might hinder their performance. It is required to invest in data cleansing, standardization, and interoperability to provide AI algorithms with reliable and complete datasets.

Regulatory and Ethical Considerations: AI applications in healthcare must navigate complex regulatory contexts and handle ethical issues about patient privacy and bias. It is required that we consult with regulatory organizations early.

User Acceptance: Healthcare personnel may be hesitant to utilize AI due to concerns about job loss or distrust in technology. There is a need to prioritize education and training to showcase AI's potential to complement, not replace, human expertise. Involve physicians in the development process to ensure that the technology satisfies their requirements.

Transparency and Explainability: Clinicians may struggle to trust and employ black-box AI algorithms effectively. There is a need to prioritize developing explainable AI systems to enhance decision-making (Aliferis & Simon, 2024).

BEST PRACTICES FOR INCORPORATING AI IN THE HEALTHCARE INDUSTRY

Collaborative Development: Collaborate extensively with diverse teams, including physicians, data scientists, and IT professionals, to ensure AI solutions are practical and user-friendly. For instance, IBM Watson and Memorial Sloan Kettering Cancer Centre collaborate to improve oncology applications with clinicians and AI engineers. Implement continuous learning methods in AI systems to adapt and improve with fresh data and user feedback. Mayo Clinic uses AI for predictive analytics, updating algorithms with new patient data to improve accuracy.

Pilot Programmes and Scaling: Begin with small-scale pilot programmes to test AI solutions, gather feedback, and perfect technology before expanding.

Patient-Centred Design Practice: Design AI applications with a focus on enhancing patient outcomes and experiences, ensuring that technology boosts care quality and accessibility. Babylon Health's AI chatbots offer instant access to medical advice, leading to increased patient engagement and satisfaction.

Robust Evaluation Metrics: Establish unambiguous measures to evaluate AI systems' effectiveness and impact, such as healthcare results, efficiency gains, and user happiness. Kaiser Permanente uses AI for population health management, regularly assessing health outcomes and cost savings.

Ethical Frameworks: Create and follow ethical frameworks for bias, openness, and patient consent (Esmaeilzadeh, 2024).

FUTURE DIRECTIONS FOR AI IN HEALTHCARE

The future of AI in healthcare promises to bring about significant improvements in patient care, clinical practice, and healthcare management. Below are some promising directions:

AI in Precision Medicine

AI will increase precision medicine by analysing genetic, environmental, and lifestyle data to build personalized treatment recommendations for each patient. AI systems, such as IBM Watson for Genomics, are evolving to provide more accurate and complete insights into patient treatment alternatives. AI can improve disease detection and prediction by recognizing patterns in medical imaging, electronic health data, and wearable devices. AI models can identify illnesses like Alzheimer's years before symptoms arise, enabling early intervention and care. AI-based surgical robots will execute procedures with less human interaction, and the outcome would be extremely accurate with a much faster recovery pace. Next-generation technologies, such as the da Vinci Surgical System, will apply advanced AI algorithms to assist surgeons.

Wearable Health Monitors: AI-integrated gadgets will continuously monitor vital indicators, delivering real-time data and early alerts for potential health risks. An example would be the advancement of smartwatches and fitness trackers to achieve medical-grade accuracy in detection and monitoring.

AI-Powered Drug Discovery and Development: AI will accelerate drug development by identifying potential candidates, predicting their efficacy, and their level of safety. For instance, some companies like Insilco Medicine and Benevolent AI utilize AI systems to come up with new medicinal compounds for drugs as well as enhance the design of drugs.

Repurpose Existing Drugs: AI can find new uses for drugs currently in use, thereby giving quicker and cheaper treatments to many diseases. AI platforms can browse through large databases for existing drugs that can effectively fight new diseases in the system. Engage more patients and foster self-management. Health virtual assistants will be stronger; they will give personalized advice regarding health, remind patients to take their drugs, and most importantly, offer psychological counseling. Babyl-on Health and Buoy Health chatbots will continue to evolve to become even more conversational and more human, thus engaging patients even further.

Chronic Disease Management: AI would manage chronic disease by analyzing the data from patients with suitable lifestyle recommendations and therapies. AI systems can read the data of diabetes patients to suggest appropriate dosages of insulin.

AI in Epidemic Prediction and Management: AI has a major role in epidemic predictions and management. This is by evaluating the data from numerous sources to find patterns and possible future epidemics. This could be possible with analysis of AI through social media, travel data, and health records to trace the spread of infectious illness transmission. AI will provide better healthcare to less developed areas as AI-based telemedicine centres can offer remote consultation services and give professional medical advice to the people living in remote areas that have fewer healthcare facilities (He et al., 2024). Such directions clarify the possibility of healthcare through AI, showing that it becomes more efficient, personalized, and accessible. With the disruptive environment, there is a need of competent healthcare professionals who can make efficient use of AI to enhance patient care services and bring innovative healthcare programmes, services, processes, culture in the hospital industry. This chapter discussed about the challenges in healthcare sector, essential skills to enhance healthcare professionals' competencies. It also discussed how the training programmes will help in enhancing essential skills amongst healthcare professionals. The chapter explained the curriculum design, interdisciplinary approach to AI education. The educational programme should focus on developing essential skills such as AI literacy, clinical expertise, critical thinking, collaboration, emotional intelligence, data analysis, innovation, ethics, and responsibility amongst the budding healthcare professionals. The entrepreneurial programmes in the field of healthcare sector enables students to design prototype for managing healthcare services. The case-based approach should also be one of the criteria to explain the use of AI in healthcare sector. The higher education institutions provide hands-on experience with AI tools and technologies to students. It is important to foster interdisciplinary collaboration between healthcare professionals, data scientists, and AI experts to encourage continuous learning and professional development, and finally, develop AI-related competencies and assessment frameworks. By educating and training the next generation of healthcare professionals in AI, we can improve patient care and outcomes with AI-driven insights, enhance operational efficiency and lower costs, drive innovation and entrepreneurship in healthcare, address healthcare workforce shortages and develop new career paths, assure responsible AI adoption, and address ethical concerns.

REFERENCES

Aliferis, C., & Simon, G. (2024). Artificial intelligence (AI) and machine learning (ML) for healthcare and health sciences: The need for best practices enabling trust in AI and ML. In Artificial Intelligence and Machine Learning in Health Care and Medical Sciences: Best Practices and Pitfalls (pp. 1–31). Springer International Publishing.

Amann, J., Blasimme, A., Vayena, E., Frey, D., & Madai, V. I. (2023). Explainability for artificial intelligence in healthcare: A multidisciplinary perspective. BMC Medical Informatics and Decision Making, 23(1), 1–18.

Chatterjee, S., Das, S., Ganguly, K., & Mandal, D. (2024). Advancements in robotic surgery: Innovations, challenges and future prospects. Journal of Robotic Surgery, 18(1), 28.

Esmaeilzadeh, P. (2024). Challenges and strategies for wide-scale artificial intelligence (AI) deployment in healthcare practices: A perspective for healthcare organizations. Artificial Intelligence in Medicine, 151, 102861.

Esteva, A., Kuprel, B., Novoa, R. A., Ko, J., Swetter, S. M., Blau, H. M., & Thrun, S. (2017). Dermatologist-level classification of skin cancer with deep neural networks. Nature, 542(7639), 115–118. https://doi.org/10.1038/nature21056

Esteva, A., Feng, J., van der Wal, D., Huang, S. C., Simko, J. P., DeVries, S., ... & Mohamad, O. (2022). Prostate cancer therapy personalization via multi-modal deep learning on randomized phase III clinical trials. NPJ Digital Medicine, 5(1), 71.

Gomes, P., Santana, E. A., & Ribeiro, B. M. (2024). Continuous learning in AI systems for healthcare: Ensuring relevance and accuracy. AI in Medicine, 50(2), 107–121.

Gulshan, V., Rajan, R. P., & Widner, K. (2021). Development and validation of a deep learning algorithm for detection of diabetic retinopathy in retinal fundus photographs. Journal of the American Medical Association, 325(24), 2446–2454. doi:10.1001/jama.2016.17216

Hachoumi, N., Eddabbah, M., & El Adib, A. R. (2023). Health sciences lifelong learning and professional development in the era of artificial intelligence. International Journal of Medical Informatics, 178, 105171.

Haddad, A., Habaebi, M. H., Islam, M. R., Hasbullah, N. F., & Zabidi, S. A. (2022). Systematic review on ai-blockchain based e-healthcare records management systems. IEEE Access, 10, 94583–94615.

Haidegger, T., Speidel, S., Stoyanov, D., & Satava, R. M. (2022). Robot-assisted minimally invasive surgery—Surgical robotics in the data age. Proceedings of the IEEE, 110(7), 835–846.

He, Y., Huang, F., Jiang, X., Nie, Y., Wang, M., Wang, J., & Chen, H. (2024). Foundation model for advancing healthcare: Challenges, opportunities, and future directions. arXiv preprint arXiv:2404.03264.

Holmes, W., Bialik, M., & Fadel, C. (2019). Artificial Intelligence in Education: Promises and Implications for Teaching and Learning. Center for Curriculum Redesign.

Huselid, M. (2015). Workforce analytics for strategy execution. The Rise of HR: Wisdom from, 72, 309–316.

Jiang, F., Jiang, Y., Zhi, H., Dong, Y., Li, H., Ma, S., & Wang, Y. (2017). Artificial intelligence in healthcare: Past, present and future. Stroke and Vascular Neurology, 2(4), 230–243.

Johnson, K. W., Torres Soto, J., Glicksberg, B. S., Shameer, K., Miotto, R., Ali, M., & Dudley, J. T. (2018). Artificial intelligence in cardiology. Journal of the American College of Cardiology, 71(23), 2668–2679.

Khan, S. D., Hoodbhoy, Z., Raja, M. H. R., Kim, J. Y., Hogg, H. D. J., Manji, A. A. A., & Sendak, M. P. (2024). Frameworks for procurement, integration, monitoring, and evaluation of artificial intelligence tools in clinical settings: A systematic review. PLOS Digital Health, 3(5), e0000514.

Kökver, Y., Pektaş, H. M., & Çelik, H. (2024). Artificial intelligence applications in education: Natural language processing in detecting misconceptions. Education and Information Technologies, 1–32.

Le, L. H., Nguyen, H. D., Crane, M., & Mai, T. T. (2024, June). Multimedia learning analytics feedback in simulation-based training: A brief review. In Proceedings of the 1st ACM Workshop on AI-Powered Q&A Systems for Multimedia (pp. 25–30).

Lera, M., Taxtsoglou, K., Iliadis, C. K., Frantzana, A. A., & Kourkouta, L. (2020). Nurses' attitudes toward lifelong learning via new technologies. Asian/Pacific Island Nursing Journal, 5(2), 89.

Logasakthi, K., Madhur, P., & Prasad, G. (2023). Exploring the role of emotional intelligence (EI) to strengthen the artificial intelligence (AI) for sustainable hr practices in the post covid-19 era. Korea Review of International Studies, 16(06), 72–81.

Mendez, R. M., Ching, T., & Honeywell, E. P. (2020). Hackathons as an Informal Learning Platform for Active Learning in Artificial Intelligence. In Proceedings of the 2020 Conference on Artificial Intelligence Education (pp. 101–106).

Merchant, Z., Goetz, E. T., Cifuentes, L., Keeney-Kennicutt, W., & Davis, T. J. (2014). Effectiveness of virtual reality-based instruction on students' learning outcomes in K-12 and higher education: A meta-analysis. Computers & Education, 70, 29–40.

Nguyen, E., Poli, M., Durrant, M. G., Kang, B., Katrekar, D., Li, D. B., ... & Hie, B. L. (2024). Sequence modeling and design from molecular to genome scale with Evo. Science, 386(6723), eado9336.

Obermeyer, Z., Powers, B., Vogeli, C., & Mullainathan, S. (2019). Dissecting racial bias in an algorithm used to manage the health of populations. Science, 366(6464), 447–453.

Pauling, C., Kanber, B., Arthurs, O. J., & Shelmerdine, S. C. (2024). Commercially available artificial intelligence tools for fracture detection: The evidence. BJR| Open, 6(1), tzad005.

Rajkomar, A., Dean, J., & Kohane, I. (2019). Machine learning in medicine. New England Journal of Medicine, 380(14), 1347–1358.

Rajpurkar, P., Irvin, J., Ball, R. L., Zhu, K., Yang, B., Mehta, H., & Ng, A. Y. (2018). Deep learning for chest radiograph diagnosis: A retrospective comparison of the CheXNeXt algorithm to practicing radiologists. PLoS Medicine, 15(11), e1002686.

Roehl, A., Reddy, S. L., & Shannon, G. J. (2013). The flipped classroom: An opportunity to engage millennial students through active learning. Journal of Family and Consumer Sciences, 105(2), 44.

Sadiku, Matthew N. O. Olaleye, Olaniyi D., & Musa, Sarhan M. (2020). Emotional intelligence in healthcare, International Journal of Trend in Research and Development, 7(1), ISSN: 2394-9333.

Sadiku, M. N., Olaleye, O. D., & Musa, S. M. (2020b). Emotional intelligence in relationships. International Journal of Trend in Research and Development, 7(1), 318–321.

Sallam, M., Barakat, M., & Sallam, M. (2024). A preliminary checklist (METRICS) to standardize the design and reporting of studies on generative artificial Intelligence–Based models in health care education and practice: Development study involving a literature review. Interactive Journal of Medical Research, 13(1), e54704.

Sharma, V., & Kumar, H. (2023). Emotional intelligence in the era of artificial intelligence for medical professionals. Journal for International Medical Graduates, 2(2), 1–2.

Topol, E. J. (2019). High-performance medicine: The convergence of human and artificial intelligence. Nature Medicine, 25(1), 44–56.

Van der Vegt, A. H., Campbell, V., Mitchell, I., Malycha, J., Simpson, J., Flenady, T., & Scott, I. A. (2024). Systematic review and longitudinal analysis of implementing artificial intelligence to predict clinical deterioration in adult hospitals: What is known and what remains uncertain. Journal of the American Medical Informatics Association, 31(2), 509–524.

Wang, D., Khosla, A., Gargeya, R., Irshad, H., & Beck, A. H. (2016). Deep learning for identifying metastatic breast cancer. arXiv preprint arXiv:1606.05718.

Whittaker, M., Hodge, N., Mares, R. E., & Rodney, A. (2015). Preparing for the data revolution: identifying minimum health information competencies among the health workforce. Human resources for health, 13, 1–12.

Wilmink, G., Dupey, K., Alkire, S., Grote, J., Zobel, G., Fillit, H. M., & Movva, S. (2020). Artificial intelligence–powered digital health platform and wearable devices improve outcomes for older adults in assisted living communities: Pilot intervention study. JMIR Aging, 3(2), e19554.

12 Artificial Intelligence (AI) Adoption and Governance *Frameworks and Best Practices*

Narayanage Jayantha Dewasiri, Mananage Shanika Hansini Rathnasiri, Kiran Sood, and Rubee Singh

INTRODUCTION TO ARTIFICIAL INTELLIGENCE ADOPTION AND GOVERNANCE

Artificial intelligence (AI) has become an essential aspect of the growth of organisations and can be called a contemporary technological paradigm with diverse potential outcomes for various business industries and societies (Dewasiri et al., 2023a). Looking at its origin in the early mid-20th century, AI has come a long way, especially with the recent advancements in machine learning, neural networks, and natural language processing even though the initial attempts to create AI were, for the most part, targeted towards achieving morphological computation and comprehension—which is in transition now. However, in the last few decades, capabilities have been proven to explode due to getting used to more sophisticated computing power and tremendous data. In today's context, AI systems become essential to many functions, from transportation and medicine to marketing and finance (Lu, 2019). These improvements highlight a concern about contemporary AI technology and its direction in the future. There are many reasons for AI adoption from a business and society perspective. AI also foresees effectiveness increments, cost controls, and new business solutions, which gives a competitive advantage amidst an ever-dynamic marketplace (Wamba-Taguimdje et al., 2020). Machine learning can execute and modify simple and repetitive procedures; big data enables essential conclusions to be drawn, and new and innovative products and services can be developed. Societal imperatives pushing AI are equally strong, with AI assuming a pivotal role in solving various issues ranging from climate change to increased accessibility of healthcare and optimisation of public services. This can save time, diagnose diseases early, recommend appropriate treatment, and even design treatment plans based on the patient's needs (Alowais et al., 2023). Equally, climate change interventions can benefit from AI applications in modelling and managing energy consumption (Ohalete et al., 2023). AI governance (AIG) is an essential framework for addressing these implications. AIG is different from conventional IT or data management, and it is a strategic and ethical concept that includes AI's responsibility, legal, and liability issues. AI Governance enables AI implementation so that no person will be harmed through unfair discrimination while ensuring their

DOI: 10.1201/9781003531272-12

privacy remains intact without any negative consequences for the society. It sets out measures that define how it will embrace the culture of openness and integrity in engineering the public's confidence. Comparing AIG with other forms of governance provides an understanding that is exclusive to AI technologies to the extent of the impact on societal morality. This chapter aims to present AI adoption and governance in more detail. The objectives are to define the need for the governance framework for AI and discover the opportunities and threats resulting from efficient and inefficient AIG. Further, it examines AI considerations and governance factors likely to inform the development of those frameworks. It also provides AI cases and success stories across industries. The chapter also highlights potential challenges organisations may encounter in AIG development and implementation, identifies the expected future trends, and briefly evaluates their impact on organisations and society. Through this study, readers can understand the fundamental tenets, approaches, and structures in AI that will assist them in effectively and responsibly reining in AI.

METHODOLOGY

This chapter adopts a systematic literature review (SLR) approach without compromising the strength of the synthesis of currently available knowledge, as pointed out by Bandara et al. (2025), Chathuranga et al. (2025), Dewasiri et al. (2024), Karunarathne et al. (2024), and Vijerathne et al. (2025), following the Preferred Reporting Items for Systematic Reviews and Meta-Analyses (PRISMA) guidelines. This approach allows for a more systematic and credible way of categorising, appraising, and systematic literature searching and review, thus aiding in gathering information, deciding what might have been overlooked and providing a more extensive view of the phenomenon from various sources. The PRISMA framework, applied to enhance the transparency and reproducibility of the review process, involves four key stages: recruitment, selection, access, and entry. During the identification stage, (1) Scopus and Google Scholar databases were searched, and keywords used while searching were AI adoption, AIG frameworks, ethical AI, regulatory compliance, and stakeholder engagement. Other sources were industry reports, white papers, and current conference proceedings. In the first step of the screening stage, every duplicate study was removed, and in the second step, the non-relevant studies were removed by the titles and abstract. Screening was done in the eligibility stage at the article level when searching for a study that overlapped with other studies that we were eligible for in title and abstract screening and full-text review based on inclusion and exclusion criteria. Last but not least, in the synthesis stage, all the studies that met the above-stated criteria were included in the final synthesis. First, a priori inclusion and exclusion criteria were set to identify appropriate studies. The inclusion criteria were centred on papers which treated organisations that had adopted AI technologies within the health sector and financial and production industries. Governance structures being proposed within these studies must consider AI and its governance concerning ethical issues, restrictions put in place by legal requirements, and how to consider stakeholders who may be affected by AI decisions or implementation structures being put in place. Positive results for increased efficiency of AI systems, greater trust of stakeholders, and the achievement of regulatory goals were critical. Further, to capture recent developments and discourse, only articles published in the last ten years and only studies in English were included in the review. Such filter criteria excluded papers specifically discussing technical AI aspects, the lack of proposed or discussed governance frameworks, and papers that did not include any comparative analysis or distinguish between outcomes regarding the effectiveness of different governance frameworks. Published papers over a decade or those written in languages other than English were also removed where no translation was possible. The PICO model of categorising the research questions was applied by dividing the questions into population, intervention, comparison, and desired Outcomes (Eriksen & Frandsen, 2018). The population element consisted of organisations and sectors implementing AI technologies in healthcare, finance, and manufacturing. The intervention concerned adopting the AIG policies, principles, and requirements organisations adopt. The comparison element compared various governance structures and their efficiency. The outcome element focused on better AI systems performance in claims, higher stakeholder confidence, and regulatory requirements. Thus, this study follows the SLR approach to synthesise extant literature on AI adoption and its governance by applying the PRISMA framework and using the PICO format. The papers selected for the final analysis totalled 37, providing solid ground for synthesising the findings and recommendations.

IMPORTANCE OF GOVERNANCE FRAMEWORKS IN AI ADOPTION

As AI integrates into various aspects of business and society, establishing robust governance frameworks becomes increasingly crucial. These frameworks are the backbone for aligning AI projects with organisational goals and ethical standards, ensuring that AI technologies are deployed responsibly and effectively.

Role of Governance in AI

Governance frameworks relating to AI are central in helping an organisation align AI-related projects with its strategic goals and ethical principles. They offer a systematised framework for approaching AI as an innovation through which AI solutions align with the organisation's vision and mission. The fact that AIG is a comprehensive process dictates the production of general regulations and standards regarding the implementation of AI in various organisations (Díaz-Rodríguez et al., 2023). This alignment is crucial to create sustainable advancement of AI to address both technical requirements and business needs and reflect ethical and social standards. Besides, governance frameworks contribute to developing AI projects' accountability and transparency (de Almeida et al., 2021). In this case, role and responsibility frameworks enable all stakeholders to understand their tasks and their work's ethical consequences. This clears up confusion over how and when a creation can and cannot be used and is, therefore, practical in discouraging abuse and encouraging proper development. Moreover, governance frameworks help make sound decisions since they outline the guidelines and best practice checklists that can be adopted in assessing AI systems and ensure that all decisions are systematic.

Benefits of Effective AI Governance

Management should note that effective AIG comes with countless advantages. First, trust among stakeholders grows as one of the primary sources of benefit (Kuziemski & Misuraca, 2020). Customers, employees, and regulators trust an organisation's AI programmes most when they observe that the organisation is serious about adopting responsible AI. Another essential advantage is adherence to the law and regulations if the relevant rules of AI governance are correctly implemented. With various governments continuing to set standards for AI's ethics and social impacts, organisations must ensure that their systems observe the standards. Enormous pressure comes from different and sometimes even conflicting regulations, which makes governance frameworks worthwhile for organisations to give them structure and describe how to adhere to the rules. It reduces the chances of legal consequences and improves the organisation's standing in the eyes of the public as a good actor in AI. It also attests that good governance enhances AI systems' effectiveness (Young et al., 2019). Governing structures for the usage of AI advocate for the appropriate usage of AI by stewarding the processes through testing, validation, and checking. They assist the organisation in achieving the targeted goal and its outcomes because of their reliability. Moreover, ethical concerns and opportunities for being biased are learned and preempted in fostering equitable solutions during AI construction, provoking organisational improvement in such organisations' performance and social responsibility.

Risks of Poor Governance

This study shows that the lack of appropriate governance in AI presents several major threats. One of the most significant challenges is algorithmic bias, which is the problem of AI bias that generates unfair or discriminative results (Varona & Suárez, 2022). It is the kind of prejudice that results from training on datasets that share this bias, faulty algorithms, or other inadvertences of AI system development. Some biases are unnoticed and unrepaired without adequate governance; organisations face severe ethical and legal repercussions. Privacy violation is another danger associated with inadequate AIG, as pointed out by Murdoch (2021). Many AI systems are built based on the data, and such data can be one's personal information or even secrets. When there is no effective compliance to govern the use of data in an organisation, it becomes easy for an organisation to experience a data breach of information, which is very costly regarding reputation and may lead to fines when the law is breached. Components of suitable governance structures relate to the governance and management of data, which must be shared, stored, and protected for privacy. Liability issues are also a notable concern when the governance of AI is not well handled, as highlighted by Wirtz et al. (2022). Since the guidelines regarding AI are still changing, organisations that are not compliant with these standards may suffer significant penalties and lawsuits. In addition, a lack of good governance usually leads to an inability to explain these systems' decisions and actions. This aspect can worsen legal and ethical concerns, where their invisibility weakens organisational objectivity and public trust.

Ensuring Ethical Use of AI

Principles of Ethical AI

The principles of ethical AI are fundamental to the development and deployment of AI systems. Key principles include fairness, accountability, and transparency (Schrader & Ghosh, 2018; Singhal et al., 2024):

Fairness: It must be ensured that AI systems everywhere are not programmed to be biased and do not discriminate against any group. This includes choosing and preparing the data appropriately, constantly evaluating the data fed into the system, and analysing it to reduce or eliminate biased inputs.

Accountability: Clear roles and responsibilities should be established for developing, deploying, and overseeing AI systems. This ensures that individuals and organisations can be held accountable for the outcomes of AI systems.

Transparency: AI systems and their decision-making processes should be as transparent as possible. This includes clear documentation of how AI systems are designed and operated and explanations for decisions made by AI systems.

Preventing Bias and Discrimination

Non-biased introduction of the datasets and avoiding discrimination in the value addition is now a challenge to AI systems' successful, ethical implementation (Lin et al., 2020; Ntoutsi et al., 2020). This type of discrimination occurs for various reasons, including inadequate datasets during model development or improper methods used in the model design (Tejani et al., 2024). For example, physical security systems such as facial recognition have been found to perform significantly worse for specific demographic categories because the training data used is skewed. Organisations should put the following best practices in place to manage these risks.

Diverse and Representative Training Data: The AI system must ensure that the training data is diverse and should represent the population.

Regular Audits and Testing: Regular audits and testing are required to address biases and inaccuracies in AI systems.

Algorithmic Fairness Techniques: Applying fairness constraints and reweighting to algorithms is required to reduce bias.

Promoting Fairness and Inclusivity

Fairness and bias mitigate the adverse effects of AI technologies on selected groups and favour other groups in society (Akinrinola et al., 2024). As highlighted below, several strategies exist for inclusive AI development.

Stakeholder engagement: Engaging the population in a society that has not mainly focused on AI technologies by including them and allowing them to participate in developing the technology.

Inclusive design practices: Finally, the practices for implementing better designs focus on people with impairments in order to make AI helpful for everyone.

Impact assessments: Carrying out a risk analysis to assess the relationship between AI systems' impacts on different groups within the population and taking necessary action to solve or minimise the harmful effects.

Therefore, this study emphasizes the need for governance frameworks in AI adoption. These frameworks contain the fundamental structure and direction necessary for sustainable development to guarantee that AI technologies are created and implemented according to an organisation's values and ethical norms. The consequences of effective AI regulation are far higher in terms of trust, adherence to the norms established by legal entities, and the effectiveness of systems compared to the risks posed by ineffective regulation. To make AI sustainable, applying fairness and accountability principles, ensuring the absence of bias, and promoting inclusiveness are crucial. Reflectively, the future of AI will pinpoint the need for authoritarian formation and regulation of its applications since innovation in this area will not stop.

KEY CONSIDERATIONS IN DEVELOPING AI GOVERNANCE FRAMEWORKS

Formulating practical AIG frameworks helps establish, maintain, monitor, and enforce responsible and ethical AI practices. This chapter discusses why AIG can be considered practical, considering its key attributes and how stakeholders can be engaged. It also offers practical suggestions for creating solid policies and procedures.

Foundational Elements of AI Governance

The governance framework should consist of principles, rules, and recommendations (Aguilera & Cuervo-Cazurra, 2004, 2009), which offer a framework for AI technologies. These are vital components that constitute the foundation of good practice governance frameworks in AI that guarantee the organisation's goals and compliance with ethical principles of the AI systems. Figure 12.1 indicates the components of a good governance framework for AI.

Policies: AI policies are documented guidelines for people in an organisation outlining procedures and laws regarding creating and applying AI solutions. They cover data protection, ethical issues, legal requirements, organisational risks, and compliance. Setting proper AI policies entails organisations understanding the numerous AI technologies and executing their governance policies unifiedly and effectively.

Guidelines: Standards offer specific information and suggestions on how to enforce AI policies. AIG offers practical recommendations regarding implementing policies within specific contexts, such as data dealing, algorithms, and systems implementation. Frameworks are also crucial in breaking down goals set at the top-down actionable steps that the developers, data scientists, or any other participant in the project may undertake.

Best Practices: Best practices refer to well-known practices that pertain to the administration of AI technologies. These practices include all nano

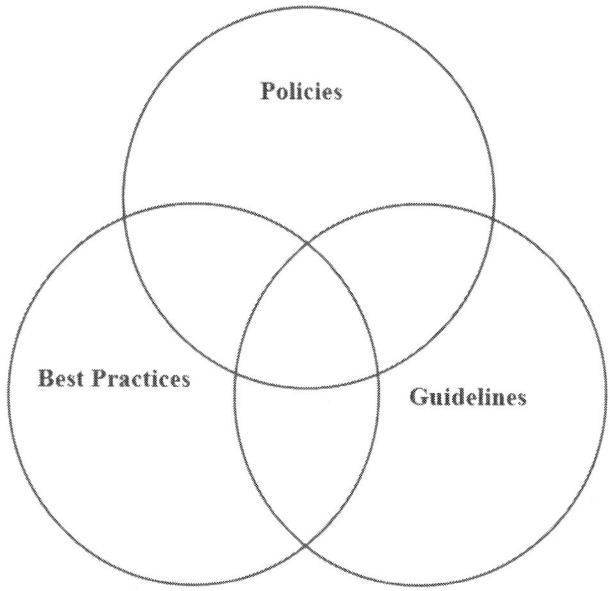

FIGURE 12.1 AI governance (AIG) framework.

Source: Authors' own.

detonation processes, including data acquisition and preparation, model learning, and assessment. Thus, best practices allow organisations to address concerns about the reliability, fairness, and transparency of AI systems. Best practices have also been modified from previous projects, and improvements have been made in AI studies.

Stakeholder Involvement and Collaboration

In order to be fully effective, AIG needs diverse stakeholders from various fields of work, starting with technologists and ethicists, and with the regular citizens, the end-users, NGOs and, last but not least, representing the state or the regulatory authorities.

Technologists: AI implementers, data scientists, and engineers power most of the technical aspects surrounding AIG. They must be involved in compliance, support the development of policies and guidelines for using AI systems in all spheres of life, and solve any technology issues.

Ethicists: Ethicists give us excellent ideas of the moral and ethical aspects of the development of AI technologies. The parties could include data subjects, customers, or consumers through organisations such as Consumers International, social scientists, or ethicists, as well as any autonomous AI system to guarantee fairness, accountability, and transparency. Ethicists can also search for possible ethical issues and recommend ethical standards and theories.

End-Users: Engaging the end-users in the governance process means that the institutions facilitate the principles of their AI systems to incorporate the users' preferences. Users can give their perceptions on the usefulness and accessibility of AI systems and their acceptability to justify the development and usage of the technologies in addressing particular challenges.

Regulatory Bodies: This study estimates that regulatory bodies and policymakers play critical roles in shaping the legal and regulatory environment for AIG. Their participation formalises AI's adherence to the set laws and regulations and minimises the legal consequences associated with AI.

Establishing Policies and Procedures

Creating effective AIG policies and procedures involves several key steps. Figure 12.2 outlines a step-by-step approach to developing robust governance frameworks; every step is interconnected.

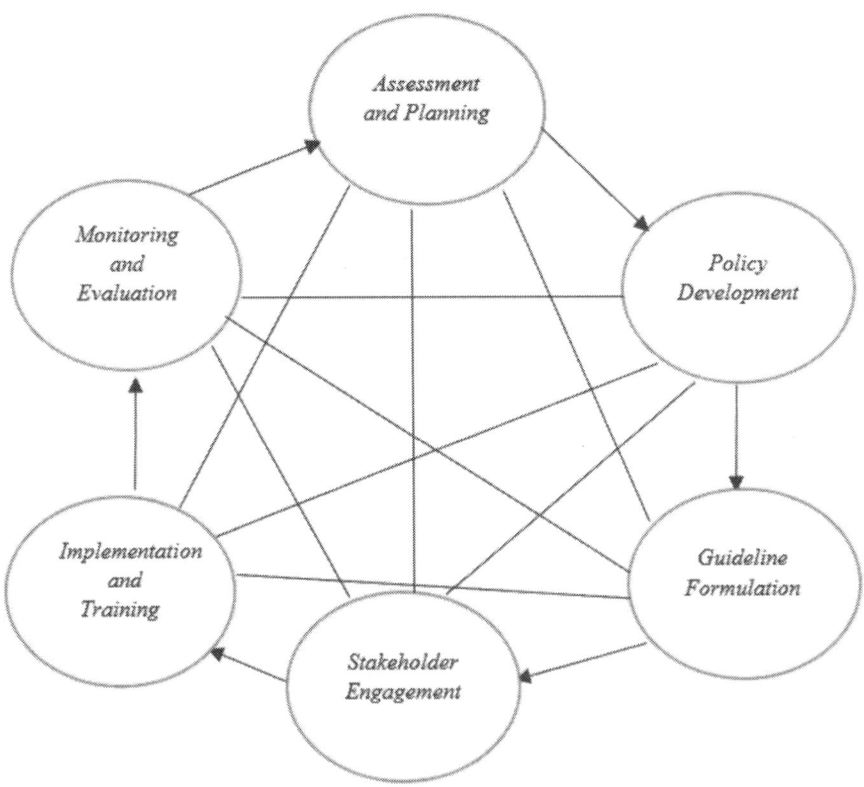

FIGURE 12.2 Establishment guidelines.

Source: Authors' own.

Assessment and Planning

The first step is a diagnostic scan of the organisational readiness, AI opportunities, threats, strengths, weaknesses, and requirements for AIG. This assessment assists in defining the areas that require governance most urgently and what kind of difficulties the organisation meets. After the assessment, the next activity is identifying the scope and goals of AIG at a particular organisation. This entails coordinating the organisation's and stakeholders' existing characteristics to provide for all the aspects captured in the framework.

Policy Development

AI policies are necessary to fill critical governance gaps in data protection, AI ethics, compliance, and risks. Such policies should ideally conform to the organisation's strategic plans and moral standards. Accordingly, AIG can be anchored to corporate strategy to ensure the different decisions and actions in the organisation are consistent as per the incorporation of AI.

Guideline Formulation

The next step is to develop implemental procedures that offer finer directions on implementing these policies. Such guidelines should cover numerous recommendations and practices applicable to general or specific stages of AI, from data gathering to model implementation. The guidelines are also crucial for ensuring the policies are implemented accordingly. Hence, every step of this stepwise guideline is mutually exclusive and interrelated.

Stakeholder Engagement

Stakeholders who are usually left out of the policy and guideline development process should be involved. This is the case with technologists, ethicists, end-users, and regulatory bodies. Organisations may also help conduct workshops, consultations, or feedback and guarantee that the policies and guidelines do not omit anything. Stakeholder engagement also assists in gaining commitment to the governance framework because of its support.

Implementation and Training

Figure 12.2 shows the actual process of applying the framework of AIG within an organisation. It entails that all the stakeholders understand and are in a position to perform their duties. Much importance should be placed on the training and availability of resources to ensure the effectiveness of the noted policies and guidelines. The training should follow the type and level of stakeholders involved with governance to empower all stakeholders in applying the governance framework.

Monitoring and Evaluation

The last phase is the creation of tools for awareness and assessment of the efficiency of the AI governing framework. This means periodically revising the measures regarding contents and approaches for policies, guidelines, and models followed regarding the feedback received, existing knowledge and work currently available, and standard guidelines prevalent in the field. In this case, the evaluation assists the organisation in discovering other areas that require enhancement and changes that need to be made to the governance structures. Consequently, building adequate policy frameworks for AIG encompasses an analytical method involving identification and evaluation, policy development, guideline standardisation, strategy formulation, stakeholder management, policy and guideline implementation and training, and policy evaluation and feedback. By following the stepwise guideline, organisations can develop suitable methods of AIG to ensure that they adopt any AI without compromising ethical factors.

Transparency and Accountability

Transformative transparency and accountability are significant to technology regulation and governance (Diakopoulos, 2020). These principles make sure that AI systems are transparent and accountable for how they perform their roles so that their risks do not affect others. Owing to the earlier conclusion and recommendation, it is possible to affirm that transparent practices enhance the understandability of AI and its decision-making patterns to stakeholders, as Felzmann et al. (2020) stated. That is, while governance structures regulate who acts on behalf of whom and monitor the general use of AI systems, accountability structures ensure that a specific individual or organisation is responsible for certain results from these systems.

Mechanisms for Ensuring Transparency

Transparency involves tools and practices that make AI systems more understandable and accessible to stakeholders (Larsson & Heintz, 2020). One such practice is the implementation of open data practices that allow transparency. Making raw data and algorithms available means that all the interested people can see and analyse the data and steps used during AI development. This openness facilitates trust and allows for outside validation of the specific impact of any AI solution. This chapter considers clarity and honesty as two critical pillars of transparency. In general, providing contextual information and algorithms supporting the outputs of AI systems enables users to increase their trust. This means avoiding using technical terms, diagrams, coloured illustrations, graphics or instructional aids when explaining technical matters.

Accountability Structures

Role and responsibility assignments within AI governing structures guarantee that the user and other stakeholders are liable for the results generated by the AI systems (Janssen et al., 2020). Accountability structures consist of role clarification, the technical power of decision, and ethical review committees. Another issue that deserves consideration is the related responsibilities of all the involved stakeholders: developers, data scientists, project managers, and those who, in one way or another, govern and oversee AI projects. The organisational differentiation of decision-making responsibilities also means only qualified and authorised individuals make decisions. Forming ethical oversight committees to review and monitor AI projects ensures they adhere to ethical standards and governance policies, further reinforcing accountability.

Reporting and Audit Trails

Record keeping of the activities in developing and implementing AI remains crucial for oversight and responsibility. Several practices include effective reporting and audit trails (Falco et al., 2021). The indexing of information in AI systems with information sources, system design, training and recognition processes, and detailed specifications on criteria that are employed in making choices provides a straightforward way of documenting how AI systems were developed and the information developed can be used in auditing purposes should the need arises. It is also essential to propose periodic reporting tools to help AI systems owners and users assess their efficacy, compliance with the principles of ethics, and outcomes. Instead, these reports should be communicated to stakeholders, governance bodies, regulating entities, and the end consumers. Further, data trails generated that record all the essential activities and choices associated with the AI systems are guaranteed to be safe, alterable, and retrievable for audit purposes. Therefore, effective strategies are needed for AIG policies and guidelines, including providing general policies and guidelines, stakeholder mapping and engagement, and policy and procedural development. A particular emphasis should be placed on the principles and practices regarding open data and the availability of clear communication structures, roles, reporting, and auditing mechanisms as critical elements to effective risk management targeting trust and accountability. Based on the above cardinal principles, organisations can set and exercise proper governance standards to ensure accurate and proper uptake of AI.

CASE STUDIES OF AI ADOPTION AND GOVERNANCE FRAMEWORKS

Investigating real-world examples of AI adoption and governance frameworks offers invaluable insights into best practices and common challenges. This section presents case studies on different industries, including healthcare, finance, and manufacturing, and an overview of best practices and possible pitfalls.

Overview of the Selected Case Studies

Healthcare Industry

AI has been applied in industries for predictive analysis and the development of custom medication and process management in the health sector. The expansion of Google's AI-based solutions, such as for radiology at the Mayo Clinic, was an excellent example of AI implementation in the healthcare sector (Zhang et al., 2021). This study shows the effectiveness of AI in medicine by analysing how the technique improves diagnostic results, streamlines procedures, and ultimately improves patient care, as revealed by the example from the case study. The partnership between engineers who work on the AI platform and doctors and intense updates about the development of AI systems are significant for using advanced technologies in the healthcare industry to enhance new and improved practices and outcomes in the future.

Finance Industry

AI supports financial industry applications in fraud detection, risk management, and customer care. The AI use case employed at JPMorgan Chase was an automated fraud detection tool, COiN (Contract Intelligence), which examines legal papers and extracts significant points that help identify deceptive and risk-prone situations (Kaswan et al., 2023). It has made financial document processing faster and less costly while improving the accuracy of detecting fraud, thus improving efficiency and building customer trust.

Manufacturing Industry

AI technologies are incorporated in manufacturing to help in decision-making to increase production efficiency, guarantee product quality, and ensure a timely and efficient supply of products. Under the industrial equipment segments, General Electric (GE) has adopted AI-based maintenance prediction systems. These systems are used to observe equipment performance over time, and they use machine learning techniques to identify future failures. Ironically, while breakdowns would otherwise slow production lines and increase maintenance costs, GE has reduced downtime and its costs since these unanticipated mechanical failures do not occur.

Success Factors and Lessons Learned

As given below, several common themes emerge from these case studies that contribute to successfully implementing AIG frameworks.

Clear Objectives and Goals: For any AI project to be successful, it should first be anchored on its objectives or goals. Companies will be in the best place to synchronize their AI strategies with the business vision, mission, and objectives framework of what they intend to accomplish with AI.

Stakeholder Engagement: Several phases also identify relevant stakeholders such as technologists, ethicists, regulatory authorities, and end-users. This approach guarantees adequate insights into the beneficial and detrimental possibilities of applying AI systems while designing them.

Robust Policies and Guidelines: This is fundamental since defining rules and regulations to be followed when developing and implementing an AI emanates hitches that would otherwise cause vulnerability and unethical practices. These policies include privacy and security on data, bias, and regulation.

Transparency and Accountability: More transparent AI activities and decisions can improve stakeholder trust. Such transparency means explaining how the AI system functions and the reasoning process used in decision-making by the systems. Furthermore, clarifying and assigning prerogatives is essential to avoid the generalisation of responsibilities at all levels.

Continuous Monitoring and Evaluation: Organisations integrate a framework for continuous monitoring and assessment of the AI systems used. Continual evaluation and adjustments, in addition to the feedback received, newly published literature, and changes in practice, contribute to the currency of AIG frameworks.

As mentioned above, several significant lessons can be learned from the case studies. Prevention is better than cure; early intervention in AI development through governance frameworks enables organizations to control or eliminate risks before they escalate, resulting in significant challenges for the organizational integration of AI systems. Availability is also crucial since AI technologies and their associated solutions are ever-changing. The governance structures must always accommodate new developments and issues as they emerge. Further, continuous training and education for all stakeholders participating in AI solutions development are mandatory. Hence, policymakers have improved their understanding of the governance framework, followed by roles within this system and ethical concerns of these emerging technologies to improve moral compliance. Therefore, through the case studies of the healthcare, finance, and manufacturing industries, it has been shown that the elements of goals and objectives, stakeholders, efficient policies, openness, responsibility, and audit are significant in the good governance of AI. From these cases, organisations can learn how to establish and use AIG structures to accomplish suitable and moral AI use.

CHALLENGES AND OPPORTUNITIES IN IMPLEMENTING AI GOVERNANCE FRAMEWORKS

Applying good AIG frameworks contains implantation challenges and the prospect of new opportunities. Today, different organizations encounter several challenges that prevent them from adopting and effectively governing AI systems.

Common Obstacles Faced by Organizations

Organisations face a few common challenges when adopting AIG frameworks. AI technologies are complex and often require and depend on high-quality data, leading to structural challenges. The most common technical challenge is integrating AI systems into existing structures. Some of these technical barriers negatively impact the implementation process of AI and can lead to errors. Some organisational factors include a lack of organisational support, fear of changes, poor organisational skills, and lack of coordination, which arise from different functional areas of an organisation. Most organisations face challenges in achieving both alignments of AI with overall organisational objectives and AI culture change. Regulatory issues arise mainly due to the changing contours of the legal framework of AI. It is often not easy to navigate through numerous rules and regulations, and today, organisations must meet data privacy requirements, ethical criteria, social acceptance, and sectorial norms.

Strategies to Overcome Challenges

A few practical solutions and organisational best practices regarding the abovementioned challenges can be followed. From a technical perspective, a sound approach towards data management is needed because the quality of our data is paramount to good investment decision-making. Organisations should use a modular approach when adopting AI, with some preliminary projects used to weigh the potential risks and benefits the organisation will encounter. From an organisational point of view, there is a need to promote creativity and learning. At present, a learning culture and targeted education support the development of essential competencies and counteract change resistance (Dewasiri et al., 2023b). However, evidence also proves that the involvement of other departments and stakeholders may also improve the focus of AI initiatives. To overcome the legal risks, organisations should keep abreast of changes in the legal environment and interact with legal authorities. Finding the best strategies and ethical standards necessary for compliance work to manage today's compliance challenges can be crucial.

Leveraging Opportunities for Improvement

Nevertheless, organisations can have considerable opportunities to enhance AI policies and governance standards. Organisations can improve their AI systems' capabilities and productivity by applying the recent developments in AI sciences. Another critical factor is to review and update the governance policies and procedures frequently—but in practice, this has to be done in the light of new research, feedback, and experience or what might be considered best practice in the field. In the same way, organisations should also engage external experts, industry consortia, and regulatory bodies to capture emerging trends and standards. This proactive approach towards AI governance, where monitoring, evaluation, or iteration are activities that we engage in daily, can help roll out better forms of AI governance. This approach minimises risks and enhances stakeholders' confidence, thus creating a favourable culture. Therefore, as much as applying AI governance frameworks appears to have potential difficulties, organisations must overcome these difficulties by effectively planning and learning the strategies and proactively engaging with regulatory developments. Hence, organisations can implement sound AI governance practices to support appropriate AI deployment by optimising improvement prospects and remaining constantly flexible.

FUTURE TRENDS IN AI ADOPTION AND GOVERNANCE

According to a study, the landscape for AI technology adoption and governance will change as the technologies evolve. Familiarising ourselves with emerging trends and their positive or negative impact on organisations may contribute to better preparing management and advancing the creation of appropriate forms of governance.

Emerging Technologies and Their Impact on AI Governance

Emerging approaches to AI platforms like quantum computing, edge AI, and federated learning are set to change how new AI systems will be built and operated. Quantum computing integrates computation capability so that it helps to develop more advanced AI models and faster results in data processing. AI capability is progressive; this advancement will call for new forms of proper governance due to the risks and ethical challenges that are bound to arise with advanced AI systems. Local intelligence, or edge AI, implies that no data is sent to data centres for processing because the results can be obtained almost instantly. However, it opens new governance questions about data protection and security and how standards will be achieved across decentralised systems. It allows training AI models across several decentralised devices even though the raw data never has to be shared. It brings enhanced data protection requirements but weakens the ways of defining the model's accuracy and stability. All these technologies will create new work relationships that require innovative and future-oriented governance systems to deal with such relations.

Anticipated Changes in Regulatory Landscapes

It can also be predicted that AI's regulation policies will tighten and be more inclusive in the future. The specific and more extensive governing rules relating to AI's ethical, societal, and economic effects will probably be instituted by such governments and global organisations. For example, the European Union's AI Act is meant to regulate AI, provide safety, and require applicable actors to be transparent and accountable. These regulations will act as a challenge that organisations must address to improve compliance approaches and incorporate regulatory issues into AIG frameworks. Some of these are obvious, such as the rising global trends on data privacy and protection, and others, which may include regulations requiring ethical standards to be placed on AI and other trends concerning AI decision-making. Such changes may present a challenge to the organisations, and it becomes the organisation's responsibility to ensure it keeps updating on any changes and incorporates the new changes into its governance structures to avoid non-compliance and to increase the level of assurance to the stakeholders.

Long-Term Implications for Businesses and Society

AI presents long-standing prospects equally to business people and societies at large. AI is poised to revolutionise industries through increased innovation, competition, and productivity. However, the findings unveil profound ethical and social ramifications. Companies need to pursue AI-related opportunities while managing related risks, including lack of employment for AI-driven job profiles, violation of people's privacy, and bias created in the AI models. Findings highlighted that AI will remain a growing phenomenon in the future and impact different facets of our lives, such as healthcare, learning, transport, and financial services. This will be important for AI advancements, which will benefit a broad population and reduce negative externalities. In addition, opacity, governance, and ethical implications will assume even greater significance as these technologies advance from adoption to deployment. Organisations that place such aspects into their governance structures will thus be better equipped to achieve trust and legitimacy for their AI endeavours. Consequently, future advancements concerning AI adoption and AIG will occur in response to both continuous improvements in technology and shifts in available regulation, as well as the understanding and effects of AI on society. Thus, flexibility and activity are essential prerequisites for organisations, which should modify their governance to counterbalance such threats and benefit from novel opportunities. In doing so, they can integrate responsible and ethical AI, which will help boost the business's general performance and, at the same time, positively impact society.

CONCLUSION

In the current AI environment, there is a greater demand for effective AI implementation and regulation standards. This chapter highlighted various perspectives of AI governance and has underlined its relevance in maintaining the consistency between AI initiatives and business objectives, values, and policies. In this study, by critically analysing the characteristics of AI governance frameworks, it is possible to understand how vital these frameworks are for constructing sustainable and responsible AI development in the future. This chapter focused on the outcome of good AIG, which consists of the prominence of the stakeholders' trust, fulfilment of legal requirements, and optimisation of the AI system. On the other hand, the associated poor governors consist of algorithmic bias, privacy infringement, and legal consequences that call for appropriate organisational governance. Understanding the principles of fair and excellent AI is critical to these initiatives. There are three principles: fairness, accountability, and transparency. Rather than risk developing flawed AI marked by bias, organisations can create creative, fair, and open social and technical systems.

Several essential factors must be examined when creating AI governance frameworks: the set of basic policies, the role of the stakeholders, and the procedures regarding the disclosure of AI actions. The specific real-life examples from healthcare, finance, and manufacturing discuss how these three sectors implemented AIG. Although there exist many barriers to AIG jurisdiction, such as technical barriers, organisational barriers, and regulatory barriers, practical solutions to AIG jurisdiction are not difficult to come by. The organisations able to have opportunities for change, regulation updates, and adoption of learning and innovation in AI are going to be the masters of an AI-challenged world.

Therefore, future trends in AI governance will be shaped by progress in AI technology, rules, and laws. New technologies encompassing quantum computing, edge AI, and federated learning will be other areas that will present new governance challenges, and thus, new frameworks will be needed. This new direction will require compliance and ethical standards that are higher than before and are proactively designed to meet anticipated changes in the regulatory environment. By the very nature of how it is being adopted and integrated into businesses and people's lives, its effects on businesses and society will be lasting. AI will fundamentally change industries and aspects of people's lives. While turning to AI is a move forward, questions of morality and ethics must be addressed.

REFERENCES

Aguilera, R. V., & Cuervo-Cazurra, A. (2004). Codes of good governance worldwide: What is the trigger? Organization Studies, 25(3), 415–443.

Aguilera, R. V., & Cuervo-Cazurra, A. (2009). Codes of good governance. Corporate Governance: An International Review, 17(3), 376–387.

Akinrinola, O., Okoye, C. C., Ofodile, O. C., & Ugochukwu, C. E. (2024). Navigating and reviewing ethical dilemmas in AI development: Strategies for transparency, fairness, and accountability. GSC Advanced Research and Reviews, 18(3), 050–058.

Alowais, S. A., Alghamdi, S. S., Alsuhebany, N., Alqahtani, T., Alshaya, A. I., Almohareb, S. N., Aldairem, A., Alrashed, M., Bin Saleh, K., Badreldin, H. A., & Al Yami, M. S. (2023). Revolutionising healthcare: The role of artificial intelligence in clinical practice. BMC Medical Education, 23(1), 689–699.

Bandara, C. M. Y. S. S., Rathnasiri, M. S. H., Dewasiri, N. J., Chathuranga, B. T. K., & Singh, N. (2025). Greening the economy for a sustainable future: Opportunities and perceptions. In S. Grima, K. Sood, E. Özen, & R. D. Gonzi (Eds.), Science of sustainable systems: Greening our economy for a sustainable future (pp. 197–213). Elsevier. https://doi.org/10.1016/B978-0-443-23603-7.00016-9

Chathuranga, B. T. K., Rathnasiri, M. S. H., Dewasiri, N. J., Jayarathne, P. G. S. A., Bandara, C. M. Y. S. S., & Bakari, M. A. (2025). Direct and indirect effect on industries and services (A). In S. Grima, K. Sood, E. Özen, & R. D. Gonzi (Eds.), Science of sustainable systems: Greening our economy for a sustainable future (pp. 215–226). Elsevier. https://doi.org/10.1016/B978-0-443-23603-7.00017-0

de Almeida, P. G. R., dos Santos, C. D., & Farias, J. S. (2021). Artificial intelligence regulation: A framework for governance. Ethics and Information Technology, 23(3), 505–525.

Dewasiri, N. J., Dharmarathna, D. G., & Choudhary, M. (2024). Leveraging artificial intelligence for enhanced risk management in banking: A systematic literature review. In R. Singh, S. Khan, A. Kumar, & V. Kumar (Eds.), Artificial intelligence enabled management: An emerging economy perspective (pp. 197–213). De Gruyter, Berlin. https://doi.org/10.1515/9783111172408

Dewasiri, N. J., Karunarathne, K. S. S. N., Menon, S., Jayarathne, P. G. S. A., & Rathnasiri, M. S. H. (2023a). Fusion of artificial intelligence and blockchain in the banking industry: Current application, adoption, and future challenges. In A. Saini & V. Garg (Eds.), Transformation for sustainable business and management practices: Exploring the spectrum of Industry 5.0 (pp. 293–307). Emerald Publishing Limited, Leeds. https://doi.org/10.1108/978-1-80262-277-520231021

Dewasiri, N. J., Pigera, A. K. M., Karunarathne, K. S. S. N., & Rathnasiri, M. S. H. (2023b). Financial services employee engagement and attitude toward artificial intelligence: Evidence from Sri Lanka. In A. Saini & V. Garg (Eds.), Transformation for sustainable business and management practices: Exploring the spectrum of Industry 5.0 (pp. 231–245). Emerald Publishing Limited, Leeds. https://doi.org/10.1108/978-1-80262-277-520231017

Diakopoulos, N. (2020). Accountability, transparency, and algorithms. The Oxford Handbook of Ethics of AI, 17(4), 197–213.

Díaz-Rodríguez, N., Del Ser, J., Coeckelbergh, M., de Prado, M. L., Herrera-Viedma, E., & Herrera, F. (2023). Connecting the dots in trustworthy artificial intelligence: From AI principles, ethics, and critical requirements to responsible AI systems and regulation. Information Fusion, 99, 101896.

Eriksen, M. B., & Frandsen, T. F. (2018). The impact of patient, intervention, comparison, outcome (PICO) as a search strategy tool on literature search quality: A systematic review. Journal of the Medical Library Association, 106(4), 420–431.

Falco, G., Shneiderman, B., Badger, J., Carrier, R., Dahbura, A., Danks, D., Eling, M., Goodloe, A., Gupta, J., Hart, C. & Jirotka, M. (2021). Governing AI safety through independent audits. Nature Machine Intelligence, 3(7), 566–571.

Felzmann, H., Fosch-Villaronga, E., Lutz, C., & Tamò-Larrieux, A. (2020). Towards transparency by design for artificial intelligence. Science and Engineering Ethics, 26(6), 3333–3361.

Janssen, M., Brous, P., Estevez, E., Barbosa, L. S., & Janowski, T. (2020). Data governance: Organizing data for trustworthy artificial intelligence. Government Information Quarterly, 37(3), 101493.

Kaswan, K. S., Dhatterwal, J. S., Kumar, N. & Lal, S. (2023). Artificial intelligence for financial services. In S. Grima, K. Sood, & E. Özen (Eds.), Contemporary studies of risks in emerging technology, part A (emerald studies in finance, insurance, and risk management) (pp. 71–92). Emerald Publishing Limited, Leeds. https://doi.org/10.1108/978-1-80455-562-020231006

Kuziemski, M., & Misuraca, G. (2020). AI governance in the public sector: Three tales from the frontiers of automated decision-making in democratic settings. Telecommunications Policy, 44(6), 101976.

Larsson, S., & Heintz, F. (2020). Transparency in artificial intelligence. Internet Policy Review, 9(2), 1–16.

Lin, Y., Hung, T., & Huang, L. T. (2020). Engineering equity: How AI can help reduce the harm of implicit bias. Philosophy & Technology. https://doi.org/10.1007/s13347-020-00406-7

Lu, Y. (2019). Artificial intelligence: A survey on evolution, models, applications and future trends. Journal of Management Analytics, 6(1), 1–29.

Murdoch, B. (2021). Privacy and artificial intelligence: Challenges for protecting health information in a new era. BMC Medical Ethics, 22, 1–5.

Ntoutsi, E., Fafalios, P., Gadiraju, U., Iosifidis, V., Nejdl, W., Vidal, M.E., Ruggieri, S., Turini, F., Papadopoulos, S., Krasanakis, E. & Kompatsiaris, I. (2020). Bias in data-driven artificial intelligence systems—An introductory survey. Wiley Interdisciplinary Reviews: Data Mining and Knowledge Discovery, 10(3), e1356.

Ohalete, N. C., Aderibigbe, A. O., Ani, E. C., Ohenhen, P. E., Daraojimba, D. O., & Odulaja, B. A. (2023). AI-driven solutions in renewable energy: A review of data science applications in solar and wind energy optimisation. World Journal of Advanced Research and Reviews, 20(3), 401–417.

Schrader, D., & Ghosh, D. (2018). Proactively protecting against the singularity: Ethical decision making AI. IEEE Computer and Reliability Societies Review, 16(3), 56–63.

Singhal, A., Neveditsin, N., Tanveer, H., & Mago, V. (2024). Toward fairness, accountability, transparency, and ethics in AI for social media and health care: Scoping review. JMIR Medical Informatics, 12(1), e50048.

Tejani, A. S., Ng, Y. S., Xi, Y., & Rayan, J. C. (2024). Understanding and mitigating bias in imaging artificial intelligence. RadioGraphics, 44(5), e230067.

Varona, D., & Suárez, J. L. (2022). Discrimination, bias, fairness, and trustworthy AI. Applied Sciences, 12(12), 5826.

Vijerathne, D. T., Wahala, W. M. P. S. B., Rathnasiri, M. S. H., De Silva, V., & Dewasiri, N. J. (2025). Literature review on sustainability. In S. Grima, K. Sood, E. Özen, & R. D. Gonzi (Eds.), Science of sustainable systems: Greening our economy for a sustainable future (pp. 33–45). Elsevier. https://doi.org/10.1016/B978-0-443-23603-7.00004-2

Wamba-Taguimdje, S. L., Wamba, S. F., Kamdjoug, J. R. K., & Wanko, C. E. T. (2020). Influence of artificial intelligence (AI) on firm performance: The business value of AI-based transformation projects. Business Process Management Journal, 26(7), 1893–1924.

Wirtz, B. W., Weyerer, J. C., & Kehl, I. (2022). Governance of artificial intelligence: A risk and guideline-based integrative framework. Government Information Quarterly, 39(4), 101685.

Young, M. M., Bullock, J. B., & Lecy, J. D. (2019). Artificial discretion as a governance tool: A framework for understanding the impact of artificial intelligence on public administration. Perspectives on Public Management and Governance, 2(4), 301–313.

Zhang, Z., Citardi, D., Wang, D., Genc, Y., Shan, J., & Fan, X. (2021). Patients' perceptions of using artificial intelligence (AI)-based technology to comprehend radiology imaging data. Health Informatics Journal, 27(2), 1–13.

13 AI in Healthcare
Unveiling Economic Potential and Strategic Insights

Harjit Singh, Manita Arora, and Avneet Singh

INTRODUCTION

The cost of medical treatment, especially hospitalization, has risen in recent years, resulting in unaffordable treatment for larger populations worldwide. The reason may be an increasing population, disease prevalence, a growing number of patients, an increased aging population—especially after COVID-19—and inflation (Smetherman et al., 2022). Artificial intelligence (AI) is widely used in various industries, and healthcare is no exception (Lee & Yoon, 2021). Linking AI to healthcare systems promises to revolutionize patient care, improve outcomes, and optimize operational efficiencies. However, significant economic implications must be considered alongside these potential benefits (Hawkins et al., 2015). This chapter aims to elucidate the multifaceted impact of AI on healthcare outcomes, revenue generation, cost-effectiveness, and resource allocation. The chapter comprehensively explains how AI adoption influences healthcare spending, reimbursement models, and financial sustainability by synthesizing existing literature, analyzing industry use cases, and examining recent research studies (Singla and Kumar 2024). The objective is to offer insights that inform decision-making processes for healthcare professionals, stakeholders, financial analysts, and policymakers, highlighting the economic dynamics of integrating AI into healthcare services (Singla et al., 2024).

The study's originality lies in its inclusive analysis of the economic dimensions of AI integration in healthcare. Unlike other studies focusing solely on clinical outcomes or technological advancements, this research emphasizes the financial aspects, offering valuable insights for various stakeholders involved in healthcare policymaking processes. To investigate the economic implications of AI in medical care, this study employs a multi-method approach, including a literature review, industrial use cases, and data analysis.

INCREASING ROLE OF AI IN HEALTHCARE

Undoubtedly, AI-enabled applications have the potential to enhance 'operational efficiency' significantly within healthcare systems. AI can reduce administrative costs and streamline medical, investigation, and billing processes by programming repetitive administrative tasks (Cheng et al., 2021). For instance, AI-powered

DOI: 10.1201/9781003531272-13

systems can handle patient scheduling, billing, and claims processing more efficiently than traditional methods. This automation not only cuts down on labor costs but also minimizes errors, leading to more accurate billing and faster reimbursements. Moreover, AI can optimize 'supply chain management' processes in healthcare (Singh & Singh, 2023). Further, predictive analytics can forecast demand for medical supplies, ensuring that inventory levels are maintained appropriately, thereby reducing wastage and saving costs. For example, AI algorithms can predict the required quantities of drugs and medical equipment based on historical data and current trends, allowing for more precise procurement and inventory management (Gupta et al., 2015).

Further, virtual or digital fitness tools offer medical providers a more all-inclusive view of the patient's health by allowing them to access patient data. Additionally, these tools provide accurate health information from their physicians to patients (Muehlematter et al., 2021), resulting in improved therapeutic consequences and efficacy. However, there are worries that such modalities might also have a more significant mental impact, specifically with the massive use of social media and instant imaging applications by sufferers, the general public, and experts. Moreover, gathered facts from a couple of resources, which include health facts structures, wearable gadgets, telemedicine, eHealth, telehealth, mobile internet devices, and other AI-enabled clinical generation, generate extensive records that boost the usage of AI and machine learning (ML) in healthcare systems (Davenport et al., 2019; Shahin et al., 2017).

In addition, digital health data encompass diverse healthcare information of hospitalized patients. Such datasets can be linked to innovative AI technology to take benefit of precise insights into affected person care (Gheflati et al., 2021). Therefore, AI has emerged as a foremost option for big-data applications. Furthermore, massive statistics analytics allow healthcare practitioners to expand their clinical offerings using analytical algorithms to enhance electronic health records (EHRs). These analytics also use the advanced versions of AI to filter out vast amounts of information on diverse grounds for better evaluation of facts (Khanna et al., 2022). In developed countries like the United States, the United Kingdom, and Germany, AI is extensively utilized in various healthcare sectors to strengthen patient health outcomes and reduce healthcare cost (O'mara-Eves et al., 2015; Price & Cohen, 2019; Thrall et al., 2018; Van Leeuwen et al., 2022); this study reveals AI's functions in healthcare, focusing on the subsequent vital factors:

i. virtual patient care
ii. scientific imaging and diagnostics
iii. scientific studies and drug discovery
iv. patient engagement and compliance,
v. predictive analytics and personalized medicine, and
vi. timely detection and prevention of diseases

Similarly, the authors cope with a few challenges related to using AI in Medicare, extending the scope of related literature on the use of AI in healthcare and allied areas (Figure 13.1).

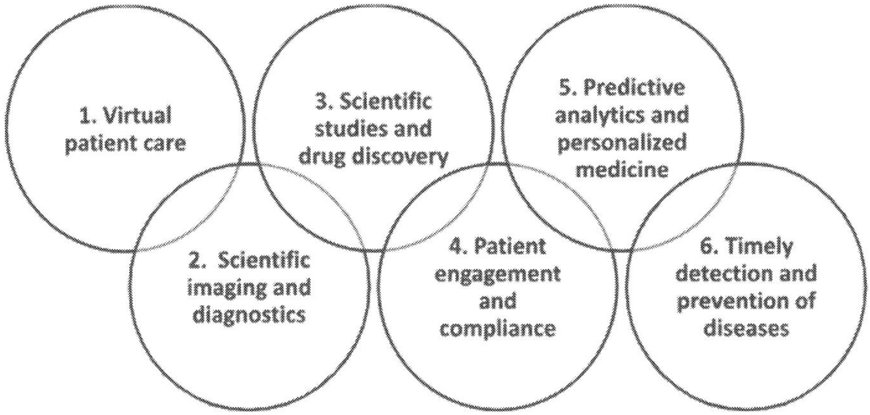

FIGURE 13.1 Applications of AI in Healthcare domain.

Source: Compiled by authors.

BACKGROUND LITERATURE

The development of man-made reasoning (computer-based intelligence, commonly called AI) in the medical field has been momentous, reshaping how the healthcare industry analyzes, treats, and cares for patients (Weissler et al., 2021). Such innovations further develop medical care exploration and lab testing reports by delivering prompt, accurate, customized therapies (Voets et al., 2021). The applications of AI to quickly analyze vast information of clinical samples aid medical practitioners in identifying rare diseases and controlling their further spread (Gomez Rossi et al., 2022). The expected uses of AI and medical services are expansive and sweeping, from checking radiological images for an early location to anticipating results from electronic well-being records (Kourou et al., 2021). Adopting AI and allied applications in hospitals, clinics, lab testing units, and research centers can facelift healthcare worldwide. Consequently, technology adoption in healthcare offers real-time data, better patient care, improved diagnosis, and digital consultations (McKee & Wouters, 2023).

AI is revolutionizing the healthcare industry by solving highly complex health issues. Linear networks and autoencoders, two cutting-edge AI methods, can produce statistics that incorporate actual situations (Ramessur et al., 2021). The pharmaceutical sector has also recognized and demonstrated AI's potential, significantly affecting modern businesses (Sunarti et al., 2021). AI models combine medication data and a patient's medical history to produce suggestions and recommendations. Numerous medical speacialists can benefit from this approach, from diagnosis to treatment planning (Ruamviboonsuk et al., 2021). AI helps provide personalized solutions for patients' novel necessities by incorporating the patient's medical history and day-to-day activities into a customized treatment plan. As a result, AI caters to diverse patient needs (Topol et al., 2019). One thing that needs to be noted is that AI is a compilation of advances rather than a single innovation. Numerous innovations directly concern healthcare, each supporting specific instruments and errands. A couple of imperative AI advances in healthcare are point by point as follows:

Virtual Patient Care

Today, there are not enough doctors, surgeons, pediatricians, and nurses to care for ill patients. As a result, patients have no option except to wait for extended hours, resulting in delays in their recovery. Health practitioners and medical professionals also struggle to treat and offer consultations during their prescribed office hours (Kourou et al., 2021). AI can automate routine hospital tasks such as doctors' appointments, lab testing slots, X-rays, and diagnostics appointments per patients' requirements just with the click of a mouse or telephonically (Gerke et al., 2020). Baig et al. (2017) opined that the recent development of wearable technologies and the adoption of generative intelligence in healthcare are no longer new. Similarly, monitoring and controlling disabled people through virtual care with live and realistic wearable technology contrasts are all pervasive and a part of patient care requirements. Further, AI can control contagious diseases, including chronic bronchial asthma, diabetes mellitus, hypertension, and sleep disorders, using wearable non-invasive sensors. Patel and Tarakji (2021) also mentioned that an affected individual with traumatic atrial inflammation as the main reason had a stroke after a widely negative workup. Later, her electrophysiologist confirmed these recorded signals and the idea that consumer wearable digital devices support precise diagnosis.

AI with predictive modules applying big data and ML can assist in predicting the spread of diseases, such as SARS-CoV infection and diabetic nephropathy, in the transplant of solid organs (Parwani et al., 2014). Voets et al. (2022) highlighted the significance of linking AI to medical care during COVID-19 and upcoming pandemics after exploring success with new AI-enabled applications. Additionally, the need for digital healthcare services has mushroomed, especially after the outburst of COVID-19. Digital metaverse applications can provide customized patient care compared to traditional OPDs (Singh & Singh, 2023). A recent study reported that telemedicine's growth with the metaverse's development increased at least 40 times during COVID-19 (Arora & Arora, 2022).

Scientific Imaging and Diagnostics

AI is an effective tool for image analysis. Radiology professionals increasingly use this to diagnose exclusive sicknesses early and decrease diagnostic mistakes in the context of prevention (Krittanawong et al., 2019). AI can precisely become aware of and examine the signs of X-ray images such as CT scans, X-rays, ultrasounds, and various MRIs. AI-enabled applications help with fast scanning and diagnosis of disorders. AI accumulates statistics about an affected person, prognosis histories, testing manners, and billing records (McKee & Wouters, 2023). AI-enabled techniques can, therefore, be used to improve the care layout and the pleasure of ill patients. Besides, AI is intelligent and capable of analyzing echocardiography movements and graphs cardiologists use to make quick decisions (Secinaro et al., 2021). One such advanced platform, 'Ultromics,' used in an Oxford clinic, integrates AI to investigate echocardiography scans to sense the disturbed and changed patterns of heartbeats and detect coronary heart diseases. Using body imaging modalities, AI has proven early detection of illnesses, including skin and breast cancers, eye ailments, and pneumonia. AI gear examines speech styles to forecast psychotic disorders and display the capabilities of nervous sicknesses in the case of Parkinson's disease – a brain disorder. Some recent studies successfully examined diabetes using ML modes. The results confirmed that the elegance augmented choice tree became a high-quality version for predicting diabetes variables (Dave & Patel, 2023). Their consequences pronounced that each one of the deep neural networks, handcrafted feature mastering, and hybrid methods could be expecting COVID-19 instances (Wahl et al., 2018).

Gheflati et al. (2021) confirmed higher efficacy in classifying breast photographs when compared with convolutional neural networks (CNNs). Besides, AI encompasses the applications of synthetic neural networks, i.e., insight-getting-to-know strategies named generative adverse networks (GANs), which impact radiological imaging. The GANs' artificial neural networks (i) are generators synthesizing snapshots similar to actual pictures and (ii) are discriminators that exhibit the distinction between artificial and actual images, producing exceptional unsupervised learning. Regarding radiological imaging, the multiplicative version can steadily duplicate pictures with new images using the capabilities of the photographs in the dataset training. The AI version can categorize the images, for instance, whether or not a radiograph is displayed.

Furthermore, synthetic control groups were created by modeling historical information, reducing the requirement for actual existence, lowering costs, and expanding treatment options in scientific trials. Recently introduced ChatGPT is a language model the general public utilizes for scientific research, academics, and consultancy. By replacing specialized clinical advice, the general public will be interested in using any such model to determine diagnoses primarily based on medical features or benefit remedy pointers. Recent studies (O'mara-Eves et al., 2015; Price & Cohen, 2019; Van Leeuwen et al., 2022) have observed that thirty percent of adults required net-based clinical advice for self-diagnosis, while over fifty percent preferred to consult their health practitioner online.

Also, X-ray scans are thoroughly accumulated and stored temporarily, and they are freely accessible to train AI systems. The AI structures can reduce the time and value of examining scientific scans and doubtlessly permit more excellent scans for enhanced focused control. AI additionally affects scientific decision-making and ailment prognosis. It can procedure, investigate, and file statistics across exceptional modalities for ailment prognosis and scientific decision-making. Thus, doctors make accurate and prompt medical decisions or even update humanoid choices in healing areas.

Scientific Studies and Drug Discovery

AI algorithms are used to do scientific studies and reduce drug discovery time (Hukunda et al., 2018). AI improves parts of the discovery process, making it quicker, safer, and affordable (Khanna et al., 2022). It can help discover new compounds that could cure diseases. It can also identify the application and state of previously tested compounds. For example, the two widely discussed drugs used to treat the Ebola epidemic in West Africa were recognized usage-fit with AI in a single day, which otherwise would have taken some months to years. AI can thus be combined with in-memory computing for drug discovery and creation (Khanna, 2020).

AI applications are best suited to study large datasets used for medical research. It is also used for literature reviews, finding research gaps, and integrating different data types to innovate drugs (O'mara-Eves et al., 2015). Pharmaceutical agencies focus on making AI more efficient for drug creation. Scientists and researchers use predictive analytics to identify appropriate candidates for clinical and medical trials to develop accurate biological processes (Weissler et al., 2021). ML combined with AI contributes to theme selection, clinical trials, research organization, data collection, and analysis. It can enlarge the patient-centered view, conclusive statements, and effectiveness and reach clinical trials. However, AI must emphasize all of its obstacles only during clinical trials. Future research efforts can include methods for improving participant management (Arora & Arora, 2022). In clinical research, generative AI can augment various datasets and intensify diversity. In addition, research efforts can be extended to conduct trials in an immersive mode using the application metaverse. The advantage of using metaverse is that it facilitates alliance between physically distant investigators.

Metaversion allows them to explore in a simulated space comparable to other researchers who have indulged in similar research. Similarly, recently introduced ChatGPT can be used in clinical studies to support data collection and provide information on clinical trials. It can help condense relevant publications, recognize significant results, and support medicine researchers in navigating massive Internet-based evidence competently (Kourou et al., 2021). In addition, a chatbot using ChatGPT helps translate the medical language for clinical scholars and researchers. However, using ChatGPT may result in ethical issues when using chatbots in medical and allied research.

Patient Engagement and Compliance

Patient engagement is a collaborative approach between patients and clinical professionals engaging patients in their healthcare processes and treatments (De Vos et al., 2022). It has become a key reason for value-based healthcare. When applied in the true sense, patient engagement improves the quality of care while reducing medical costs (Khanna et al., 2022). Doctors who keep their patients engaged in their healthcare using information technology will likely be proactive in their health management and understanding of their condition. They are more likely to make the necessary behavior changes to positively impact their quality of life (Davenport et al., 2019). It is not the responsibility of just doctors and clinicians to reach out to their patients and offer them information and indulge options. If patients are not responding and contributing to managing their health, the objective of patient engagement will be defeated (Anyodha R, 2017). Similarly, today's patients are not expected to gather information and ask their doctors questions. Patient engagement objectives will not be achieved if doctors do not educate their patients, inspire healthy habits, and win patient confidence. For patient engagement to thrive, both parties must communicate regularly with confidence and honesty (Gomez Rossi et al., 2022; Khanna et al., 2022; McKee & Wouters, 2023). AI can be very supportive in enhancing patient engagement. AI-based healthcare workflow techniques are thus applied to manage the line of treatment, future composite interventions, and the spectrum of care (Davenport et al., 2019). Sending messages, reminders, and appropriate, custom-made material that currently supports behavior is a growing, favorable field of research (Singh & Singh, 2023).

Predictive Analytics and Personalized Medicine

Resource allocation in healthcare is changing due to AI and personalized medicine (Singh & Singh, 2023). Patterns and trends that human analysts might miss are identified by analyzing large datasets (Jiang et al., 2021). Predicting patient outcomes and resource needs can be more accurate with this capability (Jiang et al., 2017). Healthcare providers can identify high-risk patients and intervene earlier, preventing the progression of diseases. AI can predict which patients are at risk of developing enduring conditions, such as Parkinson's disease and heart ailments (Pifer, R. 2023). The need for expensive treatments and hospitalizations can be prevented with early intervention in such cases (Reddy et al., 2018).

Individualized medicine uses AI to design customized treatments for patients based on their genetics and health history. This approach improves treatment outcomes. AI can analyze genetic facts to identify cancer patients' most successful treatment options, reducing the trial-and-error approach associated with traditional cancer treatments (Sunarti et al., 2021; Topel, 2019).

Timely Detection and Prevention of Diseases

AI can analyze vast amounts of data quickly and accurately, enabling the timely detection and prevention of diseases (Thrall et al., 2018). Early detection of diseases can significantly reduce treatment costs and improve patient outcomes (Sahni et al., 2023). For example, AI algorithms are widely used to analyze medical images to detect early signs of conditions such as cancer. This allows prompt treatment and reduces the need for extensive and expensive treatments later (Singh & Singh, 2023). In addition to early detection, AI can be crucial in disease prevention. By analyzing lifestyle data and health records, AI can detect patients who are at risk and can develop certain diseases and recommend timely preventive measures (Van Leeuwen et al., 2022). For example, AI can analyze data from wearable devices to monitor physical activity, diet, and other health indicators, providing personalized recommendations to prevent conditions such as obesity and hypertension.

Challenges and Ethical Considerations

Despite the ample possibilities, the usage of AI-enabled applications in healthcare is limited to some advanced countries and lines of treatments. The reason may be the presence of technical and methodological flaws in addition to privacy concerns.

Some of the most widely challenges and ethical considerations are discussed as follows:

Absence of Value Clinical Information

Healthcare professionals require reliable and up-to-date datasets for clinical and specialized approval of computer-based intelligence models. Because of the discontinuity of clinical information across a few EHRs and programming stages, gathering patient data and pictures to test computer-based intelligence calculations becomes testing (Wahl et al., 2018). Another obstruction is that the clinical information from one association may not be viable at different stages because of interoperability issues (Weissler et al., 2021). To build how much information is accessible for testing simulated intelligence frameworks, the medical care area should focus on procedures for normalizing clinical information.

Clinically Unimportant Execution Measurements

The metrics used to evaluate the performance of an AI model may not always apply to clinical situations (Al Kuwaiti et al., 2023). The disparity between the clinical adequacy shown in reality and the specialized accuracy of simulated intelligence tests is the man-made intelligence gap (Ali et al., 2023). Healthcare professionals should work together to understand and comprehend how AI algorithms enhance the quality and delivery of patient care. They can evaluate AI models for precision utilizing choice bend investigation (Berwick et al., 2008). They can assess a prediction model's clinical utility by comparing datasets and estimating the likelihood of an AI model's success in the actual circumstances.

Flaws in the Research Methodology

AI in healthcare lacks sufficient peer-reviewed studies, prospective research, and established methodologies (Bohr & Memarzadeh, 2020). Most studies have been reviewed because of verifiable patient clinical records. However, physicians must conduct prospective research on current patients over time to comprehend the value of AI-based diagnosis (Davenport et al., 2018). Additionally, physicians must integrate physical examinations with online consulting and remote monitoring technologies (such as trackers and sensors) for reliable prospective research (Gomez Rossi et al., 2022).

Protection and Security of Information

As AI depends on endless sums of quiet information, it is crucial to guarantee its security. Strict conventions and encryption procedures should be in place to secure quiet data from unauthorized get to or breaches (Guan, 2019). Second, the tendency to commit cybercrimes and breach of information is a significant ethical concern. Healthcare organizations must execute strong cybersecurity measures to protect against potential dangers (Obermeyer & Emanuel, 2016). AI frameworks should be outlined with security in intellect, and standard checking and upgrades should be performed to address rising vulnerabilities (Krittanawong et al., 2021).

Inclination and Decency in AI Calculations

AI calculations can incidentally sustain inclinations shown within the information they are prepared on, driving to unjustifiable results (Sahni et al., 2023). Moderating inclination requires assorted and agent datasets, thorough testing, and continuous observing to recognize and amend any inclinations that may develop—further moderating incongruities in healthcare results (Price & Cohen, 2019; Secinaro et al., 2021). AI ought to be utilized to address healthcare aberrations or maybe compound them. Endeavors should guarantee even-handed access to AI advances, consider social determinants of well-being, and ceaselessly assess and alter the calculations to play down aberrations in healthcare results (Ruamviboonsuk et al., 2021).

Regulatory Framework Required for AI in Healthcare

Developing appropriate regulations for AI in healthcare is essential to create a comprehensive and relevant regulatory framework that addresses unique challenges (Table 13.1). These policies must ensure patient safety, confidentiality, and ethical standards (Ramessur et al., 2021). Further, the framework should ensure compliance with existing legal and ethical standards. AI healthcare applications must comply with laws such as data protection regulations and patient consent requirements (Petersson et al., 2022). Furthermore, compliance with ethical standards such as transparency, accountability, and informed consent is also essential.

TABLE 13.1
Article Mapping for AI Challenges Facing the Healthcare Industry

Sl. No	Absence of Value Clinical Information	Clinical Settings	Flaws in Research Methodology	Information Security	Inclination and Decency in AI Calculations	Need for Regulatory Framework	Article Mapping
1	√		√		√	√	6, 32, 44
2		√	√	√		√	5, 11, 48
3			√		√		9, 17, 23, 38, 41
4	√	√		√	√		1, 7, 23, 42, 46
5			√	√		√	38, 42
6	√	√	√	√	√	√	2, 13, 23, 29, 46
7		√	√		√		4, 11, 28, 39

Source: Compiled by authors.

ECONOMIC IMPACT OF AI IN HEALTHCARE

The economic impact of AI on medical services is critical given the increasing medical services costs worldwide. To guarantee the affordable usage of medical services assets, it is pivotal to fathom both the expenses and advantages of executing simulated intelligence frameworks (Narendra et al., 2022). AI decreases medical services costs when contrasted with regular strategies. AI's cost savings in treatment have been more effective than diagnosis (Obermeyer & Emanuel, 2016). AI lessens time in conclusion and treatment when contrasted with routine techniques. High exactness in determination and treatment can be accomplished in a brief time frame (Singh & Singh, 2023). AI works on demonstrative exactness by disposing of bias and subjectivity. AI-based clinical findings lessen the probability of erroneous assessment. Patients might feel calmer seeing a specialist due to man-made intelligence innovation (Gheflati et al., 2021). Algorithm-based intelligence channels use such information to determine which treatments deliver the best outcomes. Not only can carrying out man-made intelligence innovation in medical services decrease costs, but it can likewise assist associations with augmenting their return for capital invested (Hukunda et al., 2018).

Experts opine that economic challenges related to AI in healthcare can be complex, potentially affecting investment choices. However, health economic evaluations (HEEs) keep records for evaluating the financial impact of AI-enabled applications. However, some HEEs currently suffer from procedural limitations, requiring complex procedures for assessing and making sound decisions (Benjamens et al., 2020). Therefore, challenges comprise not only health-related issues but also the capacity to introduce changes in clinical practices, carrying substantial costs (Challen et al., 2019). In short, the availability of funds, high start-up costs, and rigorous financial considerations are the key hindrances hampering the growth of healthcare skills. On the contrary, AI promises to save costs if applied realistically and with proper planning and implementation. It is estimated that the United States could save $250 to $400 billion when implemented across various healthcare sectors (Narendra et al., 2022; Pifer et al., 2023).

The financial implications of adopting AI in healthcare necessitate critical deliberations (Lee & Yoon, 2021). Though such issues and topics remain unattended in academic works and literary compilations, this study aims to bridge the gap by compiling extensive literature in one place, making it easy for future researchers to study the long-standing and sustainable economic impact of the adoption of AI. It would also equip stakeholders with extensive and updated information for strategic planning and thoughtful investment options. Identifying areas where AI can perform better, maximize cost-effectiveness, and elevate patient care will enable more precise resource allocation (Parwani et al., 2014). Additionally, researching its extended financial significance can reveal substantial returns on AI spending, offering investors a transparent financial overview backing such endeavors (Yuan et al., 2020).

The proposed financial implications of AI adoption may extend beyond initial infrastructure cost considerations but consider the long-term paybacks, including better-quality patient care, affordable healthcare expenditure, and enhanced revenue streams through value-based care models (Xuan et al., 2014). Additionally, AI-driven advances in healthcare can attract huge investments, fuel economic growth, and foster entrepreneurship in the healthcare industry. Adopting AI in healthcare services presents substantial financial opportunities and challenges (Singh & Singh, 2023). Strategic scheduling, evidence-based decision-making, and stakeholder collaboration are essential to maximize the financial paybacks while addressing potential obstacles to adoption (Muehlemattwr et al., 2021). By leveraging AI technologies responsibly, the healthcare industry can achieve economic sustainability while advancing the excellence and convenience of patient care (Gupta et al., 2015; Hawkins et al., 2015).

Long-Term Economic Impacts

While the underlying expenses of incorporating computer-based intelligence into medical services frameworks can be huge, the drawn-out monetary advantages are significant. Simulated intelligence-driven upgrades in functional productivity, prescient examination, and illness anticipation can prompt tremendous expense reserve funds and improved income streams (Retson & Eghtedari, 2020). The potential for value-based care models is one of the main long-term advantages. Esteem put together consideration centers to convey significant consideration while controlling expenses. Man-made intelligence can work with this by giving exact information and examination to gauge patient results and recognize regions for development (Shahin et al., 2017). For instance, man-made intelligence can examine patient information to recognize holes in care and prescribe medications to develop results further, prompting better patient fulfillment and decreased medical services costs (Smetherman et al., 2022). Additionally, man-made intelligence can improve income streams by empowering new action plans and administrations. For example, AI-fueled telemedicine stages can increase admittance to medical care administrations, producing extra income for medical service suppliers. Moreover, AI-driven developments, such as remote checking and virtual consideration, can set new openings for the income age. The reconciliation of computer-based intelligence in medical care can draw in critical speculation and fuel monetary development. The medical services area is a significant driver of monetary movement, and the reception of simulated intelligence innovations can invigorate development and business ventures (Weissler et al., 2021). AI-driven progress in medical care can prompt the improvement of new items and administrations, setting open doors for new businesses and laying out organizations the same (Retson & Eghtedari, 2020). For instance, healthcare providers may commercialize and adopt AI-powered diagnostic tools and treatment algorithms, generating new revenue streams for technology companies. Additionally, AI's impact on the economy is not limited to the healthcare industry (Cheng et al., 2021). By further developing medical services results and decreasing expenses, computer-based intelligence can improve labor force efficiency and contribute to, by and large, financial development. Better populaces can prompt lower non-attendance and higher efficiency, helping the more extensive economy (Gerke et al., 2020).

Economic Opportunities and Challenges

AI in healthcare presents significant economic opportunities, including cost reduction, improved efficiency, and enhanced drug discovery. AI-powered diagnostics and automation help reduce operational expenses while increasing accuracy and speed in medical decision-making. Predictive analytics optimize hospital resource allocation, reducing waste and improving patient flow (Pifer, 2023). Additionally, AI accelerates drug discovery, cutting down research and development costs. The expansion of AI-driven telemedicine and personalized healthcare makes medical services more accessible, particularly in remote areas. Moreover, AI-driven innovations foster economic growth by creating high-paying jobs in AI development and bioinformatics (Singh & Singh, 2023). However, despite these benefits, AI adoption comes with economic challenges. High implementation costs, especially for smaller healthcare providers, can hinder adoption. Ethical and regulatory barriers, such as compliance with privacy laws like Health Insurance Portability and Accountability Act (HIPAA) and General Data Protection Regulation (GDPR), add complexity to AI integration. Additionally, AI automation poses risks of job displacement, requiring healthcare professionals to adapt and upskill. Data security concerns also present significant risks, as AI systems rely on vast patient datasets vulnerable to cyber threats. Legal and liability issues surrounding AI-driven medical decisions further complicate widespread implementation. To fully realize the economic potential of AI in healthcare, a balanced approach that includes regulatory compliance, investment in secure AI infrastructure, and workforce training is essential (Khanna et al., 2020; Narendra et al., 2022). Adopting AI in medical care and allied areas presents opportunities and challenges for the entire world. Essential preparation, proof-based direction, and partner-coordinated efforts are fundamental to boost the monetary advantages while addressing possible deterrents to reception. One of the most critical financial opportunities is the potential to cut healthcare costs through enhanced operational efficiency and resource allocation. AI can potentially reduce operational costs and increase healthcare systems' overall efficiency by automating administrative tasks and optimizing supply chain management. In addition, personalized medicine and AI-driven predictive analytics may improve patient outcomes and lower treatment costs. Nonetheless, there are additional difficulties to consider. The underlying expenses of coordinating man-made intelligence into medical services frameworks can be significant, remembering speculations for foundation, innovation, and preparation (Khanna et al., 2020). Healthcare providers must carefully evaluate AI initiatives' return on investment and devise plans to reduce the financial risks associated with their implementation. In addition, there are likely moral and administrative difficulties to consider. Using AI in medical services raises significant issues about patients' data protection, secrecy, and the ethical ramifications of computer-based intelligence-driven direction (Khanna et al., 2022). Medical services suppliers and policymakers should address these worries to guarantee the mindful and moral utilization of simulated intelligence innovations. e to economic expansion as a whole. Better populaces can prompt lower non-attendance and higher efficiency, helping the more extensive economy (Pifer, 2023).

Leveraging AI Responsibly

Medical service suppliers should use simulated intelligence innovations mindfully to accomplish monetary maintainability and advance the nature of patient consideration (Singh & Singh, 2023). Creating a culture of innovation and collaboration, investing in the necessary infrastructure and training, and developing a clear strategy for AI adoption are all part of this. One of the critical techniques for dependable simulated intelligence reception is zeroing in on proof-based direction (Retson & Eghtedari, 2020). Medical care suppliers ought to utilize information and investigation to illuminate their simulated intelligence drives, guaranteeing that they depend on solid proof and are lined up with clinical objectives. This includes directing pilot studies and clinical preliminaries to assess the viability of simulated intelligence arrangements and assemble evidence of their effect (Yuan et al., 2020). Furthermore, medical services suppliers should put resources into the fundamental framework and prepare to help the reception of computer-based intelligence. This includes enhancing IT systems, guaranteeing data interoperability, and instructing healthcare professionals on using AI tools effectively (Muehlematter et al., 2021). By building the essential foundation and providing preparation, medical care suppliers can guarantee that computer-based intelligence arrangements are coordinated consistently in their work processes and used to their maximum capacity (Lee & Yoon, 2021). Finally, encouraging a culture of development and coordinated effort is fundamental for fruitful simulated intelligence reception (Gerke et al., 2020). Medical services suppliers should support coordinated efforts between clinicians, information researchers, and innovation specialists to create and execute simulated intelligence arrangements. This requires forming multidisciplinary teams and providing collaboration and knowledge-sharing opportunities (Gupta et al., 2015).

CONCLUSION, DISCUSSION, AND IMPLICATIONS

Integrating AI into healthcare presents significant financial implications, offering opportunities and challenges. By enhancing operational efficiency, enabling predictive analytics and personalized medicine, and facilitating timely detection and prevention of diseases, AI results in significant cost-cutting and improved patient care. Moreover, AI can attract investment, fuel economic growth, and foster innovation and entrepreneurship in the healthcare business. To maximize the financial benefits of AI adoption, healthcare providers must develop clear strategies, invest in the necessary infrastructure and training, and foster a culture of innovation and collaboration. By leveraging AI technologies responsibly, the healthcare industry can achieve financial sustainability while advancing the quality and convenience of patient care.

In the last few years, especially during COVID-19, the healthcare sector has seen a surge in AI-related applications. AI-enabled healthcare applications can analyze data faster than traditional methods or human attendants. Further, the literature depicts that AI applications offer accurate clinical studies, real-time data, and genetic information, which helps healthcare professionals provide precise diagnoses at the right time. Further, AI-enabled technology can automate repetitive tasks like keeping records, data entry, and scan analysis.

Nevertheless, uncertainties concerning the efficiency and cost of AI persist, underlining the requirement for execution strategies. Therefore, stakeholders must conduct health technology assessments extending to AI applications in healthcare settings to augment healthcare resources. The limited research, scarce available literature, and dearth of understanding concerning the impact of such applications present challenges for clinicians, health workers, medical facilities, and policymakers. Further, despite technological advancements, AI-enabled applications are offered or applied minimally. Standard AI tools comprise natural language processing, ML for data classification, speech recognition technology, and predictive analytics to improve healthcare professional-patient dialogue, enabling clinicians to predict future health trials, suggest treatments, and explore novel genetic associations.

Considering all the prevalent issues and challenges, the study offers directions regarding the financial effect of AI in health and allied care. While literature-based findings reveal that implementing AI has the potential to save money in the healthcare industry, it also faces some regulatory and procedural challenges. This necessitates a holistic approach to educating stakeholders about the potential benefits that hinder its growth and adoption efforts. The resistance by healthcare professionals to replacing manual processes with AI-based technical processes requires complete change management, training, and development. To conclude, decisively tending to these difficulties and directing examination on the effect of simulated intelligence in settings and nations will decide the amount we can saddle its capability to make a medical services framework that is both feasible and esteem situated. These experiences are critical for partners like medical care suppliers, payers, and policymakers as they assess the advantages of putting resources into AI advancements. This research is necessary because it can help people make better decisions and make it easier to use healthcare resources as costs increase. As a result, this review adds to the ongoing debate regarding AI's potential impact on healthcare and the economy.

AI ought to be viewed as an instrument to improve human potential. It gives usefulness as opposed to supplanting it. A person-centered approach to healthcare must be maintained. Medical care experts use computerized reasoning frameworks to settle on informed choices. Artificial consciousness advancements should be upheld and empowered by medical services experts. Makes use of expertise while still providing compassionate care to patients. Resolving these issues and moral contemplations is capable and advantageous for AI in health care services. To develop and implement guidelines, all the prospective stakeholders, such as healthcare professionals, researchers, policymakers, and technology developers, must work together. Practical standards and governance structures address such issues and promote ethical AI practices.

REFERENCES

Ali, O. et al., (2023). A systematic literature review of artificial intelligence in the healthcare sector: Benefits, challenges, methodologies, and functionalities. Journal of Innovation & Knowledge, 8(1), Article ID: 100333. https://doi.org/10.1016/j.jik.2023.100333.

Al Kuwaiti, A. et al., (2023). Review of the role of artificial intelligence in healthcare. Journal of Personalized Medicine, 13(6):951, Article 951. https://doi.org/10.3390/jpm13060951.

Arora, A., & Arora, B. (2022). Generative adversarial networks and synthetic patient data: Current challenges and future perspectives. Future Healthcare Journal, 9, 190–193. https://doi.org/10.7861%2Ffhj.2022-0013.

Baig, M. M. et al., (2017). A systematic review of wearable patient monitoring systems–current challenges and opportunities for clinical adoption. Journal of Medical Systems. 2017, 41, 115, https://doi.org/10.1007/s10916-017-0760-1.

Benjamens, S., Dhunnoo, P., & Meskó, B. (2020). The state of artificial intelligence-based FDA-approved medical devices and algorithms: An online database. npj Digital Medicine, 3, 118. https://doi.org/10.1038/s41746-020-00324-0.

Berwick, D. M., Nolan, T. W., & Whittington, J. (2008). The triple aim: Care, health, and cost. Health Affairs, 27, 759–769. https://doi.org/10.1377/hlthaff.27.3.759.

Bohr, A., & Memarzadeh, K. (2020). The rise of artificial intelligence in healthcare applications. In: Bohr, A. and Memarzadeh, K., Eds., Artificial Intelligence in Healthcare, 25–60. Academic Press (Elsevier). https://doi.org/10.1016/B978-0-12-818438-7.00002-2

Challen, R., Denny, J., Pitt, M., Gompels, L., Edwards, T., & Tsaneva-Atanasova, K. (2019). Artificial intelligence, bias and clinical safety. BMJ Quality & Safety, 28, 231–237. https://doi.org/10.1136/bmjqs-2018-008370.

Cheng, J. Y., Abel, J. T., Balis, U. G., McClintock, D. S., & Pantanowitz, L. (2021). Challenges in the development, deployment, and regulation of artificial intelligence in anatomic pathology. The American Journal of Pathology, 191, 1684–1692. doi: 10.1016/j.ajpath.2020.10.018.

Dave, M., & Patel, N. (2023). Artificial intelligence in healthcare and education. British Dental Journal, 234, 761–764. https://doi.org/10.1038/s41415-023-5845-2

Davenport, T & Kalakota, R. (2019). The potential for artificial intelligence in healthcare. Future Healthcare Journal, 6(2):94–98. https://doi.org/10.7861%2Ffuturehosp.6-2-94.

Davenport, T. H., Hongsermeier, T., & Mc Cord, K. A. Using AI to improve electronic health records. Harvard Business Review. 2018. Available online: https://hbr.org/2018/12/using-ai-to-improve-electronic-health-records (accessed on 28 December 2022).

De Vos, J., Visser, L. A., de Beer, A. A., Fornasa, M., Thoral, P. J., Elbers, P. W. G., & Cinà, G. (2022). The potential cost-effectiveness of a machine learning tool that can prevent untimely intensive care unit discharge. Value in Health, 25, 359–367. https://doi.org/10.1016/j.jval.2021.06.018

Gerke, S., Babic, B., Evgeniou, T., & Cohen, I. G. (2020). The need for a system view to regulate artificial intelligence/machine learning-based software as medical device. Npj Digital Medicine, 3, 53. doi: 10.1038/s41746-020-0262-2.

Gheflati, B. (2021). Vision transformer for classification of breast ultrasound images. https://doi.org/10.48550/arXiv.2110.14731.

Gomez Rossi, J., Feldberg, B., Krois, J., & Schwendicke, F. (2022). Evaluation of the clinical, technical, and financial aspects of cost-effectiveness analysis of artificial intelligence in medicine: Scoping review and framework of analysis. JMIR Medical Informatics, 10, e33703. https://doi.org/10.2196/33703.

Gomez Rossi, J., Rojas-Perilla, N., Krois, J., & Schwendicke, F. (2022). Cost-effectiveness of artificial intelligence as a decision-support system applied to the detection and grading of melanoma, dental caries, and diabetic retinopathy. JAMA Network Open, 5(3), e220269. https://doi.org/10.1001/jamanetworkopen.2022.0269

Guan, J. (2019). Artificial intelligence in healthcare and medicine: Promises, ethical challenges, and governance. Chinese Medical Sciences Journal, 0(0), 99. https://doi.org/10.24920/003611.

Gupta, A., Kesavabhotla, K., Baradaran, H., Kamel, H., Pandya, A., Giambrone, A. E., Wright, D., Pain, K. J., Mtui, E. E., & Suri, J. S. (2015). Plaque echolucency and stroke risk in asymptomatic carotid stenosis: A systematic review and meta-analysis. Stroke, 46, 91–97. https://doi.org/10.1161/STROKEAHA.114.006091.

Hawkins, R. E., Welcher, C. M., Holmboe, E. S., Kirk, L. M., Norcini, J. J., Simons, K. B., & Skochelak, S. E. (2015. Implementation of competency-based medical education:

Are we addressing the concerns and challenges?. Medical Education, 49, 1086–1102. https://doi.org/10.1111/medu.12831.

Hukunda, B., Rau, A., & Upadhyay, P. Reimaging healthcare opportunities with artificial intelligence. Infosys Navigate Your Next. 2018. Available online: https://www.infosys.com/industries/healthcare/featuresopinions/Documents/reimaginingheathcare-opportunities.pdf (accessed on 10 January 2023).

Jiang, F., Jiang, Y., Zhi, H., Dong, Y., Li, H., Ma, S., & Wang, Y. (2017). Artificial intelligence in healthcare: Past, present and future. Stroke and Vascular Neurology, 2(4), 230–243.

Jiang, L., Wu, Z., Xu, X., Zhan, Y., Jin, X., Wang, L., & Qiu, Y. (2021). Opportunities and challenges of artificial intelligence in the medical field: Current application, emerging problems, and problem-solving strategies. The Journal of International Medical Research, 49, 1–11. https://doi.org/10.1177/03000605211000157

Khanna, D. (2020). Use of artificial intelligence in healthcare and medicine. International Journal of Innovations in Emerging Research and Technology, 5(12). 10.31221/osf.io/eshm9

Khanna, N. N., Maindarkar, M. A., Viswanathan, V., Fernandes, J. F. E., Paul, S., Bhagawati, M., Ahluwalia, P., Ruzsa, Z., Sharma, A., Kolluri, R., Singh, I. M., Laird, J. R., Fatemi, M., Alizad, A., Saba, L., Agarwal, V., Sharma, A., Teji, J. S., Al-Maini, M., Rathore, V., & Suri, J. S. (2022). Economics of artificial intelligence in healthcare: Diagnosis vs. treatment. Healthcare, 10(12), 2493. https://doi.org/10.3390/healthcare10122493.

Kourou, K., Exarchos, K. P., Papaloukas, C., Sakaloglou, P., Exarchos, T., & Fotiadis, D. I. (2021). Applied machine learning in cancer research: A systematic review for patient diagnosis, classification and prognosis. Computational and Structural Biotechnology Journal, 19, 5546–5555. https://doi.org/10.1016/j.csbj.2021.10.006

Krittanawong, C., Johnson, K. W., Rosenson, R. S., & Wang, Z. (2019). Deep learning for cardiovascular medicine: A practical primer. European Heart Journal, 40(25), 2058–2073.

Lee, D., & Yoon, S. N. (2021). Application of artificial intelligence-based technologies in the healthcare industry: Opportunities and challenges. International Journal of Environmental Research, 18, 271. https://doi.org/10.3390/ijerph18010271.

McKee, M., & Wouters, O. J. (2023). The challenges of regulating artificial intelligence in healthcare comment on "Clinical decision support and new regulatory frameworks for medical devices: Are we ready for it?—A viewpoint paper. International Journal of Health Policy and Management, 12, 1–4. https://doi.org/10.34172/ijhpm.2022.7261

Muehlematter, U. J., Daniore, P., & Vokinger, K. N. (2021). Approval of artificial intelligence and machine learning-based medical devices in the USA and Europe (2015–20): A comparative analysis. The Lancet Digital Health, 3, e195–e203. https://doi.org/10.1016/S2589-7500(20)30292-2.

O'mara-Eves et al., (2015). Using text mining for study identification in systematic reviews: A systematic review of current approaches. Systematic Reviews. 2015, 4, 5, https://doi.org/10.1186/2046-4053-4-5.

Obermeyer, Z., & Emanuel, E. J. (2016). Predicting the future—Big data, machine learning, and clinical medicine. The New England Journal of Medicine, 375(13), 1216–1219.

Parwani, A. V., Hassell, L., Glassy, E., & Pantanowitz, L. (2014). Regulatory barriers surrounding the use of whole slide imaging in the United States of America. Journal of Pathology Informatics, 5, 38. https://doi.org/10.4103/2153-3539.143325.

Patel, & Tarakji, K. G. (2021). Smartwatch diagnosis of atrial fibrillation in a patient with embolic stroke of unknown source: A case report. Cardiovascular Digital Health Journal 2021, 2, 84–87. https://doi.org/10.1016/j.cvdhj.2021.01.001.

Petersson, L., Larsson, I., & Nygren, J. M., et al. (2022). Challenges to implementing artificial intelligence in healthcare: A qualitative interview study with healthcare leaders in Sweden. BMC Health Services Research, 22, Article No. 850. https://doi.org/10.1186/s12913-022-08215-8

Pifer, R. (2023). Artificial intelligence could save healthcare industry $360B a year. Healthcare Dive. https://www.healthcaredive.com/news/artificial-intelligence-healthcare-savings-harvard-mckinsey-report/641163/

Price, W. N., & Cohen, I. G. (2019). Privacy in the age of medical big data. Nature Medicine, 25(1), 37–43. https://doi.org/10.1038/s41591-018-0272-7.

Ramessur, R., Raja, L., Kilduff, C. L. S., Kang, S., Li, J. O., Thomas, P. B. M., & Sim, D. A. (2021). Impact and challenges of integrating artificial intelligence and telemedicine into clinical ophthalmology. Asia-Pacific Journal of Ophthalmology, 10, 317–327. https://doi.org/10.1097/APO.0000000000000406.

Reddy, S., Fox, J., & Purohit, M. P. (2018). Artificial intelligence-enabled healthcare delivery. Journal of the Royal Society of Medicine, 112(1), 22–28. https://doi.org/10.1177/0141076818815510.

Retson, T. A., & Eghtedari, M. (2020). Computer-aided detection/diagnosis in breast imaging: A focus on the evolving FDA regulations for using software as a medical device. Current Radiology Reports, 8, 7. https://doi.org/10.1007/s40134-020-00350-6.

Ruamviboonsuk, P., Chantra, S., Seresirikachorn, K., Ruamviboonsuk, V., & Sangroongruangsri, S. (2021). Economic evaluations of artificial intelligence in ophthalmology. Asia-Pacific Journal of Ophthalmology, 10, 307–316. https://doi.org/10.1097/APO.0000000000000403.

Sahni, N., Stein, G., Zemmel, R., & Cutler, D. M. (2023). The potential impact of artificial intelligence on healthcare spending. NBER Working Paper No. 30857. https://doi.org/10.3386/w30857

Secinaro, S., Calandra, D., Secinaro, A., Muthurangu, V., & Biancone, P. (2021). The role of artificial intelligence in healthcare: A structured literature review. BMC Medical Informatics and Decision Making, 21, Article No. 125. https://doi.org/10.1186/s12911-021-01488-9.

Shahin, M., Babar, M. A., & Zhu, L. (2017). Continuous integration, delivery and deployment: A systematic review on approaches, tools, challenges and practices. IEEE Access, 5, 3909–3943. https://doi.org/10.1109/ACCESS.2017.2685629.

Singh, H., & Singh, A. (2023). ChatGPT: Systematic Review, Applications and Agenda for Multidisciplinary Research. https://doi.org/10.1080/14765284.2023.2210482.

Singla, B., & Shalender, K. (Eds.). (2024). *AI healthcare applications and security, ethical, and legal considerations.* IGI Global USA. https://doi.org/10.4018/979-8-3693-7452-8

Singla, B., Shalender, K., & Stamer, K. (Eds.). (2024). *Revolutionizing the healthcare sector with AI.* IGI Global USA. https://doi.org/10.4018/979-8-3693-3731-8

Smetherman, D., Golding, L., Moy, L., & Rubin, E. (2022). The economic impact of AI on breast imaging. Journal of Breast Imaging, 4, 302–308. doi: https://doi.org/10.1093/jbi/wbac012.

Sunarti, S., Rahman, F. F., Naufal, M., Risky, M., Febriyanto, K., & Masnina, R. (2021). Artificial intelligence in healthcare: Opportunities and risk for future. Gaceta Sanitaria, 35, S67–S70. https://doi.org/10.1016/j.gaceta.2020.12.019

Thrall, J. H., Li, X., Li, Q., Cruz, C., Do, S., Dreyer, K., & Brink, J. (2018). Artificial intelligence and machine learning in radiology: Opportunities, challenges, pitfalls, and criteria for success. Journal of the American College of Radiology, 15(3), 504–508.

Topol, E. J. (2019). High-performance medicine: The convergence of human and artificial intelligence. Nature Medicine, 25(1), 44–56.

Turing, A. M. (1950). Computing machinery and intelligence. Mind, LIX, 433–460. https://doi.org/10.1093/mind/LIX.236.433

Van Leeuwen, K. G., de Rooij, M., Schalekamp, S., van Ginneken, B., & Rutten, M. J. C. M. (2022). How does artificial intelligence in radiology improve efficiency and health outcomes? Pediatric Radiology, 52, 2087–2093. https://doi.org/10.1007/s00247-021-05114-8.

Voets, M. M., Veltman, J., Slump, C. H., Siesling, S., & Koffijberg, H. (2022). Systematic review of health economic evaluations focused on artificial intelligence in healthcare: The tortoise and the cheetah. Value in Health, 25, 340–349. https://doi.org/10.1016/j.jval.2021.11.1362.

Wahl, B., Cossy-Gantner, A., Germann, S., & Schwalbe, N. R. (2018). Artificial intelligence (AI) and global health: How can AI contribute to health in resource-poor settings? BMJ Global Health, 3, e000798. https://doi.org/10.1136/bmjgh-2018-000798

Weissler et al., (2021). The role of machine learning in clinical research: Transforming the future of evidence generation. Trials 2021, 22, 1–15, https://doi.org/10.1186/s13063-021-05489-x.

Xuan, J., Jiang, H., Hu, Y., Ren, Z., Zou, W., Luo, Z., & Wu, X. (2014). Towards effective bug triage with software data reduction techniques. IEEE Transactions on Knowledge and Data Engineering, 27, 264–280. https://doi.org/10.1109/TKDE.2014.2324590.

Yuan, Q., Zhang, H., Deng, T., Tang, S., Yuan, X., Tang, W., Xie, Y., Ge, H., Wang, X., & Zhou, Q. (2020). Role of artificial intelligence in kidney disease. International Journal of Medical Sciences, 17, 970. https://doi.org/10.7150/ijms.42078.

14 Machine Learning-Based Maternal and Child Mortality Rate Prediction Using Random Forest Algorithm

Jayapandian Natarajan, Parekh Hetvi Vimal, Dikshita Sen, Cyril Lawrence, Sivaraman Eswaran, Pradeep Chintale, and Shalmali Arun Patil

INTRODUCTION

Modern-day maternal and child mortality stands as one of the most significant sources of global morbidity and mortality, especially in developing nations. However, it is saddening that a high number of deaths still occur due to complications during childbirth as well as among children under five years of age, even with the modern growth in facility of health services. A survey conducted by the World Health Organization (WHO) in 2017 estimated that nearly 295,000 women died during pregnancy or within 20 days of childbirth (Abdulla, 2020). To be precise, the global under-five child mortality rate in 2019 stands at 2 million deaths (Aheto, 2019). Such deaths require intervention, and the following statistics show that the population that needs intervention is large. Some major factors are complications during pregnancy and childbirth, severe bleeding, infection, high blood pressure, and unsafe abortion (Almond, 2012). Major killer diseases for children are neonatal deaths due to preterm birth complications, pneumonia, low birth weight due to birth asphyxia, diarrhea, and malaria (Bogale et al., 2022). Most of these deaths are perhaps avoidable if victims receive adequate and appropriate treatment on time (Cerda, 2018). Thus, it is crucial to take measures to identify populations most at risk and offer them adequate care to minimize mortality rates and have a positive, qualitative impact on the lives of women and children (Dereje, 2021). Artificial intelligence refers to the simulation of human intelligence and thinking in machines, of which machine learning (ML) is a branch that deals with the analysis of big data to find patterns and make predictions (Emechebe, 2016). To elaborate, one can note that, given a set of factors associated with women and/or children, such as demographical or health-related indicators, as well as available financial and social resources, and access to healthcare, the use of ML would allow estimating the probability of mother and child mortalities (Figley, 2022). Such predictive

DOI: 10.1201/9781003531272-14

models may be useful when shared with healthcare providers because such data can easily be used to target high-risk cases first and more preventions can be made from them. The main measure that should be achieved in this project reflects its primary goal of constructing a highly accurate ML algorithm to forecast maternal and child mortality levels. This involves several key goals: The processes include data acquisition and preparation, feature creation and reduction, model building and learning, model assessment and explanation, and implementation and oversight. Each of these goals is important to obtain accurate, credible, and efficient predictive models. Every solution starts with data collection, and in the case of creating a ML model, this is no exception. To collect information for this work, surveys and questionnaires will be administered in the hospitals, league of health facilities, and governmental agencies as well as research findings both locally and internationally. These should include the mother's age, health status, parental wealth, health and previous pregnancy details, prenatal history and details, and infant health data (Furuta, 2014). Once collected, it is important to check the data for completeness and suitability for use in data analysis. Primary data is collected through interviews or questionnaires, while secondary data is collected from companies and other reliable sources. Some of the pre-processing techniques also include missing values, duplicated entries and inconsistencies, and informational irrelevance. Another important data preparation task includes data normalization and encoding of the categorical variables that are input to ML methods (Hou, 2020).

Figure 14.1 lists the different services in healthcare by using ML. Moreover, the exploratory data analysis will be performed to describe the data in terms of distributions, correlation, and other features. Feature engineering entails the process of transforming the available dimensions within the data set into new features from the insights obtained from the exploratory data analysis (EDA) step. For instance, aggregation of a number of variables measuring individual health status can have a better predictive ability of maternal and child health as indicated by a composite health score (Ilin, 2024). Feature selection is a method frequently used to determine the features that best influence the target variable which, in this case, is maternal and child mortality (Keats, 2017). Current methods will include correlation analysis, mutual information, and model-based feature importance which include random Forest and gradient boost. Reduction techniques also prove useful in lessening the feature space, for example, the principal component analysis (PCA) (Keshta, 2021). Thus, the subsequent step from the pre-processed data and chosen features is to build and train ML models. Several methods will be considered, including logistic regression, random forest, gradient boosting, and neural networks. All of these algorithms have advantages and depend on the form of data and some properties of the problem. The next step is to select a testing dataset, which should not be used during model creation, so we will have a training dataset and a validation one. Formerly fine-tuning will be conducted with hyperparameters using such methods as grid search or random search for the best performance of the model. The models to be generated will be assessed by means of accuracy, precision, recall, F1-score, ROC-AUC, and confusion matrix to act as measures of the accuracy of the models. Model evaluation is vital during analysis to determine the merit and efficiency of the executed models. By using cross-validation methods, the models'

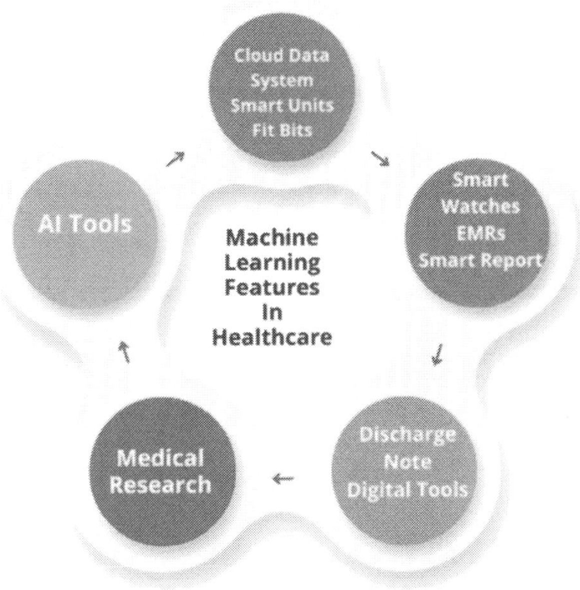

FIGURE 14.1 Machine learning in healthcare sector

Source: Authors' conceptualization.

validity and generalizability will be tested. Post-processing and model interpretability techniques such as SHAP (SHapley Additive exPlanations) and LIME (Local Interpretable Model agnostic Explanations) will be employed in the analysis of the model predictions and the features it uses (Lone, 2024). Such techniques assist in identifying the mechanisms of how factors affect the rate of mortality, as well as offering useful information to healthcare workers. Analysis of errors will be made to understand problems by deriving them from the test results of the prediction errors and misclassification. It is imperative to point out the models' limitations and ways to handle them to improve the methods' effectiveness. Once an accurate predictive model is trained and tested, it will be exported into a productive environment using Flak, Django, or FastAPI to create REST APIs or MVC architecture or be plugged into the existing healthcare systems. To address this, an interface, which could be in the form of a web or a mobile application, will be created where the professionals will feed in data to be analyzed and obtain corresponding predictions. Testing and evaluation of the result of the deployed model have to be done continually to check its performance. This entails monitoring features, measuring the shift in data distribution, and training the model when it is necessary to do so. To ensure compliance with the law, specifically HIPAA for electronic health information, security and privacy features will be incorporated to protect users' data (Nti, 2022). The concept of this ML project is to reduce the cases of maternal and child mortality using ML by predicting these rates. Therefore, this project aims to use extensive data and develop durable predictive models to offer healthcare providers with potential insights that will help in early interventions. Executing this project is very crucial to lessening the mortality rates, enhancing the status of maternal and child health, and preserving the overall health of societies across the world. The predictive models can remain valid and functional in the constantly changing healthcare environment through constant surveillance and adjustment, therefore, reducing the mortality rates as well as improving the quality of maternal and child health across the world (Odejimi, 2022).

LITERATURE REVIEW

Researchers now see predicting maternal and child deaths as a key focus. They want to use advanced ML methods to spot high-risk cases and step in to help. This review looks at new studies in this area that use ML to predict health outcomes for mothers and children. Ilin (2024) looked at how to spot health risks in kids by using data on mothers and children. The study tried different ML methods to look at health records, personal details, and money situations. It showed that finding health risks could help kids stay healthier. The work shows how important it is to bring together lots of different data and use smart prediction tools to lower health risks for children. Ilin's study shows how ML can predict many health outcomes by bringing together different kinds of data giving a strong base to help. Nti and Owusu-Boadu developed a hybrid boosting ensemble model to attempt the prediction of maternal mortality, focusing on long-lasting reproductive health practices (Nti, 2022). Their model combined algorithms that improved prediction accuracy, therefore exemplifying how ensemble methods can be effectively used to deal with tricky healthcare data. This makes the effectiveness of ML for the prediction of maternal mortality very noticeable and suggests that hybrid models offer healthcare workers very strong solutions. By design, this hybrid boosting ensemble model exploits the strong points of different algorithms to tackle the weak spots of the single algorithm approaches and hence results in more exact and dependable predictions. Bogale et al. (2022) examined perinatal mortality prediction using the health status of mothers and health insurance services using ensemble ML methods. The study used a range of predictors that included mothers' age, health history, and insurance coverage to build a predictive model for perinatal mortality. This research thus underlines the integration of different health indicators and the advantages accruable from ensemble methods in making better predictions. The authors show that ensemble methods based on combining instances of the same basic learning algorithm are able to capture many complex factors interacting to create perinatal mortality risk.

Ward et al. (2023) provided model-based estimates and projections of global, regional, and country trends in maternal mortality by cause from 1990 to 2050. In this chapter, the authors used the simulation models to obtain information on historical data and future trends in maternal mortality. The work allows valuable lessons to be learned about the actual efficacy of different health interventions. This analysis underlines a continuous process of monitoring and updating health policies that should go on if maternal mortality rates are to be brought down effectively. Medium-term projections and scenario analyses will be critical in guiding policymakers with appropriate interventions and effective allocation of resources. Dereje et al. (2021) focused on the investigation of risk factors and the prediction of neonatal and infant mortality according to maternal determinants using homogeneous ensemble methods. In the study, some of the important maternal health indicators that influence neonatal and infant mortality were identified, and with accurate models for prediction, it was shown that healthcare providers can guide timely and targeted interventions. The study supports homogeneous ensemble methods in predicting and preventing infant mortality. The identification of specific maternal health factors, such as prenatal care and nutritional status, will provide relevant variables to formulate policy and improve neonatal and infant health outcomes. To sum up, the studies presented in this overview unequivocally showed that ML serves as a key determinant for predicting maternal and child mortality. Such integration with a wide array of health data and the execution of the most sophisticated predictive models may successfully recognize high-risk cases and facilitate timely interventions that potentially reduce mortalities, improving health outcomes. Continuous development and upgrading of these models with new data sources and innovative methodologies are important in promoting better maternal and child healthcare. One common thread across all these studies is that the prediction of risk for maternal and child mortality is critically dependent on integrated data. As correctly highlighted by Ilin (2024) and Bogale et al. (2022), a good predictive model must take into account a wide variety of health indicators, among them advanced maternal age, health history, and low socioeconomic status. Machine learning algorithms work best with comprehensive datasets to capture the complex interplay of factors affecting maternal and child mortality (Ogbuoji, 2019). Another important aspect of the literature relates to the use of ensemble methods (Rajesh, 2023), which range from hybrid and homogeneous ensembles (Salih, 2024). This can result in very high improvement in prediction accuracy when combined in a hybrid ensemble model (Nti, 2022). On the other hand, Bogale et al. (2022) and Dereje et al. (2021) depict that homogeneous ensemble methods, in which several instances of the same algorithm are combined, predict perinatal and infant mortality quite effectively. Those studies thus give a clear indication of the worth of ensemble approaches in treating data that deals with health complexities and, at the same time, show an improvement in predictive performance (Singla, 2024). Ward et al. (2023) have located this in the broader perspective of policy implications for the predictions concerning maternal mortality. Based on simulation exercises, their projections give some useful insights into long-term trends and the potential impact of different health interventions (Tomašev, 2019). Such a forward-looking approach is critical for guiding policy decisions and allocation of health resources that can effectively reduce maternal mortality rates. Machine learning models for the prediction of maternal and child mortality show a high potential for improving health outcomes (Salih, 2024). Generally, a common theme emanating from the reviewed studies is that integration of data, ensemble methods, and continued monitoring with policy adjustment is necessary. To that effect, more predictive modeling techniques can be advanced by the inclusion of varied sources of data, therefore aiding researchers and health practitioners to identify high-risk cases and informing timely interventions that would reduce mortality rates of mothers and children.

PROBLEM STATEMENT

Improper care of women and children is one of the major issues in the field of public health, particularly in low and middle-income countries (LMICs), where healthcare systems proved insufficient to address the multifactorial determinants of maternal and child mortalities. There are increased rates of maternal and infant mortality amid the enhancement of equipment in the health sectors as well as improved practices. Specifically, the WHO has estimated that at least 298,000 women die during childbirth annually due to complications during pregnancy. According to the statistics of 2019, 2 million children below the age of five years died. These statistics raise a very basic question about the state of the art in the assessment of the causes and consequences of the health problems associated with such outcomes. The leading causes of maternal mortality include postpartum hemorrhage, infections, hypertensive disorders, gestational complications during and after childbirth, and unsafe abortion. Regarding child mortality, the 'big five' killer diseases are prematurity and intraneonatal conditions, pneumonia, birth asphyxia, diarrheal diseases, and malaria. Such fatalities are actually due to complications that can be easily avoided if only injured people seek the help of a qualified healthcare provider in time and get adequate treatment.

Figure 14.2 provides the working flow of the prediction model. Thus, the human aspect of the problem is to define the criteria that allow us to distinguish the most hazardous cases in advance in order to intervene in time. Defining a patient's risk using standard demographic data and medical history does not provide adequate information on the complex aspects of risk factors influencing maternal and child health. It is worth noting that people's living conditions including their social, economic, geographical location, healthcare access, nutritional status, and genetic makeup also influence outcomes. Lack of resources also adds to this problem. Resources are usually limited, especially in contemporary learning institutions. Due

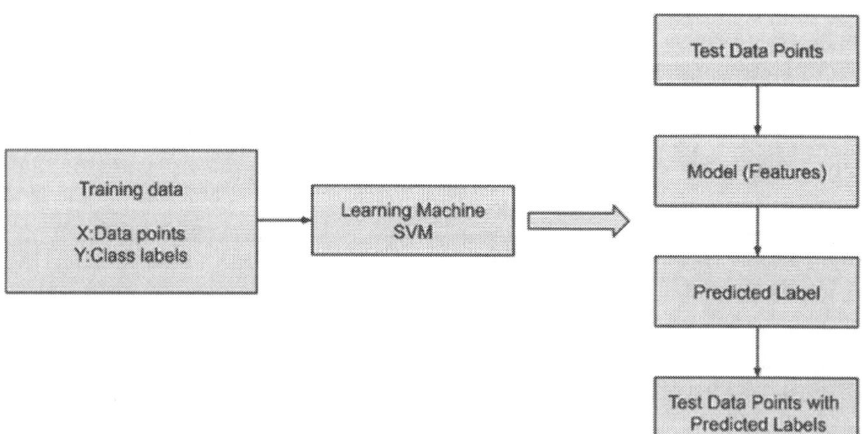

FIGURE 14.2 Machine learning prediction architecture

Source: Authors' conceptualization.

to the scarcity of personnel, medical equipment, and formal structures within health facilities, a majority of individuals in these facilities do not get adequate offers of services they require. This equally leads to a more reactive form of healthcare where correction is done once problems have occurred instead of containing them before they occur. Hence, it becomes crucial relevantly to explore methods that can help to use the currently available information to predict and prevent such adverse events before they reach life-threatening states. The great interest is applying ML because this approach essentially allows to build models that can analyze datasets containing large and complex information arrays that cannot be analyzed with the help of traditional methods to identify corresponding patterns and factors holding risk. The variables of interest can encompass demographic data, patients' medical history, socioeconomic status, and results of environmental scans, whereby the ML algorithms will determine mortality rates of mothers and children with a high degree of accuracy. When shared with healthcare providers, it is possible to organize care for specific populations, and then provide preventive and early interventional methods, which can be useful in increasing the chances of survival in numerous cases in the future. Seeking to take advantage of the possibilities that ML opens, this research seeks to revolutionize the traditional strategy for addressing the causes of maternal and child mortality by providing methods that support the identification of potential dangers and implementation of early actions. Given all these, this proactive strategy stands to enhance lower mortality rates, enhance health functionalities, enhance healthcare resource deployment, and ultimately improve global health standards.

PROPOSED MATERNAL AND CHILD MORTALITY PREDICTION

The proposed methodology for predicting maternal and child mortality using ML encompasses several key phases: The phases are data acquisition and preprocessing, feature creation and subset selection, model development and learning, model evaluation steps, and finally, model deployment and monitoring phases. Such phases are highly significant for the successful completion of an accurate, reliable and effective predictive model that will help providers in lowering mortality rates in the healthcare sector. As a fundamental step in this project, the data accumulation process is conducted in different sources in an extensive manner. Sources of data will be hospitals, other healthcare institutions, government departments, and other studies within and outside the Bowen region. These sources will, in turn, give a diverse and large sample, which is very important in enhancing the performance of the predictive models. The measurements to be used in data collection include questionnaires, interviews, and patients' records. The primary source of data shall include self-developed questionnaires/surveys to be issued to healthcare providers as well as the patients. The instruments used in this study will help in the assessment of information on the demographic variables including age, health status of the mother, parental wealth, and past pregnancy. Data pertinent to the health of the woman and her newborn will encompass prenatal history, birth history, and newborn physiologic status, respectively. Also, data pertaining to patients' demographic characteristics, medical history, socioeconomic status, and environment as well as caregivers' demographic characteristics, financial and social support available for, and patient's health insurance information will be gathered. This type of data gathering guarantees a wide range of information that reflects the complexity of the issue in question in this case, maternal and child health. Secondary data shall be gathered through record review at the medical department. This involves following up on records of prior maternal and child health outcomes in order to participate in the assessment of contributing factors of mortality. Thus, beginning with primary data and supported by secondary data, the project will have a large number of information available to create models.

Once collected, the data in question is subjected to certain procedures that make it ready for analysis. On another note, data cleaning is the initial process of the data preprocessing stage where missing records, duplicated rows, or other perturbations in the database are treated. This has to do with the nature and the degree of the missing value problem, where missing values can either be imputed or the records can be dropped. Data entry is performed to remove or clean up repeated values and organize them or make them as clean as possible to eliminate any error in the dataset. The next step is data normalization, which implies that all the values of data are to be normalized so that they can be compared between different variables. This is issued to ML algorithms that expect the input data to be in the same range. For example, metric properties like age or income can be normalized to an equal level of variation and nominal properties such as marital status or education level can be converted to numerical format by methods such as one hot encoder label encoder. Drawing on the data, EDA is carried out in a bid to describe the data distributions to reveal relationships, if any, between the variables as well as to discover other features. EDA leads to the understanding of the data; that is, it simplifies the identification of patterns and relations, which are vital when performing feature engineering. Descriptive graphical methods including histograms, scatter plots, and correlation matrices are applied to get more insight into the data characteristics.

This step is very paramount and is about feature engineering, where the collected data is transformed into features that can greatly help to advance the model. This process is done by, for instance, adding health-related variables and summarizing the results in one health index. For instance, one of the composite indicators can include prenatal care whereby different indicators of prenatal care are aggregated, or maternal and infant health can be other indicators with factors relating to them aggregated. Thus, it is logical to consider a composite score that would allow us to get a richer picture of the overall health state; this would enhance the model's prediction of mortality risks. Dimensionality reduction is applied to find out the best predictors of maternal and child mortality.

Figure 14.3 depicts the proposed workflow model. The method of determining the feature relevance includes correlation analysis and the usage of the mutual information; model-based ranking methods including, but not limited to, Random Forest and gradient boosting. Correlation analysis is used to determine if there exists a linear relationship between the features and the target variable, while mutual information quantifies the nonlinear relationships. Ranking, based on model-based feature importance, establishes feature importance by calculating the degree of impact on the model's predictability. Techniques such as the application of the PCA are used in order to dimensionalize the feature space. From the original features, PCA derives a

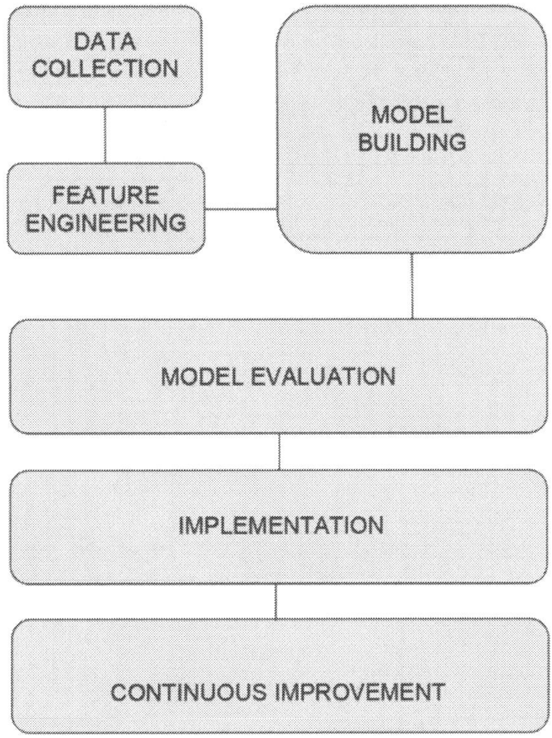

FIGURE 14.3 Proposed architecture model

Source: Authors' conceptualization.

new set of components that are orthogonal to each other and contains the majority of variability from the data. This step removes nonsignificant or less important features from the model; this process makes the model more efficient and less complex to deploy. As part of the model assessment, it was necessary to evaluate the performance of the developed models by applying the metrics usually used in the assessment of the models. Accuracy is defined as the overprediction, and precision is defined as the true positive percentage out of the total positive predictions. Sensitivity, or recall, is used to measure the ability of the model to identify the amount of actual positives out of all the positives identified by the two models. The main advantage of the chosen metric is that it synthesizes both precision and recall into a single score, which gives a proper perspective on the model's performance. The ROC-AUC evaluates the model's performance on how effectively it separates the two classes, while the confusion matrix gives the exact number of correctly predicted positive and negative classes and the number of misclassified instances.

Interpretation of the final model predictions is done by post-processing methods such as SHAP and LIME. SHAP values are important for the unified measure of feature importance and show where each feature helps in the prediction made by the model. LIME design computes local explanations regarding a particular prediction done by a model to enhance the understanding of the model functioning. Error analysis is done with the aim of identifying how those predictions went wrong and why the classifications were wrong. This step comprises splitting the confirmation cases and calculating the number of misclassifications, followed by assessing the patterns of the model's errors. Thus, by knowing the sources of errors, the model can be improved further.

The last stage is productionization, which entails building the trained models into a production environment and maintain them. The deployment process involves a framework like Flask, Django, or FastAPI for developing an interface that is friendly for healthcare practitioners. This is a user interface, in the form of a web or mobile application, through which the user enters his/her notes and gets predictions. The design concerns the versatility and reliability of the tool so that the intended audience of healthcare providers can easily apply the predictive tool into practice. However, it implies that there is constant monitoring for the model that is deployed since the model is subject to decay. Periodically, the tests and evaluations are performed to identify the changes in the distribution of data or the features. Monitoring is the process of observing KPIs, comparing actual performance with expected, and finding out the possible causes of variation. Training is required to improve the ability of the model in handling the new sampling data set. It is appreciated that the users follow legal requirements as far as their data is concerned such as Health Information Management Association of Australia Ltd (HIMAA). Security and privacy features are designed to protect the identities and medical data as well as to ensure that clients are protected. Such measures include encryption of data and proper storage of data that cannot be easily accessed by those who are unauthorized to access the information.

RESULT AND DISCUSSION

In this research predicting maternity and child mortality, our team used methodologies such us regional K-nearest neighbors (KNN), random forest classifier, decision tree, and 3D histogram equalization recursive neural network from datasets that were obtained from Kaggle and the WHO. Thus, the goal was to find out potential risk factors and causes of maternal and child mortality, so that those stakeholders who are involved in the decision-making process in the field of healthcare could make relevant decisions in order to decrease these problems. Our study focused on two powerful algorithms: Random Forest and decision tree. Participants' demographic, clinical, and environmental data were used to create three large datasets. These datasets we used were rich in information, which was crucial for our analysis. The survey data included a demographic and health survey that indicated demographic characteristics, mother's health, and socioeconomic status of the respondents. Clinical health records were used to determine the health history of the mothers and the children, including particulars of prenatal and childbirth/post childbirth treatment. Finally, Health Data summed up the actual health situation and the diseases that had been registered at a specific moment, while Environmental and Geographic Data revealed how living conditions and geographic locations could affect the health of people. Therefore, the intention of combining these sets of variables was to build a conceptual model of maternal and child health determinants. Random forest algorithm was the most useful in data analysis due to its efficiency particularly when dealing with many variables. Its particular suitability for our study lies in the fact that it is an ensemble method that constructs several decision trees and combines them to increase credentials and prevent overfitting. Random forest came out to be significantly accurate with 85% accuracy to predict survival among passengers in this case. Furthermore, its overall accuracy was at 80%, which highlighted its capacity to position the right health information on true positive situations, particularly mortality, while its specificity stood at 88%, which demonstrated its capability of identifying the negatives that are not truly negative. Such a balance between sensitivity and specificity converges with the notion of how the model is capable of offering accurate predictions. The decision tree algorithm, though basic, was useful more from the analysis point of view since results can be explained quite easily. This one forms a tree structure of decisions on one hand and the possibilities as to what could happen next on the other, which makes it appropriate to look for critical decisions and associated risk points. The aspects of the decision tree's performance identified were accuracy, sensitivity, and specificity with 78% being accuracy, 75% being sensitivity and the specificity was 80%. Even though it was, at times, slightly less accurate than Random Forest, its decision-making process was helpful in identifying main intervention points and explaining how different factors work jointly to affect mortality rates. Thus, reviewing the work of the two mentioned algorithms, one can notice that each of them has its advantages. The Random Forest model was relatively accurate on all the datasets and provided generalized output and thus ideal for broad prediction.

Table 14.1 discusses various experimental setup detail. The capacity of KNN to deal with data containing several attributes and their interactions was instrumental in discovering such factors as maternal age and health care accessibility and nutritional status. On the other hand, the interpretation of the decision tree model was helpful for gaining the point of view from factors that increased the risk or where interventions could be made. Hence, it facilitates a visual understanding of decision-making processes by the stakeholders, which makes it easier to utilize the results.

Table 14.2 is the deliberate accuracy level for the existing and proposed model. The research includes three datasets from Kaggle and the WHO to see how well Random Forest and decision tree models could predict the deaths of mothers and children. In general, it has been found that Random Forest did better than decision tree. For Sample Dataset 1, Random Forest was right 90.54% of the time beating

TABLE 14.1
Experimental Setup Details

Component	Details
Storage	20GB
RAM	8GB
Software	Python Version 3.11
Operating System	Windows 11
Graphics Card	Nvidia 3050 RTX
IDE Platform	Jupyter Notebook

TABLE 14.2
Results of Accuracy Level Prediction (In %)

Classifier	Decision Tree	Random Forest
Sample Dataset 1	81	90.54
Sample Dataset 2	89.21	97.43
Sample Dataset 3	96.50	98.23

decision tree's 81% accuracy. But for Sample Datasets 2 and 3, the Random Forest was more accurate. It scored 97.43% and 98.23%, while decision tree got 89.21% and 96.50%. Decision tree has also given a good accuracy value for the three sample datasets, Random Forest showed that it could handle different kinds of data well. It is performed across all datasets. This makes Random Forest a more reliable choice when trying to predict the deaths of mothers and children. Figure 14.4 shows the accuracy level of the decision tree.

Figure 14.5 depicts the accuracy level of Random Forest. Random Forest builds many decision trees during training and averages their outputs to make predictions. This team approach reduces the chance of overfitting, as combining multiple trees balances out biases and differences resulting in more exact and correct predictions. Random Forest can deal with missing data and stay accurate with both number-based and category-based features giving strong results across different datasets. On the flip side, a decision tree model divides the data into subsets based on the most important attribute. This creates a tree structure where each node stands for a feature, each branch represents a decision rule, and each leaf represents an outcome.

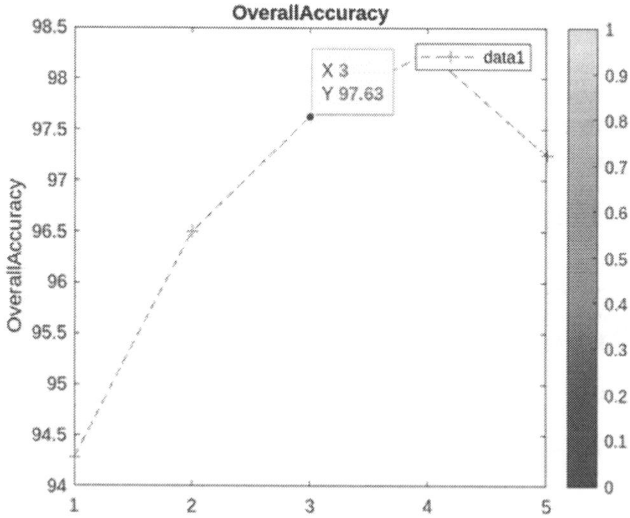

FIGURE 14.4 Accuracy level of decision tree

Source: Authors' conceptualization.

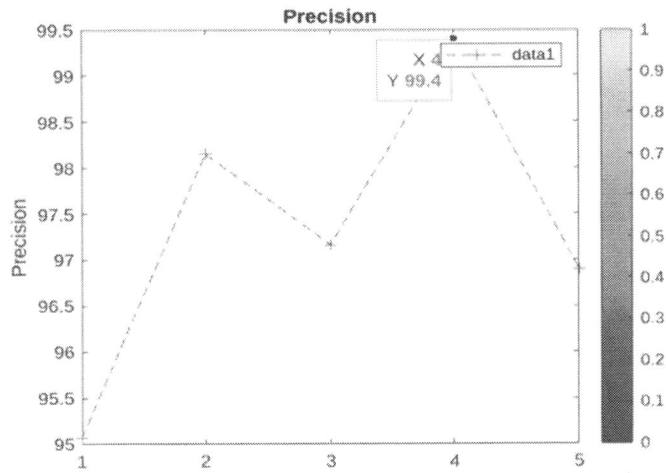

FIGURE 14.5 Accuracy level of random forest

Source: Authors' conceptualization.

While decision trees are easy to grasp and interpret, they tend to overfit with messy data. Even so, decision trees showed good accuracy in Sample Datasets 2 and 3, which points to their usefulness in certain cases. However, the ensemble nature of Random Forest ensures more reliable and accurate results. This makes it a better choice for complex data sets when trying to predict maternal and child mortality.

CONCLUSION

Healthcare promises to be greatly improved and reduced mortality by bringing ML into it. This chapter outlines a methodology for creating models that can be used for identification. While the gathering of broad information, detailed preparation, and complex feature extraction that includes composites of well-being indices will be necessary for the production of such models that are capable of predicting with great accuracy, these models include logistic regression, Random Forest, gradient boosting, and neural networks. To make the model relevant and reliable, there is a need for continuous monitoring, rigorous model evaluation, and techniques like SHARP and LIME for interpretability. The model will help healthcare professionals to make timely decisions which will enable prompt interventions and improve health outcomes. Therefore, the project's final goal is to decrease maternal and child mortality rates using ML algorithms to save lives, enhance maternal and child health, and contribute to global well-being. The goal of ongoing monitoring, adaptations, and adherence to moral principles is to produce long-lasting, beneficial effects on world health.

REFERENCES

Abdulla, E. M. Trends in maternal mortality, Al-Sadaka Teaching Hospital, Aden 2008–2018. Yemeni Journal of Medical and Health Research, 9(1&2). (2020)

Aheto, J. M. K. Predictive model and determinants of under five child mortality: Evidence from the 2014 Ghana demographic and health survey. BMC Public Health, 19, 1–10. (2019)

Almond, D., Currie, J., & Herrmann, M. From infant to mother: Early disease environment and future maternal health. Labour Economics, 19(4), 475–483. (2012)

Bogale, D. S., Abuhay, T. M., & Dejene, B. E. Predicting perinatal mortality based on maternal health status and health insurance service using homogeneous ensemble machine learning methods. BMC Medical Informatics and Decision Making, 22(1), 341. (2022)

Cerda, P., Varoquaux, G., & Kégl, B. Similarity encoding for learning with dirty categorical variables. Machine Learning, 107(8), 1477–1494. (2018)

Dereje, T., Abuhay, T. M., Letta, A., & Alelign, M. Investigate risk factors and predict neonatal and infant mortality based on maternal determinants using homogenous ensemble methods. In 2021 International Conference on Information and Communication Technology for Development for Africa (ICT4DA) (pp. 18–23). IEEE. (2021)

Emechebe, C. I., Njoku, C. O., Udofia, U. M., & Ukaga, J. T. Complications of induced abortion: Contribution to maternal mortality in a tertiary center of a low resource setting. Saudi Journal for Health Sciences, 5(1), 34–38. (2016)

Figley, C. R., Bride, B. E., & Mazza, N. (Eds.). Death and Trauma: The Traumatology of Grieving. Taylor & Francis, Washington, DC, USA. (2022)

Furuta, M., Sandall, J., & Bick, D. Women's perceptions and experiences of severe maternal morbidity–A synthesis of qualitative studies using a metaethnographic approach. Midwifery, 30(2), 158–169. (2014)

Hou, N., Li, M., He, L., Xie, B., Wang, L., Zhang, R., … & Wang, K. Predicting 30 days mortality for MIMIC-III patients with sepsis-3: A machine learning approach using XGboost. Journal of translational medicine, 18, 1–14. (2020)

Ilin, C. Early detection of pediatric health risks using maternal and child health data. Scientific Reports, 14(1), 15350. (2024)

Keats, E. C., Ngugi, A., Macharia, W., Akseer, N., Khaemba, E. N., Bhatti, Z., … & Bhutta, Z. A. Progress and priorities for reproductive, maternal, newborn, and child health in Kenya: A countdown to 2015 country case study. The Lancet Global Health, 5(8), e782–e795. (2017)

Keshta, I., & Odeh, A. Security and privacy of electronic health records: Concerns and challenges. Egyptian Informatics Journal, 22(2), 177–183. (2021)

Lone, K. J., Hussain, L., Saeed, S., Aslam, A., Maqbool, A., & Butt, F. M. Detecting basic human activities and postural transition using robust machine learning techniques by applying dimensionality reduction methods. Waves in Random and Complex Media, 34(4), 3030–3055. (2024)

Nti, I. K., & Owusu-Boadu, B. A hybrid boosting ensemble model for predicting maternal mortality and sustaining reproductive. Smart Health, 26, 100325. (2022)

Odejimi, A., Quinley, J., Eluwa, G. I., Kunnuji, M., Wammanda, R. D., Weiss, W., & Franca Koh, A. C. Causes of deaths in neonates and children aged 1–59 months in Nigeria: Verbal autopsy findings of 2019 Verbal and Social Autopsy study. BMC Public Health, 22(1), 1130. (2022)

Ogbuoji, O., & Yamey, G. How many child deaths can be averted in Nigeria? Assessing state level prospects of achieving 2030 sustainable development goals for neonatal and under five mortality. Gates Open Research, 3. (2019)

Rajesh, S. M., Chiranmai, I., & Jayapandian, N. Artificial intelligence and deep learning based brain tumor detection using image processing. In 2023 5th International Conference on Inventive Research in Computing Applications (ICIRCA) (pp. 244–248). IEEE. (2023)

Salih, A. M., Raisi-Estabragh, Z., Galazzo, I. B., Radeva, P., Petersen, S. E., Lekadir, K., & Menegaz, G. A perspective on explainable artificial intelligence methods: SHAP and LIME. Advanced Intelligent Systems, 2400304. (2024)

Singla, Babita, Shalender Kumar, and Katja Stamer, eds. Revolutionizing the Healthcare Sector with AI. Hershey, PA: IGI Global. (2024). https://doi.org/10.4018/979-8-3693-3731-8

Singla, Babita, and Shalender Kumar, eds. AI Healthcare Applications and Security, Ethical, and Legal Considerations. Hershey, PA: IGI Global. (2024). https://doi.org/10.4018/979-8-3693-7452-8.

Tomašev, N., Glorot, X., Rae, J. W., Zielinski, M., Askham, H., Saraiva, A., ... & Mohamed, S. A clinically applicable approach to continuous prediction of future acute kidney injury. Nature, 572(7767), 116–119. (2019)

Ward, Z. J., Atun, R., King, G., Sequeira Dmello, B., & Goldie, S. J. Simulation based estimates and projections of global, regional and country level maternal mortality by cause, 1990–2050. Nature Medicine, 29(5), 1253–1261. (2023)

Index

Note: Page numbers in **bold** refer to tables.

I

M

N

O

P

Q

R

S

T

V